Well-Being

Well-Being

lynda wharton

HarperCollins*Publishers*

For further women's health information, and to purchase
recommended nutritional supplements, herbs and health
products, visit www.lyndawharton.com.

Notice to readers
This book contains general information only and is
not intended as a substitute for professional advice.

National Library of New Zealand Cataloguing-in-Publication Data

Wharton, Lynda.
Well-being : an essential guide to vibrant good health for all
women / Lynda Wharton.
Includes bibliographical references and index.
ISBN 978-1-86950-618-6
1. Women—Health and hygiene. 2. Women—Diseases. I. Title.
613.04244—dc 22

First published 2007
HarperCollins*Publishers (New Zealand) Limited*
P.O. Box 1, Auckland

ISBN-10: 1 86950 618 9
ISBN-13: 978 1 86950 618 6

Cover design by Sarah Bull, Anthony Bushelle Graphics
Typesetting by IslandBridge

Printed by Griffin Press, Australia.

79gsm Bulky Paperback used by HarperCollins*Publishers* is a natural, recyclable
product made from wood grown in a combination of sustainable plantation
and regrowth forests. It also contains up to a 20 % portion of recycled fibre.
The manufacturing processes conform to the environmental regulations in
Tasmania, the place of manufacture.

All works of love are works of peace.
If we have no peace,
it is because we have forgotten that
we belong to each other.

Mother Theresa

As long as we think of peace as an absence of war, we will never have it. Peace is not a political state, it is a personal one. It begins with each of us wanting it enough to accept it fully, even if it means letting go of hatred and judgement. Even if it means loving without condition.

Peace begins with me . . .
Peace begins with you . . .
Peace begins with us.

Kate Novak

Dedication

To my beautiful daughters, Rachel and Stephanie:
you are my sunshine and my joy . . . my *raison d'être*.
May your lives ever
be filled with love and peace.

Contents

A note on units

Body levels of nutrients, and so on, are commonly measured in different ways:

g	gram
mg	milligram, 1000 mg = 1 gram
mcg	microgram, 1000 mcg = 1 mg
iu	international unit used for fat-soluble vitamins
ml	millilitre, 1000 ml = 1 litre
rad	unit of radiation, see page 217

Foreword

by Allison Roe

Women and men have at least one thing in common. Neither of them understand women! At last, *Well-being* provides a wonderful resource we've been crying out for — a book to empower women with the knowledge they need to understand their own body, and start (or further) their journey to wellness and fulfilment. And men, there's no reason to ever feel alienated, as this insightful read is the answer for any man who wishes to climb inside his woman's world and deepen his understanding of her.

My path has crossed with Lynda Wharton's many times through our mutual interest in holistic health, initially because we both had a desire to do something meaningful about the alarming numbers of women being diagnosed with breast cancer. With billions of dollars worldwide being poured into breast cancer detection, research and treatment, why are the statistics still steadily rocketing skyward? Both Lynda and I have asked these hard questions, and wondered what it will take to change the status quo? Now at last, *Well-being* provides women with the information they need to take a truly preventative approach to breast cancer, rather than merely aiming for early detection of cancer through mammographic screening. If you wonder how stress impacts on your breast cancer risk; or diet and nutrition; exercise; alcohol consumption; the pill or HRT; exposure to radiation . . . or a myriad of other everyday lifestyle factors, then this is the book for you.

I feel hugely privileged to have been invited to read Lynda's manuscript before printing. After reading *Well-being*, I can honestly say that I am excited when I think of the positive impact that this highly relevant, information-packed book will have on the health and happiness of so many women. Lynda shares practical suggestions for achieving balance in our lives — physically, emotionally, mentally, spiritually and, yes, hormonally! *Well-being* gives us the means of assuming responsibility for creating vibrant health, through eliminating the root cause of so many common female health problems. Like Lynda, I believe that we have become an overmedicated and undernourished society, and that by understanding the intelligence of our own internal 'chemistry shop'; reducing emotional, mental and physical stress; and eating the most nutritious diet possible, we can reclaim much of the responsibility for our own health destiny.

My passionate interest in health and wellness stems partly from my athletic career and a keen interest in maximising my athletic potential; but mostly from being born into a family with a long history of diabetes and heart disease. From an early age I was taught (by a medical doctor father) not to resign myself to my genetic disposition to diabetes or heart disease, but to be aware of the kinds of food and the lifestyle choices that would minimise my risk of following the family health legacy. Being raised with a 'preventative' health mentality, I appreciate the focus of Lynda's book which promotes the same truly preventative approach to well-being.

As a young athlete in my mid-teens, showing some potential as a runner, I developed chronic sciatica and lower-back pain. A leading surgeon advised that there was a congenital abnormality of the lower spine; in fact, had it been much worse, he told me, I may never have walked! After undergoing traction and wearing a hip brace for some months, I was advised in no uncertain terms to 'give up all sports'. I refused to accept the prognosis and started my own journey away from pain to wellness and robust health via complementary therapies such as acupuncture, chiropractic, massage and a range of special nutrients. I went on to win many international races, set world records and become a New Zealand champion in three different sports. My experience has taught me that when we hit a brick wall we must think outside the box in order to keep spirits high and to keep moving in the direction of our life goals.

We have a right to truthful information so that we may know the value of preventative health care and self-care, and thus make informed choices for ourselves and our families. As women we hold a special position of responsibility. As a result of our usual role as primary nurturers, we are the ones who will naturally have the most influence in bringing about a paradigm shift in health care that is so necessary to create future sustainable health systems.

In this book, Lynda shares time-honoured knowledge and modern research, along with 20 years of personal practical experience as a naturopath, traditional Chinese acupuncturist, health researcher and writer. *Well-being* is a gem that should always be close at hand; it's the kind of reference we need on the bedside table, with a spare copy on hand to pass to a friend who could benefit from it.

Well-being will positively impact on the lives of all modern women and is not only grounded in common sense and user-friendly information but will open our hearts and minds to some startling revelations! It dispels myths and introduces research not yet being widely delivered by (mainstream) health systems in the Western world! *Well-being* provides us with the knowledge and understanding to balance and heal our lives through the intelligence of nature and science working in harmony.

One realises in reading *Well-being* how the dream of a sustainable health future is possible and how the deficiencies of health systems might be tweaked in order to make good health simply achievable for all. Lynda's wonderful book helps us to value our special role in life as women and mothers; to understand ourselves better; and ultimately to help us create a healthier, happier world.

Allison Roe MBE
Won course record back-to-back Boston and New York Marathons 1981
World Marathon Record and World 20k records
Mother, wife, businesswoman, health promoter.

Acknowledgements

Thank you to so many people who have helped directly or indirectly in bringing this book to life.

First, my thanks go to my publishers HarperCollins for seeing the need for this book, and for their excited encouragement and professionalism in making it a reality.

Thanks too go to Allison Roe for taking time from her hugely busy schedule to read *Well-being* and write the foreword. New Zealand women are lucky to have you as their health advocate, Allison.

Health advocate and researcher John Appleton has (as always) been generous and enthusiastic in his willingness to share information and resources with me. Keep up the great work John, and thank you for your generosity of spirit.

Thanks to Mish McCormack (personal trainer) for her professional guidance on the exercise chapter.

To the Breast Cancer Network (NZ Inc.), many thanks for your generous permission to reproduce information from your *Upfront* newsletters. The work you do in raising the consciousness of New Zealand women in the area of prevention of breast cancer is unique in New Zealand, and invaluable.

To Martin Greenleaf, my fantastic acupuncturist . . . you have played an important role in keeping me well through the additional stresses and strains of writing this book. You are a gifted healer, and I am very grateful for two decades of your care.

My deepest gratitude goes to the special people who share their love and their lives with me . . .

My children, Rachel and Stephanie, have selflessly spent the past year seeing significantly less of their mum . . . who was constantly chained to the computer. Thank you, my darlings, for your patience, your support, and for just being the beautiful people you both are.

Mum and Dad, as always, you have been wonderful! Thank you for the school pick-ups, the cooked dinners, the house cleaning, the support and the love. I couldn't have done it without you.

To Craig, thank you for so very many things. Many hours of practical IT support, endless computer back-ups, and patience with a computer illiterate. But much, much more than that, thank you, darling, for your constancy, your encouragement and patience, and your love.

Finally, but very importantly, thank you to the many women who have shared their journey towards wellness with me, and trusted my guidance in 20 years of clinical practice. It has been an honour and a pleasure to work with each of you.

Introduction

Twenty-six years ago my life took a completely unforeseen turn, leading me unexpectedly onto the truly rewarding lifepath of holistic healing. I was a university student, studying to become a psychologist. I was completely unremarkable, living a typical student existence, complete with truckloads of stress; endless cups of coffee; sugar binges; fast foods; regular late-night studying stints; sleep deprivation; and stress-induced insomnia. By the third year of this assault, my body was screaming out for a break from these relentless insults. Chronic exhaustion marked each waking moment, and my life was a roller-coaster ride of mood swings, apathy and frequent infections. Eventually, my health challenges were threatening to get the better of me, and I was seriously considering dropping out of university. Medical investigations failed to find anything amiss, and it was strongly suggested that my malaise was 'all in my mind'.

Life-changing fate intervened in the form of a sprightly, effervescent, shockingly healthy 60-year-old woman. Mary radiated vitality, and lived life to the absolute fullest. Aware of the huge contrast between her vitality and my own, she suggested that I visit her naturopath for help. With absolutely no idea what a naturopath was, but with nothing to lose except my place at university, I dutifully presented at the naturopath's office and stepped into a previously unknown world. For a young woman with nothing but experience of the most orthodox of medicine, the visit was intriguing and memorable, and remains etched clearly in my mind to this day.

I left the naturopath's office clutching nutritional supplements and herbal potions with strict instructions for lifestyle change and a 10-day cleansing diet (and with a healthy dose of scepticism). Still, I committed to following the instructions, and awaited the arrival of the promised miracle. After months of feeling chronically unwell, within a matter of weeks I was sleeping through the night, my energy was noticeably improved, and I was feeling mentally and emotionally stable. The rest, as they say, is history.

Psychology degree in hand, I left university certain that my future lay in the realm of holistic healing, and intent upon learning more about the healing miracle I had experienced in my own life. Over the next nine years I was to complete both a Diploma in Natural Therapies and a Diploma in Traditional Chinese Acupuncture. Even now, after 20 years of holistic healing practice, I still think back to that life-changing visit to the clinic of naturopath David Duggan.

What I didn't realise at the time was that my own journey to wellness illustrated beautifully the enormous philosophical chasm separating Western allopathic medicine and holistic medicine. While seated in front of the doctor, I had recounted a list of ailments and symptoms; had had a brief physical examination (heart, lungs, and so on), and had been dispatched for a multitude of blood tests. I was, in effect, a set of 'symptoms' awaiting diagnosis. At no time was I questioned about my lifestyle, diet, or physical or emotional stresses. When my blood-test results failed to find any abnormalities, Western medicine had little to offer me. Since I could not be 'diagnosed', I could not be treated. I had joined the growing throng of chronically unwell, and had been left feeling dissatisfied and abandoned by a system of medicine adept at acute trauma intervention and symptom control, but with little to offer the 'undiagnosable chronically unwell'.

Contrast this with the seemingly bizarre, but ultimately effective, approach of the holistic practitioner. There, I was questioned in great detail about my lifestyle, diet, exercise and stress, and was asked a multitude of questions relating to the workings of virtually every part of my body . . . not just the ones presenting with symptoms of ill health. From this avalanche of information the naturopath was able to construct a 'holistic' picture of my health as a unified, integrated whole person. It was quickly evident that I was suffering from chronic adrenal exhaustion resulting from poor nutrition; a complete lack of work/life balance; caffeine and sugar addiction; and from having a hard-driving, perfectionist, type-A personality (something I am glad to say has mellowed somewhat with the passing years!). A prescription for more exercise, more rest, more fun, more balance, more nutrients, less coffee and less sugar, along with a few well-chosen herbs and nutritional supplements, was all it took to give my body the breathing space it needed to heal itself . . .

To the uninitiated patient the difference between holistic and Western medicine may appear as simple as the use of a herb or a nutritional supplement, in place of a prescription for a pharmaceutical drug. In truth, the differences are much, much deeper. Western medicine is strongly rooted in the philosophy of reductionism, which contrasts greatly with the 'holistic' philosophy underpinning the practice of holistic therapies such as naturopathy, acupuncture, herbalism, homoeopathy and osteopathy.

When a holistic practitioner sees a patient standing before them, they see an integrated human being, the result of an inseparable, indivisible communion of body, mind and spirit. Sickness manifesting in any part of the body/mind/spirit is a signal that somewhere in this integrated whole there has occurred a 'dis-harmony', which has ultimately manifested as symptoms of illness. While symptoms may manifest in a particular organ (for example, the lungs in the case of asthma), it is the level of vitality and balance within the entire organism (body, mind and spirit) which is considered of utmost importance. Of course, holistic therapy would pay special attention to improving the function of the lungs, but only within the context of raising the level of vitality of the entire body/mind/spirit.

In this particular hypothetical case, our asthmatic patient has

chronic back spasms; consumes a diet devoid of fruits and vegetables and full of processed, denatured food; has recently been
through a traumatic divorce and is consumed by grief and bitterness; is chronically exhausted and is dependent on caffeinated
energy drinks to get through the day without collapsing with
exhaustion. True healing, as opposed to symptom suppression,
can only occur when each of these underlying contributory
factors is addressed. The ultimate aim of the holistic healer is
the restoration of optimum well-being and health to the entire
organism, rather than simply the resolution of acute symptoms of
illness. All holistic therapies share the belief that it is the body's
own vital force or inherent drive towards homoeostasis (balance)
which is the true healer, with the practitioner merely clearing
away the impediments to its flow.

Contrast this with the standard Western medical approach to
asthma. Almost invariably the vital component of sound nutrition
is immediately overlooked. Rarely is enquiry made into the mental
and emotional state of the patient, and little consideration may
be given to potentially significant lifestyle factors. The lungs are
viewed in relative isolation, as the 'diseased' organ, and treated
accordingly with drugs to control symptoms and give the illusion
of 'wellness'. Not surprisingly, no true healing occurs, and the
patient commences what may be a lifetime of dependence on
suppressive pharmaceutical agents. With none of the underlying
causative factors having been addressed, the patient's vital force
remains depressed, and in some cases may actually be further
compromised by the suppressive actions of the pharmaceutical
medications. While this analytical, reductionist approach to
healing is effective in the rapid treatment of life-threatening
acute disease, in the case of more chronic conditions, it frequently
becomes so preoccupied with the intricacies of disease that it loses
sight of the whole person.

While it may sound as though I am denigrating the scientific
endeavours of Western medicine, I do in fact have a realistic
appreciation of both its strengths and its weaknesses . . . and it

does have some spectacular, often life-saving, strengths. If you have a life-threatening infection you'll be only too thankful for the pharmaceutical wonder of antibiotics. In the field of surgery, intensive care and trauma medicine, Western allopathic medicine reigns supreme. It is in the realm of chronic disease, or undiagnosable malaise, that the reductionist, analytical approach of allopathic medicine often fails spectacularly.

Holistic therapies have witnessed a huge upsurge in popularity in the last decade. One of the factors prompting this trend is the increasing awareness of the dangers inherent in Western, pharmaceutical-based medicine. 'Iatrogenic disease' is the name given to illness resulting directly from medical intervention or the use of pharmaceuticals. Almost unbelievably, in many Western countries it is the third most common cause of death, after cardiovascular disease and cancer. In America alone, nearly a quarter of a million Americans lose their lives every year as a result of the practice of Western medicine. Of these deaths, around 106,000 annually are the result of non-error negative effects of pharmaceutical drugs. An estimated 2.2 million American patients a year experience adverse drug reactions while in hospital. One in seven hospital beds is taken up by someone hospitalised because of an adverse drug reaction. America is not an exceptional case, and throughout the Western world, iatrogenic disease continues to be one of our foremost causes of death.

While popping a vitamin pill or calling in at the chiropractor's for a quick 'crunch' on the way home from work is becoming second nature for many of us, Australian studies show that around 60% of users of complementary and alternative medicines (CAM) don't tell their GP what they are doing. In some cases this is simply an act of omission, but in many others, patients fear a negative response from their doctor, and simply choose to segregate their health care into two distinctly separate camps . . . Western medicine and 'alternative' medicine.

It is the patient who has the most to lose in this unsatisfactory arrangement. As a result of this schism, they are left with fractured, disjointed and potentially dangerous health care, with no communication between health-care providers, and less than optimum results for themselves.

Integrative Medicine is a new initiative. In its simplest form, it is the practice of Western scientific medicine in combination with those complementary therapies that are strongly evidence based, and that have high-quality scientific evidence of safety and effectiveness. Professor Marc Cohen, President of the Australian Integrative Medicine Association, says of Integrative Medicine: 'IM values all aspects of a person's health — body, mind and spirit — and reaffirms the importance of an open relationship between practitioner and patient. Those who practise IM consider a patient's overall satisfaction with life, pointing to irrefutable proof that stress management and good mental hygiene positively affect healing and health.' New Zealand and Australian health-care consumers now have the option of choosing a medical doctor practising IM, and have the peace of mind of knowing that any other complementary therapies they choose to pursue can be incorporated into their overall health-care picture, with the support of their GP.

This book is the fruition of 20 years of practical experience teaching and empowering women how to take self-responsibility for creating good health, through making different choices in their daily lives. It is a self-help manual of inspiration, encouragement and sound, practical advice, giving you the tools you need for creating optimum health and well-being. I have endeavoured to answer many of the health-related questions I hear day after day in my clinic. If you are looking for an easy-to-read, practical holistic health guide to support you in your quest for optimum health, this is the book for you. It is intended to be used in conjunction with the health care offered by professionals in both the complementary and allopathic fields of healing.

I wish you well on your journey towards vibrant good health!

Lynda

Part One

Staying Well

Chapter 1

A woman's body — understanding the miracle

The female body is a living, breathing miracle of creation. While it is functional, and often aesthetically beautiful, it is also a breathtakingly complex organism. Most of us race through life inhabiting our female form with little consideration for its intricacies and wonder. In order to live a more balanced and health-promoting lifestyle, it is useful to understand the basic workings of your divine female body. By understanding its structure and function, you become more in tune with the normal rhythmic changes which occur in a healthy body . . . and in turn more aware of subtle changes which may indicate that something is amiss.

Exploring the landscape

Nature created women to procreate. It's as simple as that. As modern women we have freedoms, rights, choices and career opportunities unheard of in previous generations . . . but we still inhabit bodies designed for breeding. From the age of approximately 12 to 50, we are swept along on a wave of hormonal and physical flux, solely designed to maximise our opportunities to reproduce. We spend around 35 years of our lives either trying to avoid conception, or struggling to conceive.

Female anatomy and physiology are primarily designed to fulfil our unique roll as child bearers. The uterus, cervix, ovaries and breasts are solely designed for reproduction and nurturing the young.

On the outside

The vagina is safely tucked away behind the fleshy lips of the vulva. The *vulva* is the term given to all of the external female genitals including the lips of the vagina, the mons (the fleshy bump above the vagina, covered with pubic hair); the clitoris; the urinary opening, the opening to the vagina, the perineum (the space between the vagina and the anus), and the anus.

The *clitoris* is a small knob of exquisitely nerve-rich tissue that lies beneath the hood of skin at the top of the vaginal opening. Filled with nerve endings which produce intense sexual pleasure when stimulated, the clitoris is for many women their orgasmic 'switch'. The clitoris is purely about sexual pleasure, and has no other function or purpose.

Just beneath the clitoris, and above the vaginal opening, is the *urinary opening* through which urine from the bladder is passed. The urethra is the tube which carries urine from the bladder to the outside of the body. The female urethra is a tiny 5 cm long, in comparison with the average male urethra of 25 cm. This tiny distance between the outside world and the inside of the bladder is one of the anatomical reasons for the high incidence of bladder infections in women. The opening of the urethra is also very close to the rectum, from which bacteria can easily find their way to the urethra and bladder. Vigorous sexual intercourse can also force unfriendly bacteria from the outside of the body into the urethra.

The *vagina* has been both revered and reviled throughout history, and has been the source of both male condemnation and fascination. For women, it is the seat of our sexuality and the passage through which we confer the gift of new life. In a healthy woman it is also an incredible self-contained ecosystem, with its own intricately balanced system of self-regulation. The vagina is open to the outside world with its teeming billions of bacteria, viruses and yeast. The self-regulating ecosystem of friendly bacteria living in the vagina for the most part keeps the vagina healthy, moist and clean.

A healthy vagina maintains a pH balance of around 4 to 5, making it slightly acidic. This acidity dissuades potentially unwelcome colonisers such as bacteria and yeast. The friendly *Lactobacillus acidophilus* bacteria in the vagina (yes, the same stuff you eat in yoghurt!) help to maintain this slightly acidic environment.

The vagina is a closed-ended muscular tube about 10 or 12 cm in length, but with an amazing ability to expand to accommodate the largest of penises, or even a five-kilogram baby! The vagina is constantly bathed in a secretion from the cervix which helps to clean, balance and lubricate it. Cervical secretions are also mixed with vaginal fluids during sexual arousal. In a healthy vagina, it is normal to have a little vaginal secretion every day. Around the time of ovulation and peak fertility, the quality and quantity of mucus changes, and it becomes slippery and abundant. Healthy vaginal secretions may be clear, creamy, or slippery like egg white. They typically have a mild, non-offensive musky odour. If your vaginal secretions become green or yellow, offensive-smelling or irritating, see your doctor, as these are usually signs of a vaginal infection.

Sitting at the top end of the vagina is a hardish knob which feels like the fleshy tip of a nose. The *cervix* (which means neck) is the neck of the uterus. The cervix functions as a kind of guard, protecting the deep reproductive organs (uterus, ovaries and fallopian tubes) from invasion by marauding bacteria, viruses and yeasts. The cervix has a tiny opening which allows menstrual blood to travel out of the uterus, as well as allowing access for sperm to travel through the uterus and on to the fallopian tubes. For most of the time, the opening to the cervix is tightly closed. During ovulation and menstruation, the opening increases slightly in size. In a feat almost defying the laws of physics, this tiny gateway dilates to a massive 25 cm during childbirth, to allow the passage of a baby through the birth canal.

The cells which line the interior and exterior of the cervix are rapidly renewed and replaced by new cells. This process of cell replication sometimes goes haywire, leading to the development of abnormal, cancerous or precancerous cells. Regular Pap smears test these cells, making possible the detection (and if necessary, removal) of precancerous cells before they become more serious. (See Pap smears below.)

The cervix is the passageway to the *uterus* or womb. This hollow organ is about the size and shape of an upside-down pear, but its thick muscular walls can stretch to accommodate a fully grown foetus.

The blood-rich lining of the uterus is called the *endometrium*. Depending on the stage of your menstrual cycle, the endometrium grows and shrinks, primed by the female hormones oestrogen and progesterone. The body prepares this blood-rich lining for the potential imminent arrival of a fertilised egg; thickening the lining and forming tiny glands which secrete substances to nourish and support an implanted fertilised egg. If no egg arrives, the thickened lining is sloughed off and passed from the body as menstrual blood.

On either side of the upper uterus there are narrow, 10-cm-long tubes which extend up into the abdomen. These are the *fallopian tubes* through which an egg travels to the uterus when released by the ovaries during ovulation. They are also the super-highway through which eager sperm swim in their hunt for a waiting egg. The human egg is so tiny that it is invisible to the eye. Once the egg is ejected from the ovary, it begins its ultra-marathon six-day journey through the fallopian tubes, eventually reaching the uterus. The fallopian tubes are lined with fine hairs (cilia) which sway in reaction to tiny contractions of the tube, coaxing the egg to move down through the tube. Occasionally a fertilised egg will lose its way, setting up home in the lining of the fallopian tube, instead of in the uterus (this is termed an ectopic pregnancy). The egg then begins to grow, and if not medically detected, can cause a rupture of the fallopian tube, a situation which is a potentially life-threatening medical emergency.

One end of each fallopian tube is attached to the uterus. The other end of the tube ends with tiny finger-like projections. Suspended a small distance below these projections are the almond-shaped *ovaries*. The ovaries are not actually attached to the fallopian tubes, and when an egg is released from an ovary (which occurs monthly at the time of ovulation), the finger-like projections sway around and entrap the egg, drawing it into the mouth of the fallopian tube. If the egg is fertilised by a sperm at any point during its six-day journey from the ovary to the uterus, conception occurs. The fertilised egg anchors itself in the blood-rich endometrium, and the pregnancy test is positive! On the other hand, if an egg makes its journey to the uterus without encountering any successful sperm, the ovaries and pituitary gland (a gland at the base of the brain) begin a complex orchestration of hormones, which ends approximately 14 days later with a period.

The ovaries are located about 12 cm below the waist, on either side of the abdomen. If you have ever experienced stitch-like lower abdominal pain halfway through your cycle, you'll know exactly where your ovaries are! This is the pain of ovulation, which some women experience monthly, and others never experience. Along with the pituitary gland in the brain, it is the ovaries that are responsible for creating the female form. The hormones they secrete stimulate breast growth, female fat deposition and the onset of menstruation in adolescence. From the onset of the first period until menopause, these tiny glands work day and night to keep you female and fertile.

The ovaries are directly controlled by the *pituitary gland*. The pituitary stimulates the ovaries with a hormone called follicle-stimulating hormone (FSH). As the name suggests, this hormone stimulates the ovaries to make an egg follicle begin to ripen and grow. At the same time, the ovaries ramp up production of the female hormone oestrogen.

All of these uniquely female parts are players in an exquisite hormonal symphony. Conducting the symphony is the pituitary gland, also called the master gland because of its all-encompassing overview and control of all the bit players. Situated at the base of the brain, this tiny gland controls the timing of sexual development; controls your body during pregnancy; and decides when it's time to shift gears into the menopausal phase of life. The pituitary, in turn, is overseen by an even greater, master conductor, the hypothalamus.

Holding all the vital pelvic organs in place is a sheath of muscle called the *pelvic floor*, which is responsible for keeping everything in its right place, right up to the diaphragm. Unlike some other skeletal muscles which can atrophy and sag without causing anything more serious than a saggy appearance, weak pelvic floor muscles will make themselves heard loud and clear. Pelvic floor repair surgery is one of the most frequently performed gynaecological surgical procedures.

A weak pelvic floor will leave you battling with poor bladder control. If jumping on the rebounder, coughing violently, or taking part in an aerobics class causes involuntary leakage from the bladder, it's your pelvic floor muscles that are to blame. Inability to fully empty your bladder when you pass water is another sign of pelvic floor weakness. At its worse, a sagging pelvic floor will leave you feeling that your insides are in danger of falling out through your vagina! Indeed, if the prolapse becomes severe enough, this can actually happen.

Strong pelvic floor muscles are also important for carrying a baby to term during pregnancy, and for assisting in a normal vaginal delivery. If you don't want to end up joining the surgical list for pelvic floor reinforcement, now's the time to start adding pelvic floor exercises to your daily regime. (See Chapter 3 for information on pelvic floor exercises.)

Teenage transformation

If you have a young daughter of seven or eight, the last thing on your mind will be her eventual development into a sexually and reproductively mature young woman. And yet, it is around this time that the very first hormonal stirrings occur which orchestrate this development and the onset of *menstruation*. At seven or eight the pituitary gland is kick-starting the ovaries into producing the female hormone oestrogen. Over the next few years, increasing amounts of oestrogen, along with progesterone, will be responsible for transforming a little girl's body into the curvaceous, fertile body of a woman.

Before she begins to menstruate, the pubescent girl will have developed a fairly mature female form — her breasts will have enlarged and the nipples darkened; the external genitals will have enlarged and become thicker and covered with pubic hair; the vagina will have become deeper and its walls thicker; the uterus and cervix will have enlarged and the lining of the uterus (endometrium) will have begun its cycle of thickening. The ovaries, too, will have enlarged, and become primed to the hormones produced in the pituitary gland.

Most adolescent girls begin menstruating at some time between the ages of 10 and 16. Small or underweight girls tend to be older at the time of their first period (menarche) than heavier, more physically developed girls. Body-fat percentage is a major determinant of the age at which periods first begin, with a minimum body-fat percentage of 17% needed to trigger menarche. It's not uncommon for the first two years of menstruation to be marked by irregularity in terms of onset, duration and blood loss. This is quite normal and is not a cause for concern unless there is excessive blood loss or extreme pain.

Moon change

When the *hypothalamus* senses that the time is right, a maelstrom of hormones surge into life as the pituitary gland begins its production of the menstrual-regulating hormones follicle-stimulating hormone (FSH) and luteinising hormone (LH). FSH circulating in the bloodstream informs the ovaries that it is time to begin the menstrual cycle, prompting the ripening of several of the follicles stored in the ovaries. Only one of these follicles will mature (occasionally two or three, in the case of naturally conceived non-identical twins or triplets). Ripening follicles trigger ever-increasing oestrogen levels, which in turn trigger the lining of the uterus to thicken in readiness for receiving a fertilised egg.

Oestrogen levels peak around day 13 of a 28-day menstrual cycle. High oestrogen levels change the quality of vaginal secretions, to the more abundant, slippery, egg-white consistency seen around the middle of your cycle. Miraculously, this change in the mucus occurs because the cells actually realign themselves to make it easier for sperm to pass up through the vagina and uterus. Be warned when you see this mucus — your body is out to become pregnant! Around mid cycle, at the fertile time, the discharge also becomes quite alkaline, sugary and very hospitable to swimming sperm. Along with the fertile mucus comes a noticeable surge in libido and interest in all things sexual, designed by mother nature to encourage sexual activity at the time most likely to result in conception.

Rising oestrogen levels trigger the pituitary gland to secrete LH, in turn causing the egg follicle bulging against the surface of the ovary to burst out of the ovary and into the fallopian tube. This is the process of *ovulation*, which happens just once in every menstrual cycle. It is not uncommon for teenagers and women approaching menopause to not ovulate during a particular month, despite having a seemingly normal menstrual cycle, and bleeding every month. A young woman's body fat needs to be approximately 22% for regular ovulation to occur. Some women in their reproductive prime also fail to ovulate, as a result of hormonal imbalance such as polycystic ovarian syndrome (PCOS). Sometimes, severe stress or underweight can halt ovulation.

Once the egg begins its journey from the ovary, it lives for a mere 12 to 36 hours. However, sperm can live for up to three (and some say, five) days, so pregnancy can occur from unprotected sex anywhere from three to five days before ovulation until 36 hours after ovulation.

After the egg leaves the ruptured follicle, the follicle undergoes a miraculous transformation into a mini hormone-secreting gland, called the *corpus luteum*. As oestrogen levels decrease, progesterone levels begin to increase, triggering the lining of the uterus to begin secreting nutrients for the impending arrival of a fertilised egg. The lifespan of the corpus luteum is determined by whether conception occurs. In a non-conceiving cycle, the corpus luteum gradually degenerates over the ensuing 14 days, resulting in a slowly declining production of progesterone, and an eventual cessation of progesterone production when the corpus luteum dies around 14 days after ovulation, and a period arrives. If pregnancy occurs, the corpus luteum continues to secrete oestrogen and progesterone to maintain the lining of the uterus and keep the pregnancy viable.

The second half of the cycle, from ovulation until the arrival of a period, is marked by lower oestrogen levels and higher progesterone levels. Higher progesterone production causes changes to the breasts, such as swelling, fullness and tenderness. As progesterone is a heating hormone, the basal body temperature also rises during the second half of the month. This is called the 'thermal shift', and is the phenomenon observed on a basal body temperature chart, which indicates that ovulation has occurred.

In a healthy, balanced female body, the intricate rise and fall of female hormones occurs in perfect harmony, resulting in a regular, trouble-free menstrual cycle and mid-cycle ovulation every month. In reality, this hormonal harmony is readily disrupted by a multitude of variables, leading to menstrual problems or infertility. Changes in body-fat composition resulting from excessive dieting, over-exercise or dramatic stress-induced weight loss can completely stop menstruation and ovulation. Young body-conscious women and teenagers are particularly vulnerable to exercise-induced amenorrhoea (lack of periods). Female athletes are also at risk of fertility issues and premature bone loss resulting from abnormally low body fat.

In our Western society where the true fecund and curvaceous female form is despised, and a half-starved, bony androgyny is revered as the epitome of female beauty, impressionable young women in particular are at risk of menstrual disorders and infertility induced by underweight. Surveys show that by the age of 13, around half of all teenage girls are already unhappy with their body and body weight. By the time they reach 18, an alarming 78% are unhappy with their body image. As the mother of two daughters, one of them a teenager, I know the challenge of helping our daughters appreciate their true beauty, in the face of a bombardment of image propaganda in the media. Helping them to see the connection between their curves and their inner health is one way of encouraging a more normal, healthy body weight.

What constitutes a normal menstrual cycle varies from woman to woman. The textbook female has a period every 28 days, but real women can be healthy and yet menstruate every 25 to 35 days. The length of the period also varies from woman to woman. Some bleed solidly for seven days, while others may experience only two days of bleeding, with perhaps an additional day or two of spotting. If your periods are regular, and not painful, clotty, excessively heavy or scanty, you can consider them normal, even if they don't conform to the 28-day-cycle, 5-day-bleeding textbook scenario. More concerning is a sudden change in your normal cycle. If your periods suddenly become much longer, shorter, heavier or more painful it may be indicative of a problem. The exception to this is the years of perimenopause, when such changes are common and often just a reflection of fluctuating hormone levels.

Traditional Chinese medicine places a lot of emphasis on understanding the unique characteristics of a woman's menstrual cycle. To a trained practitioner of traditional Chinese medicine, the menses offer an invaluable insight into the health and balance of a woman's vital essences, qi and blood. For example, excessively heavy periods may indicate a condition of heat in the blood, or a weakness of spleen energy. Clotty periods accompanied by breast tenderness and irritability are a strong sign that the liver energy is blocked or impeded in some way. Very light, scanty periods often point to a deficiency of blood. It is not uncommon to see a dramatic improvement in menses-related symptoms during a course of acupuncture treatment, even when the treatment is being performed for an entirely unrelated condition.

And then comes the Meno — pause

Somewhere between your mid-forties and mid-fifties, your body will begin its transition from years of being reproductively primed. Periods rarely just stop overnight. More commonly there is a transitional time of four to five years, called the perimenopause ('around menopause'). During these premenopausal years hormone levels fluctuate wildly as the ovaries wind down and eventually run out of eggs. Periods become irregular and ovulation becomes erratic. As the ovaries stop releasing eggs, the production of oestrogen and progesterone declines — hormonal changes which can trigger a wide array of unpleasant symptoms such as mood swings, fatigue, irritability, palpitations and anxiety.

Eventually hormones decrease to a level where menstrual periods stop permanently. The very last period is officially termed the '*menopause*'. Despite the popular conception of the menopausal woman as hormonally ravaged, unstable and rapidly ageing, many woman do in fact pass through this transition with little more than the occasional hot flush and a sense of relief that

Traditional Chinese medicine and a woman's life cycle

When a woman carries a child in her womb, she bestows upon it the gift of 'jing', an essence or vitality that will see her child through its first 30 to 40 years of life. The healthier the mother is at the time of conception, and during pregnancy, the more potent her gift of 'prenatal jing' will be. This prenatal jing is gradually depleted through the process of living. Living hard with an excess of labour, inadequate sleep, poor nutrition and emotional imbalance will deplete the jing more rapidly. Along with the prenatal jing, our body produces qi (pronounced chi) and blood, to augment the life-giving properties of the prenatal jing.

Around the time of perimenopause, the prenatal jing is all but exhausted. During a menstrual period the loss of blood and qi also depletes prenatal jing. As prenatal jing stores dwindle and diminish, the woman's body begins to release less menstrual blood in an attempt to conserve remaining stores of this precious life force.

The prenatal and postnatal jing (manufactured every day from our food) is stored in the kidneys, and consequently strong kidney energy is considered vital to prevent premature or rapid ageing. Especially around the time of menopause, there is a strong emphasis on nourishing and nurturing the kidneys through 'right living', acupuncture and herbal medicine. Many of the common symptoms of menopause are considered to be a sign of weak kidney qi, and can be eased through strengthening treatments for the kidney energy. In order to keep her kidney qi strong, the menopausal woman is encouraged to ensure that she gets plenty of sleep; balances exertion and rest; exercises daily; practises calming and balancing the mind through meditation, tai chi or yoga; eats a nutritious diet and avoids excesses of eating and drinking.

the mess, pain and expense of periods is finally over. For others, however, the menopause is a bewildering time of physical and emotional discomfort. At its worse, menopause may cause severe hot flushes, chronic vaginal dryness and bladder infections, migraines, depression, anxiety, fatigue and joint pain. Check the chapter on menopause for practical tips on managing the transition naturally.

Breasts and breast self-examination

In the centre of each breast is the nipple, surrounded by the dark brown circle called the *areola* (or in younger women who have not yet been pregnant, this area is pink). The nipple is made up of erectile tissue which swells and becomes hard when the nipple is stimulated, or in the cold. The interior of the breast is made up of several lobes containing milk-secreting glands surrounded by fat and connective tissue. A network of ducts branches out from the milk-producing glands to the nipple. The whole breast is connected to the muscles of the chest wall by connective tissue.

In women of reproductive age, breasts are constantly changing in response to fluctuating hormone levels, throughout the menstrual cycle. Every month, the breasts are prepared for the possibility of conception and eventual breastfeeding. During the first two weeks of the cycle, high oestrogen levels stimulate new cells to grow in the glands, milk ducts and fibrous tissues in the breasts. At ovulation, the body starts to produce progesterone, which also affects the breasts, this time causing the cells in the breasts to start secreting and preparing for eventual breastfeeding. At this time it's not uncommon to notice an increase in breast size and tenderness, due to an increase in the amount of blood flowing to the breasts, and also an increase in fluid retention in the breasts. If you do not become pregnant, your body reverses this breast preparation, slowing down the growth of the new breast cells, and reducing the blood flow to your breasts. These cells and secretions are broken down and resorbed by your body.

Examining your breasts

Examining your breasts at the same time of your menstrual cycle every month helps you to understand what is normal, and what is not, for your own breast contours. In theory, routine checking of your own breasts every month gives you the greatest opportunity to detect lumps (which may or may not be cancerous) early on, and while they are still relatively small. In practice, though, studies have failed to demonstrate that breast self-examination (BSE) translates into a decrease in breast-cancer deaths. Dr Susan Love, in her book *Dr Susan Love's Breast Book* suggests that 'by the time you feel a lump, it's been there so long that whether you find it this month, next month or four months from now won't make a critical difference'. Studies aside, I still personally believe that BSE makes sense, and would encourage all women to check their breasts regularly.

Many women notice lumpiness and breast pain in the second half of their menstrual cycle, especially in the 7–10 days before bleeding. Sometimes referred to as fibrocystic breast disease, this condition is non-cancerous but is associated with an increased risk of breast cancer. If you suffer from 'lumpy' tender breasts, it is especially important to be vigilant in your own breast examinations, and to have a clinical breast examination annually, along with a mammogram and ultrasound when indicated.

It is best to begin examining your breasts after your first menstrual period, and certainly by the age of 25. Set aside 10 minutes (yes, that's all it takes) on one of the days straight after your period ends. Breasts are easier to examine at this time of your cycle, when hormones are at a low ebb and breasts are less swollen and hormonally lumpy. Thoroughly examining your breasts involves both looking and feeling.

Looking . . .

Stand in front of a well-lit mirror, with your arms by your sides. Look at your breasts, paying particular attention to their contour.

Look for depressions or bulges on the outline of your breasts. Look for dimpling of the skin, and check your nipples for any discharge. Repeat the inspection, but this time with your arms raised above your head. Turn side-on to the mirror so that you can see all areas of your breasts. Check again while you are pushing your palms together in front of you, or standing with your hands pressed against your hips.

. . . and feeling

Now lie down on your back. As you examine your left breast, raise your left arm above your head, with your left hand tucked in under your head and your elbow lying flat against the bed. Keep the fingers of your examining hand together, and use the flat of the fingers to perform the examination. Begin to feel your breast gently, beginning on the outside of the breast and working around on the breast in ever-decreasing, systematic circles. Also feel the upper part of your chest wall and armpit. It is probably easier to feel lumps if you use some kind of lubricant such as body lotion or oil, or perform your examination while you are soaped up in the bathtub.

Remember that when you perform BSE you should be on the alert for any *changes* in your breasts. These changes may not necessarily be lumps. You may detect a sensation of thickening or increased ropiness in your breast tissue, or there may be dimpling or puckering. Whenever you detect an abnormal change in your breasts, see your doctor immediately. Ninety-nine times out of a hundred you will have nothing to worry about — and it's worth visiting him or her with a false alarm, rather than delaying action and missing that rare lump that actually turns out to be cancer.

Pap smears

Not all types of cancer are easily preventable, but cervical cancer is. The Pap smear makes very early detection of abnormal cellular changes in the cervix possible, long before the changes become

Traditional Chinese medicine and breast health

In Chinese medicine, any breast health issue is considered indicative of an underlying imbalance of energy (qi) and/or blood. As such, breast issues such as distension, pain or lumpiness are taken seriously and treated, in the belief that remedying energy imbalance while symptoms are relatively benign will prevent more serious breast issues, such as cancer, at a later date.

Several energy lines (meridians) run up to or through the breast, including the liver, stomach, pericardium and gallbladder. Of these, it is the liver meridian which is most frequently involved in hormonal breast problems such as pre-menstrual tenderness, lumpiness or distension.

The two main functions of the liver in traditional Chinese medicine are the regulation of the smooth flow of qi and emotion in the body, and storage of blood. In the days before menstruation, the energy (qi) in the liver meridian becomes fuller and more abundant. If there are problems with stagnation or blockage of liver energy, qi circulation stagnates and in time transforms into actual physical lumps and breast distension.

What causes stuck liver qi in the first place? By far the most common causes of liver disharmony are stress, tension and

cancer. Caught at these early precancerous stages, treatment will almost always prevent the development of cervical cancer. In some cases, 'watchful waiting' is all that is required for the cells to return to normal on their own. Abnormal cell changes are usually without symptoms and are undetectable unless a Pap smear is performed. It is estimated that about 90% of cases of the most common form of cervical cancer could be prevented if women have regular smear tests at least every three years. These tests are painless and quick and there is absolutely no valid reason not to have one, especially if you are a sexually active woman.

unresolved emotional turmoil. The liver meridian is affected by suppression of emotion, and especially by excessive or repressed anger and frustration. Although anger or frustration are the primary emotions associated with the liver, the liver is like an emotional conductor, responsible for harmonising the free flow of all emotions. If there is overwhelming or intense emotional trauma, the liver is literally overwhelmed, and liver qi stagnation is one of a number of common liver pattern imbalances which can result. When stuck liver qi remains untreated for many years, the energy imbalance eventually transforms into 'stuck blood', and physical breast lumps or cysts, which may or may not be cancerous.

The spleen meridian is also often involved in the development of breast lumps. When spleen qi is weakened and prone to an energetic tendency called 'dampness', it contributes to breast-lump development. Spleen qi is weakened through excessive worry and use of the mind (such as long-term studying). An excess of cold, damp foods in the diet (such as juices, raw fruits and vegetables, dairy products and sugar) also contribute to the development of damp, as does living in a damp environment.

Cervical cancer and its causes

The good news about cancer of the cervix is that it is very preventable if you have regular Pap smears. This is because cervical cancer is usually a very slow-growing cancer, taking 10 or more years to develop from early cell changes through to full-blown cancer. There are two types of cervical cancer. Squamous cell cancer is the most common, and usually develops in the transformation zone of the cervix (the area from which cells are taken in a Pap smear). Adenocarcinoma is found in the glandular cells lining the cervix.

By far the most frequent cause of both types of cervical cancer is exposure to the HPV (human *Papilloma* virus), an extremely common sexually transmitted infection. (See Cervical dysplasia in the A–Z section in Part Two.)

Who should have a Pap smear?

The New Zealand National Screening Programme recommends that all women who have ever been sexually active have regular smears from the ages of 20 to 70. This includes single women, sexually active women (both lesbians and heterosexual), postmenopausal women, disabled women, and women who have been, but are no longer, sexually active.

What happens in a Pap smear?

A speculum is lubricated and gently inserted into the vagina to dilate it and allow unobstructed view of the cervix, sitting at the top of the vaginal canal. A tiny wooden spatula or rounded brush (like a miniature bottle-cleaning brush) is used to gently collect a sample of cells from the area of the cervix known as the *transformation zone*. This is the area where the cells covering the outside of the cervix meet the different cells which line the canal leading to the interior of the cervix. In order to have an accurate smear, it is vital that cells from this specific area are collected. The obtained cells are then smeared onto a glass slide which is sent to a laboratory for analysis. Women now have the choice of having a 'thin prep' smear, in which the obtained cells are added to a liquid medium before being sent to the lab. These tests are slightly more expensive, but studies suggest they double the rate of detection of precancerous cells, compared with conventional Pap smears.

Things to do, or not to do, before a smear

Your test results are most accurate if you avoid douching for at least five days prior to your smear (this is actually an unnecessary activity at any time, and douching can upset the delicate microflora in the vagina). It's also a good idea to avoid spermicidal creams, foams and jellies for five days before the test. Smear accuracy can also be affected if you have sexual intercourse (without a condom) in the 24 hours before the test. Don't go for a smear when you have a period as the test cannot be done at this stage of your cycle. It is best to wait at least three days from the last day of your period before having a smear.

How often should I have a smear?

The answer is different for different women. The New Zealand National Screening Programme recommends a smear every three yesrs between the ages of 20 and 70. When a woman has her very first smear, or if she has not had a smear for five years or more, it is recommended that she has two smears one year apart. This covers the small possibility that abnormal cells may be missed at the time of the first smear. Women who have previously had a high-grade abnormality are tested every year.

What do my smear results mean?

Results come back classified as any of the following:

* *Normal result.* This accounts for about 90% of all smears. You will usually be advised to repeat the test in three years' time.

* *Unsatisfactory result.* This means that the cellular sample could not be accurately read at the laboratory. There may have been too few cells in the sample, or they may have been damaged or hidden by blood or mucus. Another smear is required within 1–3 months.

* *Inflammation or infection.* This result means that there are signs of some form of infection in the vagina, causing inflammation. This has nothing to do with cancer, and is usually due to a yeast or bacterial infection in the vagina. Often no treatment is needed.

✳ *Abnormal result.* This means that some of the cells in the sample showed some kind of change away from their ideal and normal state. It does not mean you have cancer, but that you have some degree of cellular change that may be precancerous.

Can you explain what an abnormal result means?

Atypical cells (ASC-US — atypical squamous cells of undetermined significance)

This means that some of the squamous cells from the cervix show signs of small changes. This result indicates that it is difficult to tell whether the cells are normal or bordering on abnormal. You will usually be advised to have a repeat smear test in six months' time.

Low-grade changes (LSIL — low-grade squamous intraepithelial lesion)

This means that some of the cells from your cervix have been found to be mildly abnormal, usually as a result of the presence of the HPV (human *Papilloma* virus). Often these abnormal changes will right themselves without any intervention. However, your doctor will want to keep an eye on things, and will recommend a repeat smear in six months' time.

High-grade changes (HSIL)

If cells with serious changes have been detected as a result of your Pap smear, you will be referred for a *colposcopy* (an examination of the cervix with a special microscope) quickly. This result still doesn't mean you have cancer. However, it does mean that these cells have the potential to develop into cancer if not treated.

Understanding CIN

Abnormal cells are graded as CIN — *cervical intraepithelial neoplasia*. CIN means that when the cervical cells are looked at under a microscope, they appear irregularly shaped or abnormal in some way.

CIN 1 refers to mild dysplasia, or abnormal cell development, involving one-third of the cervix's covering layer. The majority of CIN 1 changes do not deteriorate further, and between a half and two-thirds of women with CIN 1 smears spontaneously revert to normal without any kind of intervention.

CIN 2 refers to moderate cell changes, more advanced than CIN 1 changes and involving two-thirds of the cervix's covering layer. Even with CIN 2 changes, there is a spontaneous return to normal in approximately 20% of women, by the time of their next smear.

CIN 3 is the most advanced stage of dysplasia, and involves changes to the full thickness of the cervix's covering layer. It is important to realise that even this most serious stage is not a cancerous condition.

A carcinoma *in situ* is diagnosed when there are cancerous cells found on the surface tissue of the cervix. The cancerous cells are confined to the area, and are not invasive. Carcinoma *in situ* is included under the CIN 3 category.

If results show CIN 1 changes, the only recommendation may be a repeat smear in six months' time. With more advanced cell changes, the next step is to have a colposcopy. A colposcope is a special microscope which allows a close-up view of the cells of the cervix, when viewed up through the vagina.

Treating abnormal cervical cells

Abnormal cervical cells are removed or destroyed using a variety of methods, depending on the location and type of your abnormal cells. A LETZ Loop procedure uses an electrical wire loop to remove the abnormal cells, with the aid of a local anaesthetic. Laser treatment removes cells with the heat from a laser beam, again using a local anaesthetic. If the cells need to be removed surgically, a cone biopsy is performed under anaesthetic. None of these treatments reduces your ability to conceive, or to carry a pregnancy to full term.

Symptoms of cervical cancer

Precancerous changes to cervical cells cause no symptoms, and can only be detected through a Pap smear. Symptoms only appear after abnormal cells have developed into cancer.

* Bleeding or spotting between periods.

* Bleeding or spotting after sexual intercourse.

* Bleeding or spotting after menopause.

* Persistent pelvic pain.

* Painful sexual intercourse.

* Unusual vaginal discharge which may be unpleasant, discoloured or blood streaked.

There are a number of different causes for each of these symptoms, and their presence does not mean that you have cervical cancer. It *does* mean that you need to see your doctor for further investigation.

Chapter 2

Diet and nutrition

Let thy food be thy medicine and
thy medicine be thy food.

Hippocrates

The best doctors in the world are Doctor Diet,
Doctor Quiet and Doctor Merryman.

Jonathan Swift

From the moment, soon after birth, when we first taste our mother's milk (or if we are less fortunate, the first bottle of formula), food and eating become firmly implanted in our psyche as one of life's supreme joys. We eat for pleasure; we eat to share social time and bonding with those we love; we eat for comfort during times of sadness and anxiety; and of course we eat to provide our body with the nutrients which are the building blocks of life.

Ironically, it is this most vital function of nourishment that we so often choose to ignore, listening instead to taste buds and emotional drives prompting us to eat dead, lifeless and nutrient-depleted 'junk' foods. When taste buds (or convenience) rule, we tend to choose foods that taste sweet or salty; or we choose fat-laden foods that supply rushes of energy and satiety. The legacy we create from making these unwise choices, day after day, is evidenced by the 'lifestyle' pandemics of the twenty-first century. Heart disease, cancer, obesity, diabetes and depression have now taken over from acute infectious disease as the leading health threats in the Western world. All of these chronic diseases can be considered lifestyle diseases, with poor nutrition a key component.

In general, New Zealanders and Australians tend to be overfed, undernourished and overweight. We consume too much dietary fat (especially animal fats); we eat too much sugar, salt and refined carbohydrate; and we drink too much alcohol.

Also, few of us manage to eat the prescribed 'five plus' fruits and vegetables every day. Our reward for such dietary choices is one of the highest incidences of diabetes, heart disease and cancer in the Western world.

If you have become one of the 'enlightened', and are making a serious attempt at dietary revolution, you have your work cut out for you. Nowhere is there more confusion, contradiction and rapidly changing advice than in the realm of human nutrition. For optimum health, should you eat a high-protein, low-carbohydrate diet? What about a diet rich in low GI carbs and avoiding high GI carbs? Is vegetarianism the way to go, or what about macrobiotics, dairy free, wheat free . . . how about food free? The opportunity for dietary extremism and resulting ill health has never been greater.

Building blocks of life

Every human being needs the basic building blocks of protein, fats and carbohydrates to stay alive. Individual requirements vary greatly, and are influenced by factors such as age, sex, lifestyle, stress levels, genetics, dietary practices (such as how much caffeine, alcohol and sugar we consume), pregnancy and lactation, and so on.

Protein

Approximately 20% of our body weight is made up from proteins. Proteins form our muscle, bones, internal organs (especially the heart and brain), skin, hair and nails. We need proteins to produce antibodies, enabling us to fight infection; and many of the hormones circulating through the body (such as insulin and thyroxine) are proteins. Proteins help us to keep the correct fluid balance in the body, preventing our cells from ballooning with excess fluids, and protein is needed for growth and maintenance of all the tissues in our body.

Unlike fats and carbohydrates, proteins are not stored in our body, and must be consumed regularly. Not all proteins are born equal. The building blocks of proteins are chains of amino acids. There are 20 different amino acids in total, 12 of which can be synthesised by our body, with the remaining 8 called '*essential amino acids*' which must be supplied through our food.

Animal products such as dairy foods, meat, fish and eggs all supply us with good-quality protein. There are also a number of different vegetarian sources of protein including legumes, grains, nuts and seeds, beans, soya products and rice. (See section on vegetarianism.)

Nuts and seeds are also a source of quality protein and when used in moderation make a useful addition to the diet — but remember they are also high in fat (although it is beneficial fat) and consequently high in kilojoules.

How much protein do you need?

Ironically, for many living in the relatively affluent West, excessive protein consumption is more of an issue than protein deficiency. The exceptions to this are women living on unbalanced weight-loss diets, or people following strict (unbalanced) vegan diets. To work out how much protein you need, multiply your ideal weight in kilograms by 0.8. This gives you an approximation of your ideal protein intake in grams. If, for instance, your body functions best at a weight of 65 kg, you need only 52 g of protein a day. In general, women need less protein than men. Growing children (especially toddlers) and adolescents need a relatively high protein intake, as do pregnant and lactating women. Pregnant or lactating women or endurance athletes need to multiply their ideal weight (in kilograms) by up to 1.8 to get an approximation of ideal protein intake in grams.

Carbohydrates

While the 'catch phrase' for protein might be 'building structure', when it comes to carbs it's all about 'fuelling energy'. Carbs are naturally occurring or synthetic chemicals made from carbon, hydrogen and oxygen. Your body burns carbohydrates as fuel to produce energy for life, and to provide energy for the brain and nervous system. That piece of bread or serving of pasta you eat is quickly converted into glucose, which is the fuel used by every cell in your body. Broadly speaking carbohydrates fall into two main groups — simple and complex carbohydrates.

Simple carbohydrates

Simple carbohydrates are represented by monosaccharides (sugar), such as glucose, fructose (found in fruit and honey) or galactose. When two of these molecules merge, they are called disaccharides, such as maltose (from cereals and grains), sucrose (cane or beet sugar) and lactose (the sugar found in cows' milk). Syrups, brown sugar and concentrated fruit juices are also simple carbohydrates. All of these sugars are considered to be 'simple carbohydrates'. They are readily broken down in the body, rapidly elevating blood-sugar levels.

When our diet contains too many simple carbohydrates it is not uncommon to develop blood-sugar problems, especially reactive hypoglycaemia or 'low blood sugar'. Simple carbs rapidly elevate our blood-sugar levels and trigger a rapid release of insulin from the pancreas (responsible for rebalancing blood-sugar levels by moving sugar out of the blood and into the body's cells). When excessive insulin is released, or when it is released too quickly, blood sugar is shunted out of the blood and into the cells rapidly, leading to a temporary lowering of blood-sugar levels.

The 'rush' which comes from a sugar hit such as a chocolate bar or biscuit is short-lived and is usually followed by an energy crash, a renewed and intensified feeling of hunger, and an urge for another sugar pick-me-up. The blood-sugar roller coaster leaves you feeling lethargic and unwell, and can eventually lead to chronic hypoglycaemia.

Complex carbohydrates

Complex carbohydrates are also referred to as *starches*. Complex carbs are formed by many glucose molecules linked together (hence they are called polysaccharides). Complex carbohydrates are found in unrefined grains such as wholegrain bread, rice, pasta, oats, rye and vegetables. Like simple carbs, complex carbs are also digested and broken down into glucose, the primary fuel needed for your body to function. In general, complex carbs contain more fibre than their simple cousins, have a lower Glycaemic Index (see below), and consequently tend to cause a slower rise in blood sugar, and a more gradual insulin response.

Fibre

The third component of carbohydrate is fibre, in the form of cellulose from fruits and vegetables and the covering of grains such as wheat bran. Fibre plays an important part in keeping the digestive tract healthy by bulking the stool (faeces) and making it easier to pass, and encouraging proliferation of healthy gut bacteria. A high-fibre diet also helps to protect us from cardiovascular disease and breast cancer. Fibre in the gut binds with oestrogen and cholesterol, helping to pass them from the body and thus preventing them from recirculating through the bloodstream and contributing to elevated cholesterol or oestrogen levels.

Understanding the Glycaemic Index (GI)

Understanding the Glycaemic Index (GI) of foods has become all the rage, especially for those trying to lose weight, or diabetics or hypoglycaemics looking for ways to balance their blood sugar.

The GI is a measure of the speed at which a carbohydrate breaks down and releases glucose into the bloodstream. The higher the GI, the more rapidly it elevates blood-glucose levels. Foods are given a rating of 1–100 on the GI scale, with glucose having a rating of 100. Broadly speaking, the more refined or processed a food is (for example, simple carbs), the higher its GI is likely to be. Foods with a high GI which cause rapid blood-sugar elevation also stimulate the greatest release of insulin, raising insulin levels quickly. Insulin has the job of maintaining a safe blood-sugar range by moving glucose out of the bloodstream and into the body's cells, especially the muscles, liver and fat cells. Lower GI foods cause a smaller rise in insulin levels, sustaining energy levels for longer, and prolonging the time until you feel hungry again. A number of popular weight-loss diets are based on the accurate premise that eating low GI carbs and avoiding high GI carbs will lower insulin levels and reduce appetite, thus leading to weight loss. Insulin also stimulates the liver to convert and store excess sugars as fats, so any diet which helps to lower insulin levels also prevents weight gain in this way.

When looking at the GI of different foods it helps to know what is considered a low, medium and high GI. High GI foods are those with a rating of 70 or more. These are the foods destined to cause blood-sugar swings and high insulin levels, and which probably contribute to weight gain. Medium GI foods have a rating of between 56 and 59. These foods can be included in your diet in moderation, without causing any problems. Low GI foods with a rating of 55 or less are those which will cause the least blood-sugar response, and will supply a longer-lasting source of energy to your body. Try to choose the majority of your carbohydrate-rich foods from the low GI list. Only those foods with a considerable carbohydrate component are given a GI rating. Non-starchy vegetables such as cruciferous vegetables (for example, broccoli, cabbage, cauliflower, Brussels sprouts, turnips, bok choy) and greens have no Glycaemic Index because their carbohydrate content is so low. Feel free to include plentiful amounts of these foods in your diet every day!

For those who are serious about exercising, understanding the different effects of varying GI foods on the body is useful. Eating a low GI food before a workout will help to sustain blood-sugar levels for a longer period when exercising. After an intense workout, having a higher GI snack with its faster-release carbohydrates will speed recovery.

Misconceptions abound in the realm of the Glycaemic Index. While the theory is interesting, the effects of differing GI foods on the body are rather more complex than most people realise. A person's blood-sugar reaction to a food is based on more than simply the GI of the food. Other influential factors include age, activity level, insulin levels, time of day, the amount of fat and fibre in the food, how refined (processed) a food is, and what other foods are eaten at the same time. The composition of a meal in terms of the ratio of carbohydrates to fat and protein will also have a bearing on how your body responds to the carbohydrates you eat. Even the cooking method you use makes a difference to GI.

While it makes sense to choose most of your foods from the low to moderate GI list, there are ways you can help to lower the insulin effect from carbohydrates you eat. Eating a protein and a healthy fat source along with your carbohydrate will tend to slow down the speed with which glucose enters your bloodstream, lowering your body's production of insulin. Mixing a low GI carb with a high GI carb at the same meal will also lower the overall GI of the meal.

The GI system of rating carbohydrates has come in for some criticism based on the fact that while it rates the blood-sugar effects of a particular carb food (quality), it tells us nothing

Glycaemic Load Table (GI per serving)

Low GI *(55 or less)*	*Medium GI* *(55–69)*	*High GI* *(70+)*
low/full-fat milk	blackberries	dates
unsweetened	citrus	prunes
yoghurt	peaches	baked white potato
soya milk	kiwifruit	corn
apples	apples	instant rice
strawberries	pears	corn flakes
plums	pineapple	rice bubbles
watermelon	raisins	bagel
grapes	popcorn	lollies
oranges	brown rice	French fries
peaches	couscous	ice-cream
yams	basmati rice	table sugar
sweetcorn	wholewheat bread	wholewheat flour
carrots	rye bread	bread
asparagus	sweet potatoes	white wheat flour
bean sprouts	aubergine	bread
broccoli	Brussels sprouts	Lebanese bread
tomatoes	peppers	Sultana Bran
cabbage	pumpkin	corn pasta
cauliflower	turnips	corn chips
spinach	carrots	microwave popcorn
lettuce	parsnip	
peas	beetroot	
red lentils	apple juice	
oat-bran bread	orange juice	
oatmeal	fruit bread	
peanuts	pita bread	
All Bran cereal	muesli	
pumpernickel	porridge	
firm pasta	Weet-bix	
lentils	white rice	
kidney beans	bananas	
chickpeas	baked beans	

about the amount of available carbohydrate within a food (quantity). The GI of a food is based on a standard measure of 50 g of carbohydrates in the food being tested. For example, a carrot contains only 4–6 g of carbohydrate, so you would need to eat approximately 10 carrots to consume 50 g of carbohydrate . . . something that few people would do in a typical meal! Many people choose to avoid foods such as carrots because of their high GI, but in reality the amount of carrot eaten in a typical meal (as opposed to the amount needed to rate its GI in testing) would do little to elevate blood-sugar levels.

To overcome this limitation, the Glycaemic Load or GL system has been developed, which takes into consideration the quantity of available carbohydrate in a serving of a particular food. The GL of a food is based on the effect of the GI of a food multiplied by its available carbohydrate content in grams, in a standard serving. Going back to the example of carrots, which have a high GI of 92, a single carrot has a low GL rating of only 5, making it a sensible food choice for those controlling blood-sugar levels. In general, fruits, vegetables, beans and whole grains have a low GL. However, when fruit is squeezed into a fruit juice, or grain made into a refined (white) flour, their GLs become very high. As a general rule of thumb, if you eat unrefined foods in their natural state (fruits, vegetables, whole grains, beans, lentils, nuts and seeds) you will be eating foods with a lower GL than those foods which have been refined and processed.

Fats

Fats are confusing, or should I say myths and misinformation are rampant in the realm of dietary fats. Confusion abounds in our fat-phobic society, in which we still keep getting fatter and fatter despite our preoccupation with the Heart Society tick and all things 'low fat'. Despite the fat phobia of some, many New Zealanders continue to have too much fat in their diet . . . and usually of the most damaging kinds.

Fats are fickle, and their effects on the human body range from detrimental to highly beneficial, depending on which type of fat we are consuming; in what quantity; and in what ratio to other fats.

Along with proteins and carbohydrates, fats make up the basic nutritional trio vital for sustaining human life. All fats are made up from a glycerol molecule with fatty acids attached to it. Fatty acids in turn are made up from a chain of carbon and hydrogen atoms with one atom of oxygen attached to it. Most fat in our bodies and in the fats we eat are in the form of triglycerides. Triglycerides are made up of three fatty acids bonded together with a glycerol molecule. A fatty acid that has two hydrogen atoms linked up to each carbon atom in the chain is called a saturated fat. When two hydrogens are missing from a fatty acid, it is a monounsaturated fat; and when there are four or more hydrogen atoms missing, the fat becomes a polyunsaturated fat.

We all need fats in our diet, every day, in order to stay well. Fats are an important source of energy, and they slow down the absorption of a meal, satisfying our appetite for longer periods. They are vital for the health of internal organs, nerves and the membranes of every single cell in our body. Without fats we cannot absorb or transport the fat-soluble vitamins A, D, E and K, and this, in time, leads to nutritional deficiency. Despite what the celebrity-hungry women's mags would have you believe, body fat is essential for well-being. Not only does body fat keep us warm, but some degree of internal fat is essential for shielding our internal organs from trauma and cold.

Ironically, dietary fats (of the right type and in the right amount) help prevent excessive weight gain and fat deposition, especially around the abdomen. Dietary fats trigger our satiety (fullness) signals much more effectively than carbohydrates or proteins. Try eating a carb-based meal with no fat, and see how quickly you are hungry again. Adding a dose of healthy fats to the same meal will quickly send a message to your brain registering that you have eaten and are now full. Fats also slow down the entry of sugars from carbohydrates into your bloodstream, in turn slowing the rise in insulin in your blood. Lower insulin levels then encourage your body to release stored body fat for energy. This mechanism may explain why, despite our obsession with 'low-fat' foods, the average weight of Westerners continues to creep upwards year after year.

Fats can be broadly divided into two main categories:

* saturated fats

* unsaturated fats:
  — polyunsaturated
  — monounsaturated.

Saturated fats

If a fat is naturally solid at room temperature, it is a saturated fat (I say 'naturally solid' because with modern food processing, liquid fats can be turned into solid fats through the process of hydrogenation, a by-product of which are troublesome trans-fats). These fats come from animal products such as meat and dairy foods, as well as the vegetable oils palm and coconut. Saturated fats carry the mantle as most maligned of all fats, with their connection with cardiovascular disease. We are constantly told that eating saturated fats equals courting heart disease. While there is ample evidence to support such a relationship, there are some contradictions to the saturated fat/cardiovascular disease hypothesis, which suggest that other types of dietary fat may be partly to blame for the rising tide of cardiovascular disease.

Before 1920, cardiovascular disease was virtually unheard of in the USA, but by the mid-1950s heart disease was the leading cause of death there. Common sense would suggest that a close look at the American diet would reveal a corresponding increase in the intake of saturated fats in that period. Amazingly, the exact converse is true. From 1910 to 1970, the proportion of animal fats (meat, butter, lard, and so on) in the typical American diet decreased from 83% to 62%, while consumption of polyunsaturated fats in the form of vegetable oils, margarine, shortening and refined oils increased by a massive 400% (along with a 60% increase in sugar and processed foods).

A look at modern-day populations around the world also uncovers some anomalies in the saturated fat/heart disease connection. One study looked at the Jewish population of Yemen with a traditional diet high in saturated fats. They were compared with Israeli Jews living on a diet containing much more margarine and vegetable oil. Contrary to expectation, the vegetable-oil group had much higher levels of heart disease and diabetes compared with the high-saturated-fat group. Interestingly, those eating the traditional saturated-fat diet were also having no sugars in their diet, compared with 25–30% of total carbohydrate sugar consumption in the other group.

The same situation occurs when looking at the diets and incidence of heart disease in India. Northern Indians eat 16 times more animal fat in their daily diets than do their Southern Indian peers, and yet their incidence of heart disease is seven times lower than that of the Southern Indians. The same anomalies are obvious when looking at Inuit people, Masai in Africa, and the Mediterranean populations. All these people eat diets high in saturated fats and yet have very low rates of heart disease.

The twentieth century saw a huge change in the fat composition of the typical Western diet. At the turn of the century, butter, lard, tallow and coconut oil were the main fatty staples, supplying predominantly saturated fats with some monounsaturated fats. Today, saturated fats are taboo, and polyunsaturates are revered as a healthier choice. This has seen a huge upturn in the consumption of omega-6-rich polyunsaturated fats such as soya, corn, safflower, and sunflower oils and margarine.

A long-term English study involving several thousand men is another one that has come up with some seemingly surprising connections between polyunsaturated fat consumption and heart disease. Half of the men in the study were asked to reduce saturated fats and cholesterol in their diet (and to stop smoking) in favour of increasing their intake of polyunsaturated vegetable oils and margarine. Just one year later those on this supposedly ideal diet had double the number of deaths of those in the control group, who were still eating their high-fat, high-cholesterol diets . . . and smoking!

Eating too much saturated fat contributes to a rise in potentially troublesome LDL (low-density lipoprotein) but focusing almost exclusively on saturates as the dietary cause of cardiovascular disease, in the face of much conflicting evidence, is short-sighted. Despite the effects of saturates on LDL levels, when the fatty plaques clogging arteries are analysed, they are found to be predominantly formed from unsaturated fats, especially polyunsaturates. Studies show that approximately 26% of the fat in arterial plaques is saturated, with the remainder made up of unsaturated fats, half of which is polyunsaturated fat.

But don't saturated fats cause cancer? For a long time, it was believed that a high intake of saturates contributed to the development of several types of cancer, including breast cancer. Many studies have failed to find a link between dietary saturated fat and increased cancer risk. In fact, there are studies which suggest that it is the rise in consumption of omega-6-rich polyunsaturates, rather than of saturates, which is linked to an increase in the incidence of cancer. Certainly, when one looks at the historical trends in fat consumption, it is the rise in polyunsaturated fat consumption which correlates with the burgeoning cancer statistics. Our ancestors — even as recently as the mid-1900s — consumed diets containing much greater concentrations of saturated fat than our own, and yet fewer of them died of heart disease and cancer.

In truth, making saturated fats the 'fall guy' of the fat world is partly unjust. Despite all the bad publicity they get, saturated fats actually have some positive things in their favour. Compared with polyunsaturated oils, saturated fat is incredibly stable and resistant to oxidation (the process which causes the fat to become rancid). They are more stable when stored and also during the cooking process. This is an important point, as rancid oils are full of cancer-causing and tissue-damaging free-radicals. Some saturated fatty acids are essential for the body to properly utilise essential fatty acids (EFAs) from the diet.

I'm not advocating that we all rush out and start gorging on hamburgers, pies and cheeses (all sources of saturated fats). It is still sensible to minimise our intake of saturates in favour of other fats which have proven health benefits. It's worth noting, though, that in obsessing about the detrimental effects of dietary saturates, we may have been turning a blind eye to the detrimental health consequences of over-consumption of polyunsaturated fats high in omega-6 fatty acids.

Coconut oil — a saturated fat with special health benefits

Coconut oil is a saturated fat with a remarkable history of health benefits dating back 4000 years in ancient ayurvedic medicine. Back then, what they didn't know was that its amazing healing qualities are linked to its high content of lauric acid, now known to be an antiviral, antibacterial and antifungal agent. All fats are described as either short-, medium- or long-chain fats, depending on the number of carbon molecules they contain. The majority of coconut-oil fatty acids are medium-chain (like human breast milk). These medium-chain fatty acids are easily digested, giving a rapid-release energy source, along with their potent antimicrobial, antiviral and immune-boosting properties.

When lauric acid from coconut oil is eaten, the body turns it into a monoglyceride called monolaurin. Monolaurin functions as a powerful antiviral, antibacterial and antiprotozoal, used to destroy fat-coated viruses such as the HIV, herpes, and influenza viruses; as well as a number of bacteria such as *Listeria*, *Helicobacter pylori* (responsible for many stomach ulcers), and protozoa such as giardia. Along with lauric acid, another of coconut oil's fatty acids — capric acid — is responsible for the oil's potent antimicrobial effects. Once ingested, capric acid is turned into monocaprin, a potent inhibitor of the HIV virus. Studies are underway into the effect of monocaprin against herpes simplex and *Chlamydia*. The medium-chain fatty acids in coconut oil have also been proven to be beneficial for heart health.

The rise of the trans-fats

While writing this chapter, I wondered exactly where I should place the section on trans-fats. Should it be under the heading of 'saturated fats', or should it sit innocuously in the 'unsaturated fats' section? You see, trans-fats are neither saturated nor unsaturated. Or more correctly, they are partially saturated fats. While I have tried to partly redeem the tarnished image of saturated fats, it is hard to find anything positive to say about trans-fats, their partially saturated cousins. I suspect that in time, we will come to see these man-made fats as the most damaging and detrimental of all dietary fats. Some are already dubbing them the 'silent killers'.

Trans-fats are produced when polyunsaturated or mono-unsaturated fats have hydrogen atoms added to them, to retard spoilage. The fats thus produced are called hydrogenated fat, or partially hydrogenated fat . . . look out for these names on food labels, and do yourself a favour — put them back on the supermarket shelf! These 'fake fats' have a bizarre molecular structure, foreign to our body, and cannot be used by the body to manufacture the long-chain fatty acids (such as EPA and DHA) used to form healthy cell membranes. While trans-fats do occur naturally in animal products, this source is extremely small compared with the level of trans-fat we ingest through consumption of processed foods.

While saturated fats are now popularly (but perhaps incorrectly) condemned for their role in fuelling the cardiovascular and cancer epidemics, a close look at trans-fats suggests that they should, in fact, assume the mantle as the most maligned of all fats. Trans-fatty-acid consumption has been correlated with increased risk of both heart disease and cancer. As if that were not bad enough, there is also evidence of their adverse effects as factors in diabetes, delayed infant growth and hormonal and immune system dysfunction.

Once in the human body, trans-fats stimulate a rise in the level of potentially troublesome LDL cholesterol, as do saturated fats, and simultaneously lower the levels of the protective, friendly HDL (high-density lipoprotein) fats (something that saturated fats don't do). This works as a cardiovascular 'double whammy', negatively affecting the all-important LDL-to-HDL ratio, an important indicator of cardiovascular risk. LDL comes in different-sized particles, and it is the smallest of these which cause the greatest problem. These tiny particles of LDL cholesterol, which readily enter the walls of the arteries and contribute to the formation of arterial plaques, are increased with trans-fat consumption. The long-running Harvard Nurses' Health Study

How to avoid trans-fats

* Buy your bread and baked goods from a local bakery instead of commercial varieties from the supermarket.

* Read labels and avoid all foods listing 'hydrogenated fat' or 'partially hydrogenated fat'.

* Avoid commercial peanut butter and either make your own or buy from a health food store. You know it has not been hydrogenated if there is a pool of oil at the top of the jar.

* If you use margarines, read labels and use those with a negligible trans-fat content, such as olive oil spreads.

* Avoid takeaways (especially French fries) from 'chain' commercial outlets.

* Avoid packaged snack foods, fried foods, 'fast foods' and hard margarine.

found that women with the highest trans-fat consumption had an almost 30% increased cardiovascular risk compared with women with the lowest consumption. The same study found a correlation between trans-fat consumption and type-two diabetes. The Harvard Nurses' Health Study was actually many studies rolled into one, and was conducted over many years. Data was collected from groups of nurses (between 70,000 and 120,000, depending on the branch of the study) and analysed.

Unsaturated fats

One of the obvious differences between saturated and unsaturated fats (be they poly- or monounsaturated) is that saturates are solid at room temperature, and polyunsaturates are liquid. Consequently unsaturates are more sensitive to the effects of light and temperature, and are more prone to rancidity.

Polyunsaturated fats

Polyunsaturated fats contain either predominantly omega-6 or omega-3 fatty acids. The omega-6-rich polyunsaturates have been strongly promoted as a healthy dietary choice, in place of saturated fats. They are mostly vegetable-based liquid oils such as safflower, sunflower, soya, cottonseed, wheatgerm, and corn oil. Omega-3 polyunsaturated fats are found in oily fish, nuts and seeds, flax oil and avocados.

Polyunsaturated oils are highly unstable and quickly become rancid when exposed to heat or oxygen, as occurs during cooking or processing of foods. Rancid oils contain huge amounts of dangerous free-radicals, which attack cell membranes, prematurely damaging or destroying cells. Free-radicals are involved in the effects of ageing, the development of cancerous cells, and the development of arterial plaques and heart disease.

Polyunsaturated oils should be kept in the fridge, or in a dark glass container in a cool cupboard. *Never be tempted to use an oil once it has developed the slightly bitter flavour of rancidity, as it will act as a carcinogen in your body.*

Omega-3 and omega-6 fatty acids

There are some polyunsaturated fatty acids which are vital for our well-being, but cannot be made by our body. These two 'essential fatty acids' or EFAs must be regularly ingested as part of our daily diet. They are *linoleic acid* (an omega-6 fat) and *alpha-linolenic acid* (ALA, an omega-3 fat). These EFAs are the vital precursors used by our body to manufacture a range of other important long-chain fatty acids such as DGLA, EPA, DHA and arachidonic acid. These fats are involved in creating healthy, flexible cell membranes, which are a vital component of optimum cellular function. Essential fatty acids are also essential for the growth and maintenance of blood vessels and nerves, and for maintaining the suppleness of skin and connective tissue. EFAs (especially DHA) are also a vital component of brain tissue.

EFAs are also needed for the production of locally functioning transmitter substances called prostaglandins and eicosanoids, which are involved in cell-to-cell biochemical functions such as energy metabolism, and cardiovascular and immune system function. Prostaglandins are a subset of a larger group of localised tissue hormones called eicosanoids. Eicosanoids are created in cells and stay within the cell working to catalyse numerous important biochemical reactions. We are still continuing to discover the myriad of vital functions that prostaglandins and eicosanoids fulfil in the human body.

The type of fats you consume strongly influence the type of prostaglandins predominating in your body. Our Palaeolithic ancestors consumed diets which supplied roughly equal proportions of omega-6 to omega-3 fatty acids, a balance which the human body is happiest with. Modern man, living on a largely processed diet with an abundance of processed polyunsaturated fats, now consumes approximately 20 times more omega-6 than omega-3 fats. This is partly because polyunsaturated fats rich in omega-6 fatty acids have become the most popular choice for cooking and food processing alike.

Prostaglandins are produced through different pathways,

depending on the type of fatty acids they begin with. Omega-6 fatty acids are used to produce series 1 prostaglandins. Prostaglandins produced from the omega-3 pathway are called series 3 prostaglandins, and start with the unsaturated fatty acid EPA, found in fish, fish oils and eggs. Finally, there's the series 2 prostaglandins produced from a starting point of the unsaturated fatty acid, arachidonic acid (found mostly in butter, meat and eggs).

Prostaglandins in the 1 and 3 series are considered to be more favourable and beneficial than those in the 2 series. This is because series 2 prostaglandins are pro-inflammatory and also increase the stickiness of blood platelets, thus increasing risk of clotting. In direct contrast, series 1 and 3 prostaglandins quell inflammation, and decrease the stickiness of the blood. An over-abundance of the omega-6 fatty acid, arachidonic acid (predominantly from animal foods and saturated fats) will lead to excessive production of series 2 prostaglandins. Beneficial 'anti-inflammatory' series 3 prostaglandins need omega-3 fats in their production. Linolenic acid is converted into EPA, which is the precursor to these 'friendly' prostaglandins. Fish oil provides ready-made EPA, and consuming a diet rich in oily fish, or taking fish oil supplements daily, helps to shunt prostaglandin production into this favourable pathway. A low dietary intake of these omega-3 fatty acids is implicated in the development of inflammatory conditions such as arthritis, eczema, asthma and migraine. A low omega-3 intake in infancy and childhood has been associated with the development of food allergies, skin conditions and some learning disorders.

Fish oil and flax oil have become popular health supplements, due to their high content of health-promoting omega-3 fatty acids. Fish is rich in the two omega-3 fatty acids EPA and DHA, which can also be manufactured by our body if we have a plentiful dietary intake of the alpha-linolenic essential fatty acid (found in flax, soya and canola oils). Vegetarians who object to supplementing with fish oil can in theory reap the same benefits by using flax oil in their diet. I say 'in theory' because the conversion of alpha-linolenic acid into EPA and DHA is not always an efficient process. For this reason, I would always recommend using fish oil supplements instead of flax supplements, unless there is an objection on vegetarian grounds.

Findings of the 2003–2004 New Zealand Total Diet Survey

This dietary analysis is carried out in New Zealand every five to six years, and tests more than 120 different foods commonly consumed in the New Zealand diet.

* Sodium (salt) intakes are well above recommended levels for all age groups.

* Iodine intake is very low.

* Women over the age of 25 are consuming only half the RDI (recommended daily intake) of iron.

* Half of 990 food samples screened contained detectable residues of pesticides.

* Lead exposure from food and environment continues to drop (since the advent of lead-free petrol) and we have some of the lowest exposures in the world.

* Intakes for most New Zealanders of arsenic, cadmium, lead and mercury are mostly well below Provisional Tolerable Weekly Intakes.

Those concerned with the fight against disease know that our bodies are designed to overcome disease processes before they become established. Our systems are readily disrupted by toxins and an absence of sufficient quantities of nutrients.

Nutritional Cancer Therapy Trust

Monounsaturated fats

Monounsaturated fats come from plant foods, and are the darlings of the fat world. They include olives and olive oil; canola oil; nuts and seeds, and avocados. Monounsaturated fats are the main component of olive oil (75%), and canola oil is also high (60%) in monounsaturated fat. Because of the multitude of proven health benefits of olive oil, I always recommend the use of extra virgin olive oil in place of canola oil. Monounsaturated fats are more stable than polyunsaturates, and less prone to rancidity and free-radical production. Monounsaturated fats do wonderful things for our health, especially the cardiovascular system. Regular consumption of monounsaturates helps to lower potentially troublesome LDL cholesterol while simultaneously increasing heart-protective HDL cholesterol. Polyunsaturates, on the other hand, lower LDL levels but do not increase protective HDL cholesterol. The Mediterranean diet is high in monounsaturates as a result of the large amounts of olives and olive oil consumed daily, and has been proven to be one of the most effective diets for optimising cardiovascular health, along with reducing the incidence of several types of cancer.

Boost your monounsaturated fat intake by cooking in extra virgin olive oil; sprinkling olives through salads; using a olive oil (or olive and avocado) spread in place of butter or margarine; making salad dressings from extra virgin olive oil and balsamic vinegar or lemon juice; sprinkling nuts and seeds through salads, porridge and muesli.

Dietary know-how

Are you one of the many people who wants to change their diet for the better, but you haven't got a degree in nutrition, and you're not quite sure how to navigate your way through the endless bombardment of conflicting nutritional information? If you have answered 'yes' to this question, read on for the simple ABCs of sound nutrition and vibrant good health.

A quick word of advice . . .

In the heat of your enthusiasm, don't be tempted to try to change every less-than-perfect aspect of your diet overnight. Remember, you are most likely trying to change the eating habits of a lifetime, and if you want the changes to be more than a temporary 'diet', you will need time to establish new routines, and accustom your body to its new nutrient-dense fuel. Take time, make gradual changes, and be proud of each small step along the way to optimum nutrition.

Change starts in the supermarket

Changing your habits at the table is only possible if you change your shopping habits at the supermarket. In the early days of change, supermarket willpower will be needed, so it's important to try to find a shopping time when you are not hungry or emotionally unbalanced. Doing the shopping at the height of a PMS chocolate craving is probably not conducive to sound judgement and good food choices!

While it's a broad and sweeping statement, the aim at the supermarket is to change the ratio of different food types in the trolley. Packaged, processed, or refined foods will become the smallest component in the trolley, to make room for the mountains of fresh fruits and vegetables you'll be eating. The rest of the trolley is allocated to whole grains, nuts and seeds, healthy fats and proteins. Whizz past the 'junk' shelves containing biscuits, lollies, soft drinks and 'pseudo' foods, to allow for loitering over the vegetables . . . and time to read some mags on the way out!

✻ Minimise intake of processed foods that usually contain added fats, trans-fats, sugars, colourings and preservatives.

✻ Eat wholefoods as close as possible to their natural state.

Nature's superfoods — fruits and vegetables

If it has been grown in the ground or on a tree, and it doesn't come wrapped in cellophane with added fats, colourings and preservatives, it's one of your greatest nutritional allies. I'm talking about fruits and vegetables, of course. While eating five-plus servings a day is your first nutritional goalpost, ultimately aim for nine. It's actually not as impossible as it sounds. Have fresh fruit or berries on morning cereal or yoghurt; snack on fruit mid-morning and mid-afternoon; invest in a juicer and sip on vegetable juices through the day; make lunch a salad, and have a mixture of steamed, stir-fried and raw vegetables at night, and you've easily met your target for the day.

Not only do fruits and vegetables supply the bulk of our dietary fibre, they are also our main source of disease-fighting antioxidants and phytonutrients. No amount of nutritional or antioxidant supplements can replace the myriad of intricately balanced, life-sustaining phytochemicals found in fruits and vegetables. All the research done tells us that people who consume generous amounts of these foods are at lower risk of all the big killers such as cancer, heart disease, diabetes, obesity . . . and other illnesses such as age-related eye disorders, digestive disorders, gum disease and even PMS!

Women who have the greatest intake of carotenoid-rich vegetables in their diet (these are, for example, carrots, kumara, red peppers, broccoli, spinach, apricots, tree tomatoes) have the lowest incidence of breast cancer. Similarly, men who eat 1.5 cups of cruciferous vegetables a week (broccoli, cabbage, cauliflower, Brussels sprouts, turnips, bok choy) reduce their risk of prostate cancer by 40%.

While all fruits and vegetables are good for you, aim for a rainbow of bright, coloured produce every day. Dark greens, bright reds, oranges, yellows, blues and purples all contain different antioxidants and phytochemicals, so variety is the spice of life when it comes to covering the nutritional bases with fresh produce.

* Eat vegetables raw, dry-baked or lightly steamed or stir-fried, as opposed to boiled to death.

* Buy small amounts regularly, store in the refrigerator, and use quickly.

* Chop vegetables at the last minute before cooking.

* Frozen vegetables are a healthy addition to fresh vegetables, if necessary due to time pressures.

* Invest in a fruit and vegetable juicer, and drink a large glass of freshly juiced vegetable juice daily. Choose from a mixture of carrot, beetroot, celery, parsley, wheatgrass, alfalfa, and spirulina powder for a nutrient-dense superfood cocktail.

* Eat 5–9 servings of fruits and vegetables daily.

* Include a daily serving of cruciferous vegetables (broccoli, cauliflower, Brussels sprouts, cabbage).

* Choose a rainbow spectrum of different, strong-coloured fruits and vegetables daily (purple, green, blue, red, orange, yellow) as they are especially rich in antioxidants.

Bread — the staff of life

'If it's white, it's light': which, translated, means all grains that are white and refined are not only light on the stomach, but also light in nutrients and fibre. Replace all your refined, denatured white grains with unrefined wholegrain products. White, cottonwool bread can be replaced with delicious (and infinitely more satisfying) wholemeal bread. Try brown rice instead of white (or if you can't get used to the chewy texture, at least choose low GI basmati rice), and wholemeal pasta instead of white.

Swapping to unrefined grains is an easy way to increase the

fibre content of your diet. It also has beneficial spin-offs such as regular bowel motions and a lowered risk of contracting a range of different cancers, heart disease, and diabetes, as well as lessening the risk of obesity. Unrefined grains also help to stabilise blood-sugar levels, minimising insulin spikes, keeping you full for longer and helping you to maintain a healthy weight.

As many nutrients are destroyed in the refining of grains, eating predominantly whole grains will boost your intake of B-vitamins, vitamin E, and zinc and chromium.

* Choose from a variety of whole grains including wheat, rye, barley, oats, millet, soya flakes, buckwheat.

* Choose wholemeal or pumpernickel bread (high in fibre and with a low GI for blood-sugar regulation).

While whole grains beat refined grains hands-down in terms of their nutritional content, not everyone does well on a diet high in grains. Many people find that wheat, or gluten (the protein component in many grains) leaves them feeling bloated, sluggish, fatigued and unwell. If this sounds like you, try eliminating gluten-containing grains from your diet for a period of several weeks, and look for an improvement in your general well-being. Gluten-containing foods include: wheat, oats, rye, spelt, barley, wheat starch, durum flour, couscous, kamut, bulgur, triticale, most cereals, grains, pastas, bread and processed foods. Corn, rice, buckwheat and millet do not contain gluten.

Fibre — facts and fallacies

Fibre is the part of our food which we cannot digest, and which is passed out virtually unchanged in our stools. Our dietary fibre comes from fruits and vegetables, grains, beans, legumes and nuts and seeds. Most Westerners don't get enough fibre in their diet, and we pay the penalty with a range of gastrointestinal disorders ranging from chronic constipation and haemorrhoids through to bowel cancer and a frighteningly high incidence of cardiovascular disease and cancer. Yes, fibre intake influences your risk for both heart disease and some forms of cancer. Some types of fibre such as pectin and gum (found in citrus fruits, apples, pears, oats, legumes, beans, peas and lentils) help lower blood-cholesterol levels.

Fibre-rich foods provide lots of appetite-satisfying bulk without supplying huge amounts of calories. Consequently, eating a high-fibre diet is usually kind to your waistline as well as your heart and your gut!

(See Chapter 6 for more information on dietary fibre.)

* Boost fibre intake by eating more fruits and vegetables, whole grains, wheat and oat bran, wheatgerm, brown rice, nuts and seeds, lentils, beans and legumes.

On the subject of fat

For detailed information on dietary fats see the Fats section at the start of this chapter, and also Chapter 6.

The typical New Zealand and Australian diet contains:

Too much

Calories	Protein	Salt
Sugar	Alcohol	Dairy products
Red meat	Phosphorus	Fat
Saturated fat	Hydrogenated oil and trans-fats	

Not enough

Fibre

Fresh fruit and vegetables

Monounsaturated fats

Nuts and seeds, legumes, beans and pulses

Nutrients including calcium, magnesium, zinc, selenium, iron, B-vitamins, vitamin E and essential fatty acids

Food sources of vitamins and minerals

Vitamin A (Retinol) Liver, fish liver oils, egg yolk, dairy products

Beta-carotene Leafy green vegetables; yellow and orange-coloured fruits and vegetables

Vitamin B1 (Thiamine) Wheatgerm, bran, wholemeal flour, brown rice, brewer's yeast, blackstrap molasses, sunflower seeds, peanuts, avocado

Vitamin B2 (Riboflavin) Brewer's yeast, organ meats, oily fish (herring, mackerel, trout), dark green vegetables, nori seaweed

Vitamin B3 (Niacin) Liver and organ meats, poultry, fish, peanuts, yeast, wheatgerm, avocado, dates

Vitamin B5 (Pantothenic acid) Organ meats, brewer's yeast, fish, chicken, peanuts, wholegrain cereals, peas, cauliflower, avocado

Vitamin B6 (Pyridoxine) Organ meats, wheatgerm, egg yolk, soya beans, peanuts, walnuts, bananas, prunes, cauliflower, cabbage, avocado

Vitamin B9 (Folacin) Green leafy vegetables, beets, asparagus, broccoli, liver, kidney, oranges, pineapples, bananas, berries, brewer's yeast

Vitamin B12 (Cobalamin) Meat, most fish, crabs, oysters, egg yolk, milk, yoghurt

Biotin Egg yolk, liver, brewer's yeast, brown rice, nuts, milk

Choline Soya beans, egg yolk, brewer's yeast, wheatgerm, fish, peanuts, leafy green vegetables, organ meats

Inositol Whole grains, oranges, molasses, liver, brewer's yeast

PABA (para-amino benzoic acid) Liver, brewer's yeast, wheatgerm, rice, eggs, molasses

Vitamin C (Ascorbic acid) Citrus fruits, rosehips, acerola cherries, melons, strawberries, broccoli, Brussels sprouts, tomatoes, cabbage, peppers

continued

Vitamin D (Calciferol)   Fish liver oils, egg yolk, butter, liver

Vitamin E (Tocopherol)   Vegetable oils (especially wheatgerm oil), seed and nut oils, wheatgerm, nuts and seeds

Vitamin F (essential fatty acids)   Dark green leafy vegetables, most green plants, alfalfa, kelp, blackstrap molasses, polyunsaturated oils (such as safflower), liver, milk, egg yolk, fish liver oils

Calcium   Green leafy vegetables, broccoli, cauliflower, peas, beans, nuts, molasses, sesame seeds, soya beans, dairy products

Chromium   Brewer's yeast, beef, liver, whole wheat, oysters, potatoes, wheatgerm, beets, mushrooms

Iodine   Fish, shellfish, sea vegetables, kelp, vegetables grown in iron-rich soil

Iron   Wheatgerm, beef, liver, pork, lamb, chicken, shellfish, clams, oysters, egg yolk, millet, oats, brown rice, dried peas and beans, nuts and seeds, green leafy vegetables, dried fruit, yellow fruits

Magnesium   Dark green leafy vegetables, nuts, seeds, legumes, brown rice, soya beans, tofu, whole grains, wheatgerm, millet

Phosphorus   Protein foods (meat and fish), sugar, soft drinks

Potassium   Spinach, parsley, lettuce, oranges (especially the skins), bananas, apples, avocados, wheatgerm, nuts and seeds

Selenium   Brewer's yeast, wheatgerm, liver, butter, fish, lamb, brazil nuts, barley, oats, brown rice, shellfish, garlic, onions, mushrooms

Sodium   Seafood, beef, celery, beets, carrots, artichokes, sodium chloride (salt) in most processed foods

Zinc   Oysters, red meat, herring, egg yolk, chicken, whole wheat, rye and oats, pecan nuts, brazil nuts, pumpkin seeds

Protein pointers

Most New Zealanders have adequate protein in their diet . . . in fact, many eat too much protein. (See the section on protein at the start of this chapter.)

If you are not a vegetarian, vary proteins widely, choosing from a range of fish, poultry, and red and white meat. Individual protein requirements vary greatly, but in general the protein component of the meal should be balanced with carbohydrate and vegetables. That means that the traditional Kiwi meal of a slab of red meat, covering half the plate, with a token blob of vegetable matter, is not a balanced meal!

If red meat is a protein staple most days of the week, reduce your saturated fat intake, and add health-giving omega-3 fats by eating fish three to five times a week. Fish is a complete protein, rich in the beneficial fatty acids EPA and DHA. These fatty acids exert a remarkable cardiovascular protective effect, helping to lower blood cholesterol, and to reduce the 'stickiness' of the blood cells (helping to prevent blood clots, strokes and heart attacks). The fish which contain the largest amounts of these fatty acids are mackerel, sardines, salmon and trout.

* Use the palm method to calculate your approximate daily protein intake. The size of the palm of your hand (including its thickness, but excluding fingers) is the size of a healthy protein serving at each of your main meals. Snack-size protein servings are one third of a palm in size.

* Eat protein little and often throughout the day to help regulate blood-sugar levels and minimise food cravings or over-eating.

* Vary proteins — fish, chicken, red meat, eggs, nuts and seeds, rice plus lentils or beans, grains plus nuts (nut butter on wholemeal bread), dairy products.

* Aim to eat three to five servings of oily fish weekly (salmon, sardines, herrings, tuna).

Balance proteins, fats and carbs

Balance the ratio of protein, carbs and fats in your meals to moderate blood-sugar levels and prevent the development of insulin resistance.

* For main meals (lunch, dinner) eat one palm-sized serving of protein (see above); include two palms of low GI vegetables. If you are eating medium or high GI carbs such as rice or pasta, reduce the carb serving to one palm; or one palm of low-GI vegetables and half a palm of higher-GI carbs; one tablespoon of high-quality fats such as olive, flax or coconut oil; avocados, nuts, seeds or nutbutter.

Drinks count, too

Do you reach for a caffeine fix every hour or so? If coffee and tea drinking is more than an occasional pleasure, you could experiment with some caffeine-free alternatives. Try some of the wide range of herbal teas available to us. They don't all look and taste like pond weed. Pleasant and health-giving teas include rosehip (rich in vitamin C and iron); peppermint (especially good for strengthening the stomach and improving digestion); chamomile (a calming and sedative tea just right for a nightcap). The fruity range of herbal teas is delicious and a tasty introduction. Why not try replacing some of your coffee with a cereal coffee, dandelion coffee, or carob drink?

If you just can't live without that coffee taste, you could alternate between cereal coffees and decaffeinated coffee, but make sure that the coffee you choose has been water-decaffeinated, to avoid chemical residues.

Remember, too, to drink plenty of fresh, filtered water, in small amounts regularly throughout the day. Aim to drink at least eight glasses of water a day, including herbal teas — but not tea and coffee.

(For the lowdown on alcohol, see Chapter 6.)

* Drink a minimum of 8 glasses of water or herbal tea daily.

* Regulate caffeine intake to no more than two or three cups of coffee or tea daily.

* Drink 2–4 cups of well-brewed green tea daily for antioxidant protection.

Regulate blood sugar

A stable blood-sugar level will sustain energy levels and regulate mood as well as helping to regulate weight within a healthy range. Avoid insulin spikes and resulting low blood sugar in the following ways.

* Choose foods from the low to medium Glycaemic Index, and avoiding high GI foods.

* Eat little and often throughout the day (breakfast, mid-morning, lunch, mid-afternoon, dinner).

* Always eat breakfast. Choose from a combination of complex carbohydrates and proteins; for example, wholemeal bread with tinned fish (salmon, sardines, herrings, tuna); or eggs, or low-fat cheese. Cooked wholegrain porridge with added oatbran, soaked linseed, nuts and seeds and fresh fruit. Add a little unsweetened natural *acidophilus* yoghurt if desired.

* Include a protein at lunch and dinner.

* Eat smaller meals to allow for a healthy snack that will sustain blood-sugar levels at mid-morning and mid-afternoon.

The choice of vegetarianism

Twenty-five years ago, when I was at naturopathic college, I became a vegetarian at a time when making such a choice was considered a sign of strong "hippy" leanings. Thankfully, such narrow-mindedness is now a thing of the past and vegetarianism in all its various forms has become a common, mainstream dietary choice. Making such a choice is usually prompted by health concerns, an aversion to meat, or a philosophical or spiritual stand. In its most extreme form, vegetarianism precludes the consumption of any animal products or derivatives. Known as *vegans*, these most extreme of vegetarians avoid all meat, fish, dairy products and eggs. Less restrictive is the choice of lacto-ovo vegetarianism, practised by the majority of vegetarians, in which meat and fish are precluded, but dairy products and eggs are included in the diet.

The vegetarian diet has been extensively researched, and has been proven to offer many health benefits. Many of these occur as a combined result of the exclusion of animal proteins such as meat, and in some cases dairy products, from the diet; and inclusion of higher than usual amounts of protective foods such as fruits, vegetables, whole grains, nuts and seeds, beans and lentils. These foods are rich in antioxidants, 'healthy' fats (omega-3 and omega-9 fatty acids — omega-9 fats are found predominantly in olive oil), fibre, phyto-oestrogens and lignans; each of which are good for our health.

In general, a vegetarian diet, when compared with an omnivorous diet (in which animal proteins are consumed) tends to be:

* lower in saturated fat

* lower in protein (many Westerners consume excessive amounts of protein, and a high protein intake is associated with kidney stones, osteoporosis and possibly heart disease and some cancers)

* higher in fibre

* higher in phyto-estrogens and lignans (associated with reduction in risk of some forms of cancer)

* higher in antioxidants from increased intake of fruits and vegetables (high antioxidant intake is associated with protection against a range of cancers, heart disease and premature ageing)

* higher in 'healthy' omega-3 and omega-9 fats (associated with protection against heart disease and cancer)

* lower in iron, zinc, and vitamins A and D

* lower in vitamin B12 (in vegan diets).

Research has consistently shown that vegetarians and vegans suffer from a lower incidence of many of the chronic diseases common to modern-day Western society, such as obesity, cancer, diabetes and heart disease. For example:

* Vegetarians are approximately 40% less likely to develop cancers compared with meat eaters. Large USA studies looking at Seventh Day Adventists (who are all vegetarian) have shown that there is a significant reduction in cancer risk among those who avoided meat. Harvard studies involving hundreds of thousands of subjects show that regular meat consumption increases colon cancer risk by approximately 300%.

* Vegetarians have a reduced incidence of cardiovascular disease, including cholesterol problems and high blood pressure. Vegetarians tend to have a much lower intake of saturated fats and cholesterol as a result of not eating meat and/or dairy products. (The exception to this, of course, are lacto-ovo vegetarians who may actually increase saturated fat consumption by over-reliance on dairy products as a source of protein.) Along with the reduced

dietary intake of cholesterol and saturated fat, the high dietary fibre content of the typical vegetarian diet further lowers levels of potentially troublesome LDL cholesterol.

* Vegetarians have a lower incidence of type-two diabetes. The typical vegetarian diet, low in fat and high in fibre and complex carbohydrates, allows insulin to work more effectively in the body.

* Vegetarians experience fewer problems with kidney stones and gallstones, as diets which are high in animal proteins increase the body's excretion of calcium, oxalate and uric acid, which are the main components in kidney-stone formation. Gallstones are usually associated with the consumption of diets high in saturated fats, and such a diet doubles the risk of stone formation in women.

* Vegetarians have a reduced risk of osteoporosis. Many vegetarian diets are lower in calcium but their diet seems to protect bones against age-related thinning. This is partly because meat is high in phosphorus and actually encourages the release of stored calcium from bones. (See Osteoporosis in the A–Z section in Part Two.)

Is a vegetarian diet for everyone?

Undoubtedly there is much to be said for the health benefits of vegetarianism, but the truth is that not everyone does well on a vegetarian diet. I myself was a lacto-ovo vegetarian for 15 years, and gave up this dietary choice when I finally faced the fact that I was simply 'failing to thrive'. I suffered from constantly low energy despite consuming a textbook-perfect vegetarian diet. Shortly after returning fish and, occasionally, chicken to my diet, the improvement in energy levels was remarkable. Throughout my 20 years in practice I have come across other vegetarians with health issues (usually centring around fatigue, menstrual disorders and low resistance to infection). Contrast these exhausted vegetarians with yet others who run marathons while living on vegan diets, and it's easy to see that individual biochemistry and genetic make-up also play a significant part in determining an individual person's optimum diet. Despite the research showing that a vegetarian diet is a healthy one, the reality is that it does not suit everyone.

My advice to those wishing to become vegetarian is to try such a diet for a period of time, but to listen to your body to determine whether it is the healthiest choice for you. I would also suggest that you don't impose a massive dietary change upon yourself (such as going from being a meat eater to a vegan) at times when your body is already faced with additional stresses — for example, during pregnancy or lactation, or when you are under severe emotional or physical stress.

To optimise your health as a vegetarian

Ensure that you have adequate protein in your diet (especially important if you are a vegan and are not consuming eggs or dairy products). Contrary to the beliefs of many, it is easy to obtain adequate protein in a vegan or vegetarian diet as long as a wide range of different grains, nuts and seeds, lentils, and beans are consumed regularly. It was once thought that food combining was essential for the body to obtain the complete range of necessary amino acids to form complete proteins. This idea has now been refuted. Amino acids obtained from food can combine with amino acids made in the body, and so it is unnecessary to eat a specified combination of foods at a particular meal. We now know that incomplete proteins can be stored in the body for many days to be combined with other incomplete proteins. As long as all essential amino acids are included in the diet, it doesn't matter whether the proteins are complete or incomplete.

Traditional Chinese medicine and vegetarianism

From the perspective of traditional Chinese medicine, the dietary regime chosen by a person should reflect the needs of their individual energy balance. In Chinese medicine, all foods have an inherent energy (cold, neutral, warm, hot) which can alter the energy of a person when consumed.

Many of the foods in a vegetarian diet, such as fruits, vegetables, juices and grains, have an inherently cold energy. This inherently cold energy is further compounded when the foods are eaten in their raw state. Traditional Chinese medicine recognises that vegetarians often exhibit qi (pronounced chi) imbalances directly related to their predominantly 'cold' energy diet. In particular, 'coldness' of the kidneys (kidney yang deficiency), stomach and spleen (stomach qi deficiency and spleen yang deficiency), and blood deficiency are commonly observed patterns in vegetarians.

Symptoms related to these imbalances include: fatigue, lethargy, sensitivity to cold, frequent urination, night urination, scanty or absent menstrual periods, abdominal bloating, loose stools.

Chinese medicine emphasises the importance of 'stoking the fire of the middle burner' for maintaining good health; for example, keeping stomach and digestive energy strong. For the vegetarian, especially those eating a predominance of raw foods, this is especially difficult. To prevent qi and blood deficiency and to strengthen the energy of the middle burner, Chinese dietary therapy recommends the following.

* Eat primarily cooked foods, or at least balance cooked and raw foods. Moderate raw/cooked balance depending on the seasons. During the winter (a cold, or yin, season), reduce intake of raw foods and increase cooked foods. During the summer (a warm, or yang, season), the body can usually tolerate more raw foods and fewer cooked foods.

* Consume more energetically warm foods than cold foods so that the overall impact on digestive energy is one of warming, not cooling. Cold foods include: raw fruits and vegetables; physically cold foods; citrus fruit and juice, peanut butter, bananas, asparagus, barley, kelp, mango, mung bean sprouts, lettuce, seaweed, salt, tomato, watermelon.

* As many vegetarians have a weakness of spleen energy, include plentiful amounts of spleen qi tonifying foods such as cooked squash, carrot, sweet potato, yam, turnip, leek, onion and pumpkin; well-cooked rice and oats, cooked peach, cherry, strawberry, cardamom, cinnamon, nutmeg, black pepper, and small amounts of cayenne and fresh ginger.

* Chew food well to make the work of the digestive fire easier.

* Avoid drinking with meals as this extinguishes the digestive fire.

* Never eat to excess as this will 'clog' the 'furnace' with sludge!

* Iced, frozen or chilled foods should be eaten rarely and sparingly as they extinguish digestive fire.

Meat is a major source of iron and zinc. However, it is still very possible to obtain adequate supplies of both of these minerals without eating meat. If you are a vegetarian woman with heavy periods, have your iron levels checked periodically to ensure that you are obtaining adequate iron from your diet, to compensate for that lost during heavy bleeding. (See the A–Z section in Part Two on anaemia, and the section on iron and zinc below.)

Vitamin B12 deficiency can be an issue for vegans, but is rarely a problem for vegetarians. Found predominantly in animal products, small amounts of this vitamin can be found in plant products due to bacterial contamination. Vegan sources of vitamin B12 include: spirulina, sea vegetables, tempeh and miso. Fortified cereals, nutritional yeast, fortified soya milk and multivitamins also supply B12. (See Vitamin B12 below.)

> There are four basic foundations of achieving and maintaining good health. These are diet, exercise, adequate rest and relaxation, and a good mental attitude.
>
> Bob Flaws (Traditional Chinese medicine author)

> The spirit cannot endure the body when overfed, but, if underfed, the body cannot endure the spirit.
>
> St Frances de Sales

For more information on dietary choices, see Chapter 6.

A look at vitamins and minerals

The human body does not live by carbohydrate, protein and fats alone. Without vitamins, minerals and trace elements there can be no life . . . and without adequate amounts of nutrients, there can be no healthy life.

Vitamins are organic compounds found in animal and plant products, most of which we must ingest regularly to stay healthy.

There are a few vitamins such as some of the B-complex nutrients which we can, in theory, manufacture for ourselves, but most of the others must be supplied through our diet. The main function of vitamins is to work as coenzymes in a wide variety of different metabolic reactions essential for growth, vitality, resistance to disease, and normal digestive functioning.

Vitamins are broadly classified as being 'water soluble' (B-complex, C and bioflavonoids) or 'fat soluble' (A, E, D, K). As the name suggests, water-soluble vitamins are not stored in the body, and are readily excreted in the urine. They are unstable and readily damaged during the cooking (or even chopping) of food. They must be supplied in adequate doses every day. Because of their easy excretion from the body, most water-soluble vitamins can be taken even in high supplemental doses without any toxic effect. Fat-soluble vitamins, on the other hand, can be stored in body fat and the liver, and so we can stay healthy for a longer period if there is an occasional day when we don't get our full complement of these. Because they are readily stored, fat-soluble vitamins have the potential for greater toxicity problems if taken in high amounts for long periods.

Will a multi a day keep the doctor away?

Ten years ago, it was a rare New Zealander who completed his or her morning breakfast ritual by gulping down nutritional supplements. Today's health-conscious baby-boomers have changed that, with 60% of New Zealanders taking some form of nutritional supplement on a daily basis. Many Kiwi kitchens host a variety of glass bottles containing multi-coloured tablets offering the promise of radiant health and well-being. The most common nutritional purchase is the ubiquitous 'multivitamin and mineral' supplement, or the 'multi'. Since it contains a wide spectrum of vitamins and minerals, many consider a multi to be a kind of nutritional insurance policy, helping to ensure that we receive all the nutrients we require on those less-than-perfect days when the alarm clock fails to ring and breakfast is a non-event; or dinner is a pie on the way home from the office. Putting aside the hype, do we really need a daily multi, or does a 'healthy diet' give us all the nutrients we need?

The mythical balanced diet

Until recently many doctors and nutritionists have used the 'balanced diet' claim to argue that multivitamins are an expensive waste of time. The research says otherwise. The US Department of Agriculture surveyed 21,500 people in 1982 and found that only 3% actually ate a healthy, balanced diet every day, and not a single one of them met the recommended daily intake of the 10 most important vitamins and minerals on a regular basis. New Zealanders are similarly existing on a variety of less than ideal diets . . . often lacking in fresh fruits and vegetables, fish and protein, and saturated with simple carbohydrates, sugars and junk foods. Deficiencies of iron, zinc, calcium, folate and even vitamin C are commonplace.

It's not just poor choices in the supermarket and at the dinner table which contribute to nutritional deficiency. The 1992 Earth Summit report showed that in the last hundred years the mineral content of soil around the world has declined dramatically. Agricultural soil is routinely fertilised with only a fraction of the 50 different essential nutrients required for optimum human health. Plants, unlike humans, can grow when trace elements such as chromium or selenium are missing from the soil. Even with an optimum diet, we can only absorb the minerals and trace elements from our food if they are present in the soil in which our food crops are grown.

Even if we make an effort to eat a healthy diet (and we make the questionable assumption that our crops are brimming with all the nutrients we need), there is still major depletion of nutrients resulting from the processing and cooking of our food. Produce is often picked green, gas ripened and kept in a cold store. Then there's the ongoing breakdown of vitamins resulting from transportation, storage under supermarket lights, refrigeration and finally chopping and cooking. The steamed carrot sitting resplendent on your plate may well contain only a fraction of the beta-carotene and vitamin C it contained while growing in the ground.

Some of the things we do on a daily basis increase our nutrient requirements, block absorption or increase excretion of nutrients. Drinking alcohol, coffee or consuming a high-sugar diet leads to depletion of a range of nutrients including B-complex, vitamin C, magnesium, zinc and chromium. Smokers require additional vitamin C, B-complex and vitamin A. Women taking the oral contraceptive pill need additional B-complex, zinc and vitamin C. Similarly, during pregnancy or adolescence nutrient requirements escalate. Breastfeeding, stress, recovery from surgery, or fighting infection all boost nutrient requirements.

After years of strenuously denying the necessity of nutritional supplementation, the prestigious *Journal of the American Medical Association* recently stated 'most people do not consume an optimal amount of all vitamins by diet alone', and 'it appears prudent for all adults to take a vitamin supplement'.

That only leaves the question of safety . . .

Most nutritional supplements have a huge margin of safety. Compared with the number of New Zealanders who die from pharmaceutical reactions, 1524 in 1998 alone (the last year of detailed official statistics available), the number of deaths recorded as a result of nutritional supplements is zero. In the past ten years New Zealanders have spent $1.3 billion on natural health products, with no fatalities and a less than 0.01% adverse reaction rate.

While taking a multivitamin and mineral tablet every day will be of benefit to most people, there are some times when supplementing the nutrients obtained from a healthy diet can be of even greater benefit:

* during pregnancy and breastfeeding (ensure that you use a supplement specifically designed for this time)

✳ during times of increased stress or emotional turmoil

✳ before and after surgery

✳ if you have a chronic illness, or lowered immunity leading to frequent infections

✳ if you are a smoker or use the oral contraceptive pill

✳ if you are on long-term medication such as steroids for asthma, tranquillisers, antidepressants or gastric ulcer medication.

The trouble with RDIs

In the nutrition section below you will see that each vitamin or mineral is followed by its RDI or recommended daily intake. It's important to understand exactly what an RDI is, and to realise their somewhat arbitrary nature.

The RDI (or RDA in some countries) is a figure set by government-appointed scientists, based on how much of a nutrient is needed to prevent serious vitamin-deficiency diseases such as scurvy (vitamin C), beriberi (B1) or pellagra (B3). There is a vast difference between the level of a nutrient required to prevent a frank deficiency, and the level required for optimum health. For example, a paltry 60 mg of vitamin C a day will prevent scurvy, but several thousand milligrams a day confer huge health benefits in the prevention of chronic disease.

RDIs are a source of controversy, and there are huge differences in the levels set by various countries, which can vary by as much as 1000%. There has been a general trend for many RDIs to gradually be set at higher and higher levels with the increasing awareness of the importance of optimum nutrition for good health.

There is another problem with RDIs. They are set for a mythical 'normal' person who is healthy, doesn't smoke, drink, experience stress, take drugs, have infections or endure hormonal imbalances. Of course no such person exists, and each of these conditions which pertain to real people drastically increases our nutrient requirements.

There is a huge amount of evidence that nutrient intakes many times higher than the RDIs improve the health of our nervous, cardiovascular, and immune systems as well as helping to reduce our risk of a variety of cancers.

Vitamin B

The B-complex vitamins

'B-complex' describes a group of water-soluble vitamins that usually occur together in nature. These nutrients need each other for effective absorption and utilisation. It is rare to find a particular B-vitamin deficiency in isolation. Because of their bio-chemical interdependence it is generally not a good idea to take any of the B-complex vitamins as a supplement on its own. For example, taking high doses of supplemental B6 over a long period of time without also taking a B-complex supplement can lead to a deficiency of vitamin B2.

When you think B-complex, think 'energy'. B vitamins work as coenzymes to catalyse many of the essential biochemical reactions in the body. B vitamins are vital for energy production, and without them your body would be unable to change dietary carbohydrates into glucose. We burn glucose to provide energy, and without B-complex vitamins we would be exhausted, apathetic slobs . . . perhaps this sounds like you? If so, taking B-complex vitamins may be a part of your return to vitality. B-vitamins are also needed in the metabolising of protein and fat, and are vital for the normal functioning of the nervous system, for healthy skin and hair, and for normal muscle tone.

Vitamin-B deficiency is especially common among people following strict weight-loss regimes or those living on diets high in refined carbohydrates, sugars, alcohol or coffee.

What are the signs and symptoms that you may need more B-vitamins in your diet, and/or a B-complex supplement?

Exhaustion, becoming fatigued easily; skin problems; hair falling out; a variety of nervous and emotional symptoms such as depression, anxiety, PMS, mouth ulcers, cracks at the corner of your mouth, poor appetite, insomnia and restless sleep are common signs of vitamin-B deficiency.

Finding Bs in your food

B-vitamins are plentiful in wholegrain (unrefined) cereals such as wholemeal bread, wholegrain oats, rye and barley, and brown rice. Nuts, beans, peas, leafy green vegetables and milk are also dietary sources of these vitamins. If you're a meat eater, liver is a B-complex powerhouse. If you're vegetarian, brewer's yeast is packed with B-vitamins and makes a useful supplemental source as long as you don't have any problems with *Candida* (yeast issues).

Even if your diet is rich in B-vitamins, there are times when deficiency is possible. Consuming a diet containing lots of alcohol, sugar or caffeine can deplete B-vitamins, and cigarette smokers destroy large amounts of B-vitamins in their body. Antibiotics, sleeping pills and the oral contraceptive pill can also lead to reduced B-vitamin uptake and utilisation. When under a great deal of emotional stress (or during pregnancy or lactation), or when fighting an infection, B-complex requirements increase dramatically.

Many female disorders, such as pre-menstrual tension, bleeding abnormalities, breast disorders, depression and minor health problems during pregnancy improve when additional B-complex nutrients are supplemented.

A look at some important Bs

Vitamin B3 (niacin, nicotinic acid and nicotinamide)

Like vitamin B2, B3 is essential for the metabolising of carbohydrates. It is also essential for a healthy nervous system, and to maintain the health of the skin and the digestive system. This vitamin also improves blood circulation and helps lower blood-cholesterol levels.

Vitamin-B3 deficiency is not particularly common. It is usually seen only in people who drink large amounts of alcohol at the expense of their food intake. The symptoms of B3 deficiency are many and varied. They include skin problems such as dermatitis; weakness and lack of energy; poor appetite and indigestion; and pronounced nervous system disorders such as depression, irritability, tension and frequent headaches.

B3-supplements are contraindicated in certain situations. If you are taking medication for high blood pressure, you should speak to your doctor before taking high doses of B3, as this vitamin can cause a substantial drop in your blood pressure (which is of course a good thing, and may mean that your medication can be reduced). Vitamin B3 can raise blood-sugar levels, and so if you are a diabetic, be wary about using high supplemental doses. Supplementary niacin has much to offer in the management of heart disease and problems related to poor circulation, such as muscle cramps and headaches; Ménière's disease; gum disease, anxiety and depression, and acne. Taken in its nicotinic acid form, B3 can lower blood pressure and blood-cholesterol levels, and help stabilise blood-sugar levels in hypoglycaemics.

RDI for niacin
* children (1–18 years): 6–14 mg
* women: 14 mg
  — during pregnancy: 18 mg
  — during lactation: 17 mg
* men: 16 mg

Vitamin B5 (pantothenic acid)
Pantothenic is derived from the Greek word *pantos* meaning 'everywhere', and indeed this B-vitamin is found in a wide range

of natural foods. If your diet contains generous amounts of whole grains and fresh fruit and vegetables, you can be fairly sure that your B5 needs are being met. Like vitamins B2 and B3, this is one of the B-vitamins that we can manufacture ourselves if we have healthy gut bacteria.

Vitamin B5 is intimately involved with our metabolism at a cellular level. It is also vital for the release of energy from our food. But first and foremost, pantothenic acid is acknowledged as being a 'stress fighter' supreme, being closely involved with the function of the adrenal cortex. The adrenal glands perch one on top of each kidney, and are involved in the 'fight-or-flight' response whenever we face stress. Vitamin B5 is an essential nutrient for the production of cortisol and other adrenal hormones secreted in response to stress.

Long-term stress can lead to adrenal exhaustion, with its symptoms of low blood sugar, chronic fatigue and an uncomfortable dull, low backache (in the kidney area). Increasing your intake of B5 through taking a high-potency B-complex supplement (perhaps with additional B5 also) can improve your adrenal health and your ability to withstand chronic stress. B5 requirements also increase dramatically when fighting infection or recovering from surgery.

It is also a good idea to use a balanced B-complex supplement, including a substantial amount of B5, whenever you are taking antibiotics. This vitamin helps to reduce the toxicity and side effects of these drugs.

RDI for pantothenic acid
   ✳ children (1–18 years): 3.5–4 mg

   ✳ women: 4 mg
      — during pregnancy: 5 mg
      — during lactation: 6 mg

   ✳ men: 6 mg

Vitamin B6 (pyridoxine)

Vitamin B6 is one of the most researched B-vitamins, with a wide range of therapeutic uses. It is essential for the utilisation of energy from all types of food. It also helps in the production of red blood cells and antibodies. Vitamin B6 is involved in the balancing of sodium and potassium in the body, and thus helps to normalise fluid balance (prevent oedema), as well as being involved in normal electrical function of nerves, heart and muscles. B6 is vital for normal immune function, as it is involved in the production of antibodies. It is also an important component in the manufacture of red blood cells, and the synthesis and function of RNA and DNA in every cell in the body.

Like vitamin B5, this vitamin occurs naturally in many foods, but is destroyed through the refining and processing of foods. It is quite common to find deficiency states in women who eat poor diets, or who frequently go on slimming diets. If you take the contraceptive pill, you should also take a daily balanced B-complex supplement containing at least 50 mg of B6.

Serious deficiencies of this vitamin are found in half of all women using the pill. Vitamin B6 requirements are markedly increased whenever oestrogen levels in the body are increased, such as occurs when using the oral contraceptive pill or hormone replacement therapy.

Similarly, during the pre-menstrual part of our cycle, and during pregnancy, B6 requirements are dramatically increased. Pregnant women who rely solely on dietary sources of B6 generally obtain only 50% of their RDA, and lactating mothers don't fare much better, with dietary intakes of only approximately two-thirds of their RDI. This is even more dramatic when you consider that much research suggests that the RDIs of B6 for pregnant and lactating women are far too low anyway.

Supplementing with B-complex and additional B6 in the range of 50–150 mg a day helps reduce many of the common symptoms of PMS, including breast tenderness, fluid retention (B6 is a natural diuretic) and mood swings.

Since vitamin-B6 supplements help so many women suffering from morning sickness, it has been postulated that this condition is partly due to a B6 deficiency, heightened by the high levels of oestrogen at this time, increasing B6 requirements.

Vitamin-B6 deficiency during pregnancy can have more serious repercussions than simply making you feel nauseous, and has been implicated as a factor in the occurrence of more serious problems in the latter part of your pregnancy, such as toxaemia, high blood pressure and eclampsia. Pregnancy-onset diabetes is also more common when B6 levels are low.

How do you know whether you need more B6 in your diet?

Common deficiency symptoms include problems with fatigue and blood-sugar fluctuations, frequent infections, fluid retention and pre-menstrual tension, emotional symptoms such as depression, anxiety and irritability. Dandruff, dry skin and a cracked sore mouth and tongue are other common B6-deficiency symptoms. If you are eating a high-protein diet, or a diet high in sugar, your need for this vitamin is markedly increased. Likewise, when taking antibiotics, the pill or hormone replacement therapy, you need to increase your intake of the vitamin.

If you fall into one of the 'high requirement' categories, include plenty of the B6-rich food sources in your diet, as well as using a balanced B-supplement supplying at least 50 mg of B6 a day. Useful dietary sources include: organ meats, whole grains, wheatgerm, fish, chicken, eggs, soya beans, peas and beans. B6 has low toxicity as a supplement when taken in doses of up to 150 mg a day. Occasionally, when used in high doses of 200 mg or more, a type of (largely reversible) peripheral nerve disorder can occur. In practice, I find that most people respond to therapeutic levels of B6, with an upper limit of 150–200 mg a day.

When taking B6-supplements, always take a balanced B-complex as well. As is the case with most nutritional supplements, adding large amounts of a certain nutrient in isolation can cause imbalances and deficiency of other nutrients. High doses of B6 taken in isolation can induce a magnesium deficiency. Supplemental B6 actually works more effectively when taken along with a magnesium complex.

RDI for vitamin B6
* ✻ children (1–18 years): 0.5–1.2 mg
* ✻ women: 1.5 mg
    — during pregnancy: 1.9 mg
    — during lactation: 2 mg
* ✻ men: 1.7 mg

Vitamin B9 (folic acid, folacin or folate)

Folic acid occurs abundantly in vegetables (especially the leafy green ones) and fruit. However, it is easily destroyed in the process of cooking, exposure to light, and also through storage. A low dietary consumption of fruit and vegetables, combined with the fragility of this B-vitamin, means that folic acid deficiency is common . . . in fact, folic acid deficiency is one of the most widely occurring of all nutritional deficiencies. Deficiency is especially common in pregnant or lactating women, and women taking the pill; in the elderly; in alcoholics; and in people using pharmaceutical drugs including antibiotics (tetracyclines) and psychiatric medications.

Common signs of a folic acid deficiency include: exhaustion, lethargy, lack of appetite and irritability, headaches and a sore or swollen tongue. Folic acid is essential for the formation of red blood cells and haemoglobin (the oxygen-carrying part of red blood cells), and without it a type of anaemia develops. Psychological symptoms include apathy, poor memory and concentration, depression and irritability. Folic acid supplements can help with the healing of wounds and leg ulcers, and with the restoration of normal, healthy cervical cells.

Folic acid is also essential for the formation of nucleic acid, which is needed in great amounts for the rapid production of new body cells which occurs during the growth of a foetus. Today, it is widely acknowledged that there is a strong correlation between a deficiency of folic acid during pregnancy and a high incidence of neural tube defects (NTD) such as spina bifida. Studies show that pregnant women receiving folic acid supplements have a massive 1900% reduction in the incidence of spina bifida babies, compared with unsupplemented mothers.

Similarly dramatic results were obtained in experiments with women who had already had cleft-palate and harelip babies. Without supplementation, 7.4% of these women went on to produce babies with similar defects — compared with a 1% recurrence in the supplemented group! The message is obvious. If you are pregnant or, better still, when you are trying to become pregnant, bump up your folate intake with generous servings of leafy green vegetables daily . . . and use folic acid supplements to supply at least an additional 800 mcg of folic acid a day. Try to use folic acid supplements for three months before conception, and continue throughout the first 12 weeks of pregnancy.

Folic acid deficiency can also contribute to the development of toxaemia of pregnancy, premature birth, and haemorrhaging after birth. Start munching on silverbeet salads and spinach pies!

Folic acid also has a part to play in preventing cancer, with its key role in building DNA, the compound which forms our genetic blueprint. Several studies have shown that people who have a higher daily intake of folic acid (either from food or from supplements) have a lower risk of developing both colon and breast cancers. Women who drink alcohol regularly have an increased incidence of breast cancer, but if they supplement with folic acid, their increased risk is markedly reduced.

RDI for folic acid
　✻ children (1–18 years): 150–400 mcg
　✻ women: 400 mcg
　　— during pregnancy: 600 mcg
　　— during lactation: 500 mcg
　✻ men: 400 mcg

Vitamin B12 (cobalamin)

Our body requires only trace amounts of this vitamin, but without it we become horribly crippled, and then die! Vitamin-B12 deficiency this severe rarely occurs, and when it does, it usually affects strict vegans who eat no meat, dairy products or eggs (the predominant dietary sources of B12); or else it occurs in people lacking an enzyme called the 'intrinsic factor' vital for the absorption of this vitamin (this usually only occurs in elderly people). Excessive use of laxatives or antacids can also compromise B12 levels in the body.

If you are a strict vegetarian, useful food sources of B12 include spirulina, tempeh and miso, and yoghurt containing live *Lactobacillus* bacteria. B12 supplements are usually only needed by strict vegans, or by elderly people with absorption problems (in which case the vitamin is administered by injection).

Ongoing lack of B12 can result in a particularly nasty type of anaemia called pernicious or megoblastic anaemia. This causes exhaustion and nervous-system problems such as weakness, numbness and tingling of the limbs. Left untreated, this anaemia can be fatal.

Chronic fatigue can sometimes be the result of low B12 levels, and B12 injections (usually along with folic acid supplements) are often used to successfully remedy this situation.

RDI for vitamin B12

✻ children (1–18 years): 0.9–2.4 mg

✻ women: 2.4 mg

   — during pregnancy: 2.6 mg

   — during lactation: 2.8 mg

✻ men: 2.4 mg

Vitamin C

Ascorbic acid, calcium ascorbate, sodium ascorbate

If this powerful antioxidant vitamin had been discovered by a pharmaceutical company and its manufacture patented, it would have been marketed as one of the true wonder-drugs of all time. I could easily fill the entire space of this book talking about the healing properties of vitamin C. As a therapeutic agent it is indicated in the treatment of a huge and varied array of ills, including: any type of infection (viral or bacterial) or immune suppression; hepatitis; allergies; any conditions of stress, be they emotional or physical; cancer and heart disease; arthritis; wound healing and recovery from surgery; gum disease; skin problems; blood clotting disorders; poisoning; drug addiction . . . and the list goes on and on . . .

As humans, we rate as biochemical oddities when it comes to vitamin C. We (along with guinea pigs and monkeys) are the only species unable to manufacture this vitamin in our gut. We are totally dependent upon dietary and supplemental sources. Interestingly, while the human RDI is set at a paltry 60 mg a day, a 70 kg goat manufactures around 7000 mg of vitamin C a day; and a monkey in a zoo needs around 5000 mg a day to stay healthy! It doesn't take much common sense to figure out that the 60 mg daily dose we need to prevent an actual vitamin-C deficiency is very well short of what we need for optimum health.

While it is true that vitamin C occurs in many of the fruits and vegetables we eat, it is also true that vitamin-C deficiency is surprisingly widespread. (See chart on pp. 71–72 for sources.) In part, this is a result of our poor diets, with a generally low intake of produce naturally rich in vitamin C; and in part it's a reflection of the fragility of this vitamin, which is destroyed by improper storage and cooking. Refrigerate fruits and vegetables to conserve maximum amounts of this vitamin. As a water-soluble nutrient, vitamin C is destroyed during the cooking process, especially when vegetables are boiled to death! Swap to a steamer and lightly steam vegetables, or eat them raw. Drink the water used for steaming (it's full of nutrients), or use it as a stock for soups.

How much vitamin C do we need? In truth, nutritional authorities still can't agree on just what constitutes an adequate intake of vitamin C. Whatever the RDI may be, it's worth pointing out that there is a world of difference between the amount of vitamin C required to prevent deficiency states, and the amount ideal for optimum health (many, many times greater). In terms of preventing deficiency (rather than optimising health), we know that there are several factors that greatly increase vitamin-C requirements. Cigarette smoking is top of the list. Every cigarette destroys 25 mg of vitamin C in the body. If you are a smoker, you should ensure that your vitamin-C intake far exceeds the paltry RDI of 60 mg. Cigarette smoke is a potent carcinogen and full of free-radicals, and all smokers would help to minimise the destructive health consequences of their addiction by supplementing with a minimum of 2000 mg of vitamin C (or more) daily — better still, why not supplement with vitamin C and stop smoking at the same time!

Regular use of steroids, for example in the control of asthma, skin conditions or joint injuries and arthritis, boosts vitamin C requirements, as do long-term courses of antibiotics such as those prescribed for acne. Are you using sulphur drugs, or taking aspirin daily for arthritic pain? You, too, need to take supplemental vitamin C.

Living with high stress levels also increases our vitamin-C requirements as vitamin C is involved in the production of the stress hormones norepinephrine and epinephrine (adrenalin).

What do we need vitamin C for in our bodies?

Many early sailors met their end with a slow and torturous death from scurvy, caused by a lack of vitamin C in the traditional seafaring diet. Bleeding, swollen gums, spontaneous bruising and dry scaly skin were the symptoms of this common killer. While few Westerners die from this condition any more, the signs of easy bleeding, gum disease and spontaneous bruising are commonplace amongst the elderly . . . and indicative of a vitamin-C deficiency. In fact, vitamin-C deficiency amongst the elderly is almost endemic; it is largely the result of a lack of fresh fruits and vegetables in their diet. Vitamin-C deficiency contributes significantly to the development of many of the ills affecting the elderly, such as impaired cognition, frequent infection, paper-thin skin and easy bruising and wounding.

Vitamin C is essential for the manufacture of the protein collagen, used to form the connective tissue in skin, hair and bones. Collagen gives us structure and support, and without it we would resemble the 'baggy, saggy elephant'. If you've ever seen a heavy smoker with saggy, deeply lined skin, looking a good ten years older than his or her chronological age, you have witnessed the end results of collagen breakdown caused by vitamin-C deficiency (and free-radical bombardment).

The formation of connective tissue is especially important after surgery or injury, and for the healing and repair of wounds and burns, and at such times vitamin C is needed in abundance. Supplementing with 5000 to 10,000 mg of vitamin C daily can speed wound healing miraculously (less if this level of supplementation causes very loose bowels).

Vitamin C is also a useful ally before surgery, as it is essential for the formation of red blood cells, and thus can reduce the risk of haemorrhage during or after surgery. Vitamin C is also essential for the body's absorption of iron and folic acid, so it's not surprising that a vitamin-C deficiency can contribute to iron-deficiency anaemia. Two early signs of vitamin-C deficiency are bleeding gums and easy bruising, either of which are a loud and clear signal that vitamin-C supplies are depleted.

Vitamin C stimulates natural immunity by activating neut-rophils (a type of white blood cell) essential for front-line defence against viruses and bacteria. Lymphocytes (another type of white blood cell) are also stimulated by vitamin C, helping to increase our production of antibodies against the 'invaders'. While self-help for recovery from a cold or flu may involve swallowing vitamin C in the range of 2000 to 10,000 mg a day, megadoses of this vitamin are also used in the treatment of some serious diseases such as cancer and AIDS, with impressive results. In these instances, intravenous vitamin C is administered regularly in doses ranging from 20,000 to 100,000 mg.

Vitamin C also plays an important role in preventing heart disease. Vitamin C supplementation is important for anyone with heart disease or raised cholesterol levels, where supplemental doses as low as 1000 mg a day can lower total cholesterol levels, and prevent the oxidation of cholesterol plaques in the arteries. It is increasingly acknowledged that it is the oxidation of these plaques (through the attack of free-radicals), and the resulting inflammation which poses the greatest risk to our cardiovascular health. Vitamin C also reduces the 'stickiness' of the blood (as do fish oil, garlic and turmeric), reducing the formation of arterial plaques and blood clots.

Vitamin C and cancer

Swallowing megadoses of vitamin C while neglecting to eat a healthy diet and to live a balanced lifestyle is no guarantee against cancer. However, in combination with a healthy lifestyle, vitamin C gives us the added benefit of its powerful antioxidant properties, protecting cell membranes and DNA from damage by free-radicals, thus helping to safeguard against potentially cancerous cellular changes. High-dose vitamin C also works as an immune stimulant as well as enhancing tissue repair and healing.

Vitamin C also has a directly toxic effect on cancer cells. Intravenous vitamin-C therapy has a long history, with some impressive evidence of its efficacy as a safe, non-toxic therapeutic agent for anyone fighting cancer.

High doses of vitamin C create peroxides (like hydrogen peroxide) in the cells. A healthy cell quickly converts these substances to inert oxygen and water, using enzymes called catalases. Cancer cells contain much less catalase than healthy cells, and are therefore unable to convert peroxides into harmless substances. Thus peroxide concentrations rise within the cancer cells, causing cellular damage or death.

Until recently, intravenous vitamin C was the only way to produce sustained increases in intracellular vitamin C at levels high enough to demonstrate the ability to be toxic to some cancer cells (without damaging healthy cells). With high-dose vitamin-C therapy, the route of administration has been an important factor in determining the therapeutic effect, with intravenous administration demonstrating plasma concentrations of vitamin C about 25 times higher than in the case of oral administration of the same dose. We can only absorb vitamin C through our stomach and intestines in levels up to approximately 4000–6000 mg a day. After that, the vitamin passes straight through the gut, and ends up causing diarrhoea. The newly available form of liposomal C is absorbed in much higher doses (see p. 102).

Vitamin C and pregnancy

During pregnancy, vitamin C requirements escalate, especially so in the third trimester, when the growth of the foetus is rapid. Many women have problems with haemorrhoids or varicose veins during pregnancy, both of which are symptomatic of vitamin-C deficiency.

It is not a good idea to take massive supplemental doses of vitamin C (5000 mg or more per day) during pregnancy, as there is some indication that when the foetus develops in an overly 'C-rich' environment, its post-birth requirements are greatly increased. However, supplements providing 1000–2000 mg of vitamin C daily are of great benefit during pregnancy, along with plentiful amounts of C-rich foods. While all fruits and vegetables contain vitamin C, especially good sources include: kiwifruit, tamarillos, citrus fruit, green peppers, tomatoes, bean sprouts, melons, berries, dark green leafy vegetables, cabbage, and broccoli.

Some pointers on how to supplement with vitamin C

The range of vitamin-C supplements available can be over-whelming. Which one you choose can dramatically effect how much benefit you get from your supplement. Whenever possible, choose a vitamin-C 'complex' containing bioflavonoids as well as vitamin C.

The three most common forms of vitamin C supplements are ascorbic acid, calcium ascorbate, and sodium ascorbate. Then there's esterified vitamin C, and liposomal vitamin C . . . each with different pros and cons.

If you suffer from hypertension and follow a low-sodium diet, you are best to avoid the sodium ascorbate form of vitamin C. If you have ever suffered from calcium oxalate kidney stones, you are best to avoid the calcium ascorbate form.

Ascorbic acid (available in powders and tablets) is economical, and contains 100% vitamin C. Such supplements are therefore the most concentrated form of vitamin C. Ascorbic acid powder can be used for 'megadosing', but tablets, which contain fillers and binders, should not be taken in megadoses. If using tablets, always swallow them whole rather than chewing them, as ascorbic acid is very corrosive to tooth enamel. Some people find ascorbic acid is irritating to their digestive system, especially those suffering from excessive stomach acid, or gastric ulcers. These people often find the more gentle calcium ascorbate form of vitamin C to be less irritating.

Calcium ascorbate is a useful source of absorbable calcium and vitamin C; it contains no sodium and is non-acidic. Because of its calcium content, calcium ascorbate should not be used as a long-term 'megadose' vitamin-C therapy, as calcium overload may occur.

Sodium ascorbate is a non-acidic form of vitamin C, and is suitable for 'megadosing' unless you have an issue with high blood pressure, in which case the sodium content of this supplement may be a problem for you.

Ester C is the name given to a patented complex of non-acidic vitamin C and metabolites. Ester C has been proven to have superior absorption compared with traditional forms of vitamin C, and to stay in high concentrations in the blood for longer periods. It is also used more efficiently by cells and connective tissues. It is non-irritating to the gut, and does not affect tooth enamel.

An exciting and innovative newcomer to the field of vitamin-C supplementation, orally administered liposomal C, provides, for the first time, an equivalent plasma concentration to intravenous vitamin C, and does not cause diarrhoea even when taken in high oral doses of 10,000–20,000 mg a day. Unlike other forms of oral vitamin C, liposomal C is able to transport almost 100% of its vitamin C content past the gastro-intestinal barrier, regardless of the size of the dose. One of the problems with traditional oral vitamin C is that the bioavailability of the C dramatically decreases as the dose increases. So much so, that with a 100 mg vitamin-C tablet, 98 g will be used by the body. In contrast, in order to deliver 2000 mg of usable vitamin C, an oral dose of 16,000 mg is required! Taking a 16,000 mg dose of liposomal C actually delivers this amount of C to the cells in your body.

Getting the most from your supplement

Whichever form of vitamin C you decide upon, there are some general rules to help you get the most from your supplement.

Vitamin C is a water-soluble vitamin and is quickly passed out of the body in urine (not so quickly in the case of ester C or liposomal C), so you get more value for your money if you take vitamin C in small, frequent doses rather than as one large dose.

If you are using high doses of vitamin C to help fight an acute infection, you may discover your 'bowel tolerance'. This occurs when you have achieved tissue saturation, and the vitamin C begins to affect your bowels, making your stools loose. This is uncomfortable rather than dangerous. At this stage, cut back slightly on vitamin C intake, until your stools return to normal.

High doses of vitamin C seem to increase the body's expectation and requirements for this vitamin. Consequently, it is best to reduce your intake gradually if you have been using high doses for several days or more. If you have been taking a few thousand milligrams of vitamin C for several days to fight a cold or flu, don't just suddenly stop your supplementation as soon as you feel better. Instead, reduce your intake by a couple of hundred milligrams each day, until you get back down to your usual supplementation rate.

RDI for vitamin C

✳ children (1–18 years): 35–40 mg

✳ women: 45 mg
   — during pregnancy: 60 mg
   — during lactation: 85 mg

✳ men: 45 mg

Bioflavonoids (vitamin P)

Do you carefully peel all the white fleshy pith from your orange and throw it away? If you do, you are throwing away a nutritional jackpot crammed with bioflavonoids. This vitamin, essential for the proper absorption of vitamin C, occurs naturally in citrus fruits, plums, blackcurrants, apricots, blackberries and cherries, and buckwheat. Green peppers, tomatoes and broccoli are also good dietary sources.

As well as enhancing vitamin-C absorption, bioflavonoids perform important functions in their own right. Bioflavonoids strengthen the walls of blood vessels and capillaries (and regulate their permeability); and without adequate supplies, blood capillaries become fragile and rupture easily. The result is easy bruising, and bleeding problems such as recurrent nosebleeds, bleeding gums, or abnormally heavy menstrual periods. If your monthly periods keep you virtually housebound because of the heavy flow, bioflavonoids (along with other nutritional supplements) may offer you relief.

Supplementing with bioflavonoids has proven to be effective in a number of conditions, including easy bruising, nosebleeds, heavy periods, bleeding ulcers, and habitual miscarriage.

RDI for bioflavonoids

None determined, but it is generally recommended that if you are using vitamin C supplements, bioflavonoids should also be supplemented in the ratio of 100 mg for every 500 mg of vitamin C.

Fat-soluble vitamins

The fat-soluble vitamins A, E, D and K are readily stored in our body, unlike water-soluble vitamins which are easily excreted. Consequently, there is more potential for toxicity if large amounts of fat-soluble vitamins are taken in supplemental form.

Vitamin A (retinol or beta-carotene)

Vitamin A occurs as both a fat-soluble and a water-soluble vitamin. Pre-formed vitamin A (also called retinol or retinoic acid), is fat soluble, and is found in animal products such as egg yolks, milk, butter, and liver. Beta-carotene (also known as pro-vitamin A) is the water-soluble precursor to vitamin A, found in dark green leafy vegetables, and yellow and orange fruits and vegetables.

Why do we need vitamin A?

When you think of vitamin A, think of your eyes, skin and mucous membranes (such as the lining of the lungs, mouth, throat, bladder, stomach, vagina, and so on). This vitamin is essential for the health of your skin, and without enough of it, your outer wrapping becomes rough, dry and covered with acne! Your inner linings also rely on vitamin A for their health. By strengthening the walls of the cells in the mucous membranes such as the lungs, this vitamin improves our resistance to infection by bacteria and viruses. Vitamin A also directly boosts immunity by stimulating the production and activity of white blood cells.

The old wives' tale about carrots helping us to see in the dark is actually not too far from the truth. If you find night driving difficult because you are blinded by oncoming headlights, then you have a clear indication that you need more of this vitamin in your diet. Other common symptoms of vitamin-A deficiency include: a range of eye problems, poor immunity, dry bumpy skin (especially on the back of the arms), acne, boils, dandruff, and periodontal disease.

Like vitamin C, vitamin A (in particular beta-carotene) is a powerful antioxidant. It was once thought that low dietary intake of vitamin A contributed to an increased incidence of a range of cancers, but a number of large trials have disproven this theory. Some studies have even shown the reverse, with beta-carotene supplements leading to an increased incidence of cancers amongst smokers.

Many of us have traumatising childhood memories of the compulsory daily teaspoon of foul-tasting cod liver oil. Despite the fact that the cod liver oil tasted like poison, mother was probably doing us a great service as fish liver oil is the richest source of pre-formed vitamin A.

Supplementing with vitamin A

When it comes to vitamin-A supplements, it's important to realise that there is a world of difference between using pre-formed vitamin A, and beta-carotene supplements. Pre-formed vitamin A is fat soluble, and consequently readily stored in the body. Taken in high doses (50,000–100,000 iu per day) for long periods, fat-soluble vitamin A can be toxic. It is inadvisable to take more than 10,000 iu daily of pre-formed vitamin A without some professional guidance.

Common signs of vitamin-A toxicity include: frontal headaches (due to a slight swelling of the brain); nausea and vomiting; irritability; dizziness; and hair loss. Your skin may itch and become flaky and you may lose your appetite. These signs of 'hyper-vitaminosis' are all reversible when you reduce your intake of the vitamin.

One more word of caution — if you are pregnant or planning to become pregnant, limit your supplementation with pre-formed vitamin A (retinol) to no more than 5000 iu a day. Some research suggests that higher doses can cause foetal abnormalities. However, you can supplement with large amounts of beta-carotene without risk to your child or yourself.

Beta-carotene can be taken in massive doses without any danger of toxicity, except the possibility of an orange tinge to the palms of your hands and the soles of the feet. However, beta-carotene is not a suitable supplementary source for everyone. If you have diabetes or a sluggish thyroid, your ability to transform beta-carotene into usable vitamin A is greatly reduced. Try to increase your natural intake of beta–carotene and pre-formed vitamin A rather than (or as well as) relying on nutritional supplements.

When including lots of beta-carotene-rich fruits and vegetables in your diet (seaweed, green vegetables, asparagus, carrots, yams, kumara, pumpkin, apricots, peaches, mango, papaya, cherries, watermelon), it's worth knowing that your ability to absorb the beta-carotene from its natural food sources is enhanced with cooking. Carrot soup gives you a greater beta-carotene hit than does munching on a pile of raw carrots.

Vitamin-A absorption and utilisation is also enhanced by the mineral zinc, so if you're low in zinc (which is an alarmingly common situation), then you're also likely to have problems with making use of your ingested vitamin A. Absorption is also reduced if you drink alcohol regularly, have a vitamin-E deficiency, take cortisone medication, or use iron supplements.

RDI for vitamin A
- ✻ children (1–18 years): 1000–3000 iu
- ✻ women: 2300 iu
  - — during pregnancy: 2500 iu
  - — during lactation: 4300 iu
- ✻ men: 3000 iu

Vitamin D (calciferol)

Dubbed the 'sunshine vitamin', vitamin D is essential for the proper absorption and utilisation of calcium, and for the normal calcification of bones. Humans can manufacture their own vitamin D with the aid of sunlight upon our skin. However, the New Zealand obsession (rightly so) with slopping on tons of sunscreen every time we're out in the sun's rays diminishes our ability to manufacture this vitamin. In general though, despite sunscreen, the average antipodean soaks up enough ultraviolet rays to ensure that vitamin-D deficiency is not a problem.

Supplementing with huge amounts of calcium and phosphorus will make no difference to bone density if we are lacking in vitamin D. The importance of this nutrient for healthy bone formation is evidenced by the old scourge of the industrial lower classes during the Industrial Revolution — rickets. This bone-deforming disease was rampant due to a combined lack of dietary vitamin D and sunshine exposure. Vitamin-D deficiency also contributes to the development of osteoporosis by reducing the absorption of calcium.

Recently vitamin D has been in the news for its ability to prevent certain types of cancers. Studies from around the world have shown that people who expose themselves regularly to the sun (and consequently have more vitamin D) are at lower risk of certain cancers including colon, rectal and breast cancers.

Sunshine aside, we can obtain vitamin D through food sources such as egg yolks, liver and fish. Milk is also enriched with vitamin D. Vitamin-D deficiency is rare amongst healthy, active

New Zealanders. However, the elderly are at risk as a result of their limited sunshine exposure and 'picky' eating habits.

Vitamin-D requirements are increased during pregnancy and breastfeeding, and also during the menopause when our calcium absorption and utilisation changes, as a result of declining oestrogen production. Infants and children with rapidly developing skeletons also need greater amounts of this vitamin.

Since it is a fat-soluble vitamin, vitamin-D supplementation can cause toxicity issues when taken in doses of more than 2000 iu daily for extended periods. Supplement with high doses of vitamin D only after consulting your health professional.

The RDI for vitamin D is 200–600 iu per day, depending on age. The currently accepted maximum safe level of supplementation is 2000 iu per day. RDIs for vitamin D are very controversial, with some researchers claiming we need much greater levels for optimum health.

Vitamin E (tocopherol)

Along with vitamin C, I consider vitamin E to have earned its accolades as a true 'supernutrient'. Vitamin E is actually not a single nutrient, but rather a family of eight different fat-soluble compounds called the tocopherols. The majority of vitamin-E supplements contain alpha-tocopherol, and of late there has been a number of studies contradicting previously favourable claims for supplementing with this nutrient. Consequently 'vitamin E' supplements have been slammed in the media. In truth, it is the mixed tocopherol supplements, containing the full range of tocopherols, which demonstrate the most impressive therapeutic effects when taken as supplements.

Vitamin-E deficiency is common. The vitamin is most abundant in cold-pressed vegetable oils, avocado, raw nuts and seeds, soya beans and the germ of whole grains . . . all foods which are sadly lacking in the average Western diet. Survey the trolleys when you next visit the supermarket, and notice the mountains of white bread and commercially denatured cooking oils, and you will see why few of us have our requirements for this vitamin met. Adding more vitamin E to your daily diet is as simple as changing to a wholemeal bread; sprinkling a tablespoon of fresh wheatgerm on morning cereals; using cold-pressed vegetable oils daily; and snacking on a variety of different nuts and seeds.

What does vitamin E do for you?

Vitamin E supplementation has been caught in a storm of controversy in the past few years, with the sensational finding of a few studies suggesting that supplementing with more than 400 iu a day of vitamin E actually increases all causes of mortality. A closer look at these studies reveals that the subjects used were all over the age of 55, and already had heart disease or diabetes; or were people who had or previously had had cancer; or people who might have been at higher risk of developing heart disease or cancer. Consequently, it is impossible to extrapolate the findings to a healthy population of people. There is, in fact, a multitude of reputable studies using healthy subjects, that demonstrate a reduction in mortality with vitamin-E supplementation.

Similarly, the benefits of vitamin E for cardiovascular health have been called into question in the past few years, based on the findings of some large and respected international studies. One of these, the widely acclaimed GISI prevention trial, showed no preventative effects after more than three years of vitamin-E supplementation among 11,000 heart-attack survivors. It's important to realise these studies again used subjects who already had heart disease, as opposed to a healthy population.

In a healthy population, the picture seems to be different. When it comes to vitamin-E supplementation for healthy women, there is strong evidence that there are cardiovascular benefits. A large study published in 2005 looked at the effects of vitamin-E supplementation on 40,000 healthy women, who received 600 iu of vitamin E every second day for a 10-year period. In contrast to the findings of studies using unhealthy subjects, this study found that there was no increased mortality in the healthy women receiving vitamin-E supplements. Instead, the researchers found a 24% reduction in cardiovascular deaths in the supplemented group. In the case of women over the age of 65, the benefits were even more pronounced, with a 49% reduction in cardiovascular deaths and a 34% reduction in heart attacks.

Vitamin E is a natural, low-toxicity 'blood thinner'. Because of this anti-clotting effect, it is unwise to take large amounts (more than 300 iu a day) of supplemental vitamin E before undergoing surgery or in the weeks leading up to childbirth. Taken in smaller doses, this nutrient will assist with healing after surgery and reduce the likelihood of post-operative problems with blood clots.

Vitamin E helps our muscle cells to breathe, and supplementing with E allows our muscle cells to function effectively on smaller amounts of oxygen. This adds up to a noticeable improvement in energy levels, endurance and stamina. Applied topically to scars and wounds, vitamin E can work miracles. If you have a scar or adhesions from surgery, pierce a 500 iu potency vitamin-E capsule (natural alpha-tocopherol source) and apply the oil twice daily for several weeks. You'll be amazed at how the adhesions soften and the scars fade.

Women and vitamin E

Vitamin E can effectively treat a wide variety of female health issues, ranging from irregular periods, scanty periods and painful periods, to itching and inflammation of the vagina and hot flushes experienced during menopause. When it comes to period pain, vitamin E is nature's alternative to prostaglandin inhibitors such as aspirin and Ponstan. The uterus produces local hormones called prostaglandins, an excess of which is partly responsible for overly fierce uterine contractions during menstruation. Non-steroidal anti-inflammatories, such as aspirin or flufenamic acid (Ponstan), slow down or stop the production of these prostaglandins, thus greatly reducing menstrual pain. Vitamin E is able to reduce these same prostaglandins. It also helps ease pain by enhancing circulation and reducing the amount of oxygen needed by working muscles in the uterus.

During a period, the powerful muscle of the uterus contracts dramatically, forcing out the menstrual blood. It is thought that it is this powerful contraction, and the resulting constriction of blood supply to the uterus, that is partly responsible for the agony of menstrual cramps. Vitamin E enhances blood supply to the uterus, and at the same time reduces its oxygen requirements, thus lessening pain.

Vitamin E has also been a godsend for many menopausal women, with its ability to reduce the intensity and frequency of hot flushes. Increase dietary vitamin E, and if necessary, add in a natural tocopherol vitamin-E supplement in doses of 200–1000 iu per day, and feel your flushes fade. Vitamin E taken orally and used locally can also improve thinning, drying and burning of the vagina. Pierce a vitamin E capsule and apply the oil to the inside of the vagina for rapid relief.

A lack of dietary vitamin E may contribute to decreased fertility in both men and women. The Greek name for vitamin E is *tocopherol*, meaning 'to bear children'. Animal studies show that diets low in vitamin E decrease fertility. Vitamin E is one of the main antioxidants involved in protecting the cell membranes of sperm from oxidation by free-radicals. Its supplementation has been shown to enhance the ability of sperm to fertilise an egg in test tubes. In doses of 600–800 iu a day, alpha-tocopherol vitamin-E supplements may increase sperm count and motility.

Vitamin E and miscarriage

Women living on a vitamin-E-deficient diet are more likely to miscarry. Vitamin E is essential for enabling the fertilised egg to attach firmly to the wall of the uterus. It is also an essential nutrient for the development of a healthy placenta. If you have a history of miscarriage, supplementing with vitamin E (under the guidance of a health professional) prior to conception and during the first four months of pregnancy may be of great benefit.

Some hints about using vitamin-E supplements

Vitamin E supplements come in d (one-molecule natural form) and dl (two-molecule synthetic) forms, of which the natural d-alpha-tocopherols are the most potent and best value for money. As most vitamin-E supplements are oil-filled capsules, they should be refrigerated after opening to help prevent rancidity developing. Vitamin-E supplements are best taken before breakfast or before going to bed, and with a fat source of some kind. Fat-soluble vitamins such as A, D, E and K should always be taken along with a meal containing fats, to facilitate their absorption.

Besides the health problems already discussed, there are certain other situations in which taking vitamin-E supplements is appropriate. Women using synthetic oestrogen in the form of the oral contraceptive pill or hormone replacement therapy should supplement with additional vitamin E, as oestrogen interferes with the absorption of this vitamin.

If you use a lot of vegetable oil in cooking or salad dressings, you will need to increase your intake of vitamin E. These fats increase the rate of destruction (oxidation) of vitamin E. It is also a good idea to use vitamin-E supplements if you are taking large amounts of evening primrose oil as a supplement. If you are taking iron supplements (especially inorganic iron such as that prescribed by doctors for pregnant women), take vitamin-E supplements 8 to 12 hours before or after the iron.

As with all fat-soluble vitamins, it is possible to have too much of a good thing with vitamin E supplementation. If you plan to use more than 500 iu of vitamin E a day, and you have high blood pressure, check with your health professional first. In fact, standard medical advice is now not to use more than 400 iu of vitamin E daily if you have pre-existing heart disease (based on the increased mortality seen with doses higher than this amongst people with heart disease). Higher supplemental doses, where appropriate, are still recommended if there is no evidence of heart disease.

If you are on pharmaceutical blood-thinning drugs such as warfarin or aspirin, check with your doctor before adding vitamin E to the mix, as the combination may lead to excessively 'thinned' blood and an increase in bleeding time.

RDI for vitamin E
* children (1–18 years): 5–8 mg
* women: 7 mg
    — during pregnancy: 7 mg
    — during lactation: 12 mg
* men: 10 mg

Coenzyme Q_{10} (CoQ_{10})

CoQ_{10} is a powerful antioxidant. It is a fat-soluble, vitamin-like nutrient. It is present in every cell of the body, and it also occurs naturally in a number of foods including organ meats, soya oil, sardines, mackerel and peanuts. In theory, our body can synthesise its own CoQ_{10} through a complex 17-step process. In reality, though, this process is often impaired, and this leads to a decrease in CoQ_{10} levels in the body. A lack of dietary CoQ_{10} or biochemical changes which cause an increased requirement of this nutrient can also lead to deficiency.

As well as functioning as a powerful antioxidant, CoQ_{10} serves as a coenzyme for several of the key steps in the production of energy within every cell. Athletes are often lacking in CoQ_{10} as their high energy production burns through huge amounts of this nutrient. With the widespread use of pharmaceutical drugs, drug-induced CoQ_{10} deficiency is also increasingly common. Statins, beta-blockers and tricyclic antidepressants all affect CoQ_{10} levels adversely.

CoQ_{10} is especially important for heart health.

Therapeutic doses of CoQ_{10} have been proven to result in:

* reduction in blood pressure and heart rate

* reduction in sweating and palpitations

* reduction in need for cardiovascular drugs

* decreased chest congestion after heart failure

* prevention of the negative effects of beta-blockers without impairing the positive effects

* improvement of mitral-valve prolapse in children.

Statin drugs are widely prescribed for cholesterol problems. These drugs interfere with the body's ability to manufacture its own CoQ_{10}, leading to a drug-induced deficiency of this vital cardiac nutrient. Heart-failure victims often have abnormally low concentrations of CoQ_{10} in their heart muscle. Some scientists believe that while statins reduce LDL and total cholesterol levels, they may also increase the risk of sudden heart failure related to CoQ_{10} deficiency.

CoQ_{10} supplementation has been shown to:

* increase energy levels

* prevent or improve cardiovascular disease

* boost immunity

* prevent or treat periodontal disease

* kill some cancer cells (in laboratory research).

Supplementing with CoQ_{10}

Research into CoQ_{10} is extensive and increasing rapidly, but as yet it is still not known exactly how much CoQ_{10} is required as an ideal 'preventative' dose. Research shows that blood levels of CoQ_{10} and heart function change with supplementation of just 30–60 mg daily. Many aware cardiologists recommend 100 mg of CoQ_{10} daily to safeguard cardiovascular health. Patients with active heart disease are often prescribed doses of between 400 and 600 mg a day. CoQ_{10} is a fat-soluble compound which is best absorbed when taken with a meal containing fat. A recent New Zealand study demonstrated that not all forms of CoQ_{10} are equally absorbable and bioavailable. Ensure that any supplement you use is in an oil-based encapsulated form rather than in tablet form, for maximum absorption.

CoQ_{10} levels can be measured with a blood test. Normal levels are 0.8 to 1.2 mcg per millilitre of blood. For therapeutic benefit, however, CoQ_{10} levels need to be increased to 2.5 to 3.5 mcg by supplementation.

Finally, if you decide to supplement with CoQ_{10} and you are taking any type of cardiac medication, it's important to let your GP know, as the effects can be dramatic, and existing medication may need to be reduced or altered. For example, blood pressure may drop significantly, leading to low blood pressure if existing medication is not reduced.

RDI for coenzyme Q_{10}
None determined.

Essential fatty acids (vitamin F)
Linoleic acid and linolenic acid are both fatty acids that must be supplied by your diet, and cannot be manufactured in the body. Thus they are termed 'essential' fatty acids (EFAs). They are found mostly in seeds, wheatgerm, corn and safflower oil, and flax seed (linseed).

Evening primrose oil, and more recently borage and star flower oil, are commonly used supplemental forms of EFAs. Dietary EFAs must undergo conversion in our body into a more usable form. This conversion process is sometimes hampered by dietary practices such as: a high intake of red meat; dietary trans-fatty acids; alcohol consumption. Deficiencies of zinc, vitamin B6 and magnesium also interfere with the EFA conversion process. In contrast to this, evening primrose and star flower oil provide 'preconverted' essential fatty acids which can be readily used by the body.

EFAs are vital for the health of every cell in our body, being essential for the creation and health of the fatty membrane surrounding every cell. They are involved in cholesterol metabolism and cardiovascular health; joint lubrication; immune function; hormonal regulation; and ensuring healthy skin, hair and connective tissue. Deficiency symptoms include skin disorders such as dry skin, eczema, psoriasis or acne; hair loss; frequent infections; sores around the corner of the mouth and in the nose.

PMS and EFAs
See PMS in the A–Z section in Part Two.

EFAs and osteoporosis
Nobody disputes the fact that adequate amounts of dietary calcium are essential in order to prevent bone degeneration and osteoporosis. Simply swallowing litres of milk or bottles of calcium supplements will still not necessarily guarantee that your bones receive all the calcium they need. Calcium is a poorly absorbed mineral, with as little as 20% of dietary calcium actually being utilised by the body. Calcium absorption is enhanced in the presence of evening primrose oil or fish oil. When taken along with calcium, the essential fatty acids in these oils increase calcium absorption from food and supplements, reduce the amount of calcium excreted through the kidneys, and increase the amount of calcium fixed into bones, where it is needed.

(For more information, see discussion of fats at the start of the chapter.)

Minerals

Minerals, like vitamins, are essential for life, but sadly mineral deficiency is commonplace. The human body cannot synthesise any of its own minerals, thus all minerals must come to us from the earth, through the food chain. Modern intensive farming practices deplete our soils of minerals and trace elements, and consequently produce mineral-depleted foods. Minerals are also more difficult than vitamins to digest and absorb, and minerals compete with one another for absorption. This is especially an issue when supplementing with minerals. For example, large amounts of zinc will reduce your absorption of iron, copper and phosphorus, while too much calcium hinders your uptake of magnesium, zinc and manganese.

Minerals are divided into two main categories: macrominerals (which we need a lot of), and trace or microminerals (which are needed only in trace amounts). Macrominerals include calcium, magnesium, potassium, phosphorus, sodium, sulphur and silicon. Microminerals include iron, zinc, copper, iodine, chromium, and several other less well-known minerals.

Calcium

Of all the essential minerals, calcium is needed in the greatest abundance. Without calcium, our bones would crumble and our teeth would fall out; our nervous system would be in tatters and our muscles would be useless.

This mineral is essential for building and maintaining a strong 'break-resistant' skeleton. The 1% of body calcium that circulates in our bloodstream (as opposed to being locked into our bones) is responsible for muscle contraction and relaxation — calcium deficiency is a very common cause of muscle cramps. Blood calcium is also essential to regulate blood pH, and to assist with blood clotting whenever necessary. The nervous system relies on calcium in the transmission of nerve impulses, and the release of 'calming' brain chemicals such as serotonin.

While it's true that dairy products are rich in calcium, they are only one source of this macromineral. There are a number of reasons why simply guzzling gallons of milk to get your daily calcium may not be a good idea. Many people find that including large amounts of dairy foods in their diet leads to excessive mucus production, abdominal bloating, and gas. Dairy intolerance is surprisingly common. A high dairy intake has also been associated with increased incidence of diabetes, prostate cancer and breast cancer.

Other useful dietary sources of calcium include: green vegetables (broccoli, kale, watercress, cabbage, silverbeet and spinach), tempeh and tofu (fermented soya bean products), calcium-enriched soya milk, bony fish such as sardines, pilchards, salmon, herrings; and almonds, sesame seeds and tahini. Even with generous dietary supplies of calcium, it is not uncommon for the body to absorb only 20–50% of dietary calcium (a problem which becomes increasingly common with age). Absorption is especially poor if you have low stomach acid; or if you frequently use antacids or medications for stomach ulcers. Calcium absorption is also hindered by a high-fat diet, or by deficiency of vitamins A, C or D. Oxalic acid found in spinach, rhubarb and chocolate also interferes with calcium absorption; as does phytic acid, from whole grains.

A diet high in salt, sugar, protein or phosphorus (found in abundance in red meat and soft drinks) increases the excretion of calcium in the urine.

How do you know if you have a calcium deficiency?

There are a number of common warning signs that you may be lacking in this important mineral. Do your muscles seize in painful cramps? Does your heart sometimes race out of control, for no particular reason? Does your family accuse you of being a nervous wreck — tense and flying off the handle at the least provocation? Are your nails brittle? Maybe your teeth feel loose, or keep you running back to the dentist for yet more fillings. Spontaneous or easy fracturing is also a loud and clear indication of calcium insufficiency (usually along with a deficiency of a range of other minerals and vitamins). If this sounds like you, then bumping up your dietary calcium intake is vital . . . and perhaps you should be using a calcium supplement as well.

Calcium and pregnancy and lactation

During pregnancy and breastfeeding, calcium requirements escalate to around 1500 mg a day. During pregnancy you are manufacturing a whole new baby skeleton inside your body, and the calcium crucial for this job has to come from your own supplies. Inadequate calcium intake at this time does not jeopardise your baby's skeleton, but it does affect your own. Your growing baby's needs come first as far as your body is concerned. If you lack sufficient dietary calcium for the job, your body simply steals stored calcium from your own bones. Too many pregnancies like this and you end up at high risk of osteoporosis later in life.

High blood pressure and toxaemia during pregnancy are dangerous to both the mother and the unborn baby. Increasing calcium levels during pregnancy reduces the risk of these complications. In studies in which pregnant women received daily calcium supplements of between 1500 and 2000 mg, the incidence of hypertension was halved, and the risk of pre-eclampsia decreased by between 45% and 75%.

Calcium supplements

(For information on how best to supplement with calcium, see Osteoporosis in the A–Z section in Part Two.)

Calcium supplementation is safe, unless taken in excess (around 4000 mg a day). Taken in these doses, calcium can precipitate out of your blood, causing problems with abnormal deposits in muscles and soft tissues. If you have a history of calcium oxalate kidney stones, it is still safe to supplement with the calcium citrate or hydroxyapetate form of calcium, if needed.

RDI for calcium

* children (1–18 years): 500–1300 mg
* women: 1000 mg (increases to 1300 mg from menopause)
  — during pregnancy: 1000 mg
  — during lactation: 1000 mg
* men: 1000 mg

Magnesium

In theory, magnesium is abundant in green vegetables and grains. I say, 'in theory', because, as is the case with all the macrominerals, the mineral content of our food is simply a reflection of the mineral content of the soil from which it springs . . . and that soil is often over-farmed, and therefore depleted. Magnesium deficiency is one of the most common nutritional deficiencies I see in my clinic. This is a reflection partly of our soil health, and partly of our low dietary intake of foods most likely to contain magnesium (raw wheatgerm, soya beans, figs, corn, oily nuts and seeds, and green vegetables).

The magnesium content of foods is further compromised by chopping and cooking. The problem is compounded by our consumption of coffee and tea, alcohol and sugar — all of which increase our magnesium requirements.

A CSIRO (Commonwealth Scientific and Industrial Research Organisation) study of Australian adults found that daily intake of magnesium was below the RDI in the case of 50% of all males and 39% of all females tested. Similar testing in America found approximately 85% of adult females to have magnesium intakes below the RDI. Magnesium deficiency is also common amongst older adults, who tend to have a lower dietary magnesium intake, coupled with reduced absorption and increased excretion of magnesium in the urine. Chronic malabsorption problems such as Crohn's disease, and gluten sensitivity reduce magnesium absorption. Magnesium deficiency is also common amongst heavy drinkers of alcohol.

Magnesium is vital for health in so many different ways. It is required in the biological function of at least 360 enzymes in the human body, and is involved in the production and transfer of energy in every cell in the body. Magnesium is also essential for the synthesis of protein, and for the proper functioning of nerves and muscles — including the most important muscle of all, the heart. It is nature's muscle relaxant and an 'anti-stress' mineral supreme. It also helps us to absorb other minerals, such as calcium and phosphorus, as well as vitamins B, C and E.

How do you know whether you need more magnesium? Think exhausted, jumpy, tense, twitchy and crampy . . . the classic magnesium-deficient personality. If you jump every time the phone rings, and the ads screaming at you from the television make you feel like screaming back . . . think magnesium. Maybe you've noticed your eyelids dancing a jig while you focus on the computer screen. You guessed it — twitches and spasms mean magnesium deficiency. Other common symptoms to look for include: fatigue, poor appetite, insomnia, memory problems, apathy, irregular heartbeat or palpitations, depression and mood swings, and PMS.

Magnesium and your heart

Observational studies show that a diet high in magnesium reduces the risk of cardiovascular disease and heart attacks, and plays an important part in regulating blood pressure.

Magnesium deficiency is involved in a myriad of cardiovascular problems, as this mineral is so essential for the normal functioning of the heart. Both calcium and magnesium are involved in the normal function of the cardiac muscle. Calcium allows muscles to contract, while magnesium allows them to relax again, preventing spasm. A lack of magnesium is often associated with heart attacks which result from spasms of the smooth muscle in the heart. Supplementation with magnesium is a common naturopathic practice in the treatment of angina, hypertension, irregular heart rhythm, and elevated blood triglycerides.

Magnesium and diabetes

Magnesium plays an important role in the metabolism of carbohydrates and the maintenance of healthy blood-sugar levels. Type-two diabetes (in which the body becomes resistant to the effects of the blood-sugar-regulating hormone, insulin), often causes sufferers to have low levels of magnesium in the blood.

Supplementing type-two diabetics with magnesium improves insulin response and helps to normalise blood-sugar levels. Studies show that amongst overweight adults, those most likely to eventually develop type-two diabetes are those with the lowest dietary intake of magnesium.

PMS, menstrual cramps and magnesium
See PMS and Dysmenorrhoea in the A–Z section in Part Two.

A word on magnesium supplementation
The most easily absorbed forms of magnesium supplements include magnesium chelate, aspartate, citrate and diglycinate. The bicarbonate, oxide or carbonate forms are less absorbable.

Magnesium supplements are best taken on an empty stomach, as taking them with your meals will reduce hydrochloric acid production and slow the digestion of your meal . . . as well as the absorption of your mineral supplement.

Take calcium and magnesium supplements on an empty stomach, along with a little ascorbic acid (or lemon juice) to maximise absorption. Just before going to bed is a good time to take them, and the natural soporific effect of magnesium and calcium will ensure a peaceful, deep sleep. Adequate B6 is also important for magnesium absorption, and if taking a combined magnesium formulation, always look for one that contains additional vitamin B6.

If you are taking high doses of calcium, your magnesium requirements are increased. If you have a high-protein diet, or consume a lot of phosphorus-rich foods such as red meat and cola drinks, or drink more than the occasional glass of alcohol, your magnesium requirements are also increased.

Magnesium should not be taken as a supplement in isolation, as it can upset the balance of other minerals, in particular calcium. Long-term, high-dose magnesium supplementation should always be combined with additional calcium, preferably in the ratio of one part magnesium to two parts calcium.

RDI for magnesium
 ✶ children (1–18 years): 80–360 mg
 ✶ women: 420 mg
  — during pregnancy: 350 mg
  — during lactation: 310 mg
 ✶ men: 320 mg

Potassium

This electrically charged mineral is found inside the blood cells, and along with sodium is classed as an 'electrolyte'. In fact, potassium and sodium have a special relationship, and must be finely balanced for good health. The combination of potassium and sodium maintains a normal balance of fluids in our body, and prevents fluid retention, oedema and an increase in blood volume, which can cause hypertension. Potassium is also important for normal muscle contraction and a regular heartbeat.

Potassium occurs in a wide range of natural foods, and our ancestors need not have worried about obtaining adequate potassium from their daily diet. They existed on a wholefood, unrefined diet, low in sodium and high in potassium-rich fruits and vegetables.

The same cannot be said for the average modern diet. Not only have we turned the natural high-potassium/low-sodium ratio on its head, but we also consume a diet of denatured, processed and potassium-depleted foods. Now we binge on a multitude of high-sodium foods (salt in any form, potato chips, snack foods, frozen and canned foods with added salt, cheese, and so on), and often eat less-than-ideal amounts of fresh fruit, vegetables and whole grains to supply the balancing potassium we need. This common imbalance in the ratio of sodium to potassium encourages fluid retention, oedema and heart problems. Diuretics are commonly prescribed to deal with fluid retention, and while they may get rid of the excessive fluid, they contribute significantly to the further depletion of potassium levels!

Even if your diet is rich in potassium foods, you may need to boost your intake during heatwaves when you lose a lot of potassium in your sweat; after a bout of diarrhoea or vomiting; or if you use drugs such as diuretics, laxatives, aspirin, digitalis or cortisone.

Also, consider increasing your dietary intake of potassium (through plentiful supplies of fresh fruits and vegetables) if you drink a lot of caffeinated beverages or alcohol, or if you eat a lot of sugar, all of which deplete potassium stores.

Early symptoms of potassium deficiency include fatigue, muscle weakness, slow reflexes, depression and mood swings, and skin problems such as dry skin or acne. Cardiac problems such as arrhythmia, high blood pressure and congestive heart disease are also associated with low potassium intake. Reducing the amount of sodium in your diet, while simultaneously increasing your intake of potassium-rich fruits and vegetables (and, if needed, taking a potassium supplement with your health professional's supervision) can help to rectify these conditions.

Potassium broth is a traditional naturopathic solution to potassium deficiency. The broth is made from potato peelings (make sure they are not green), carrots, onions, garlic, cabbage and any other green vegetables readily available. Chop the vegetables into small pieces and cover with water in a large pan. Simmer gently for 30 minutes, and then drink the liquid. Any leftovers can be stored in the fridge for a couple of days in an airtight container. It is also a good idea to drink the water used for steaming or boiling vegetables, as this nutritious water contains leached potassium and other minerals and vitamins from the vegetables.

RDI for potassium

* children (1–18 years): 2000–2600 mg
* women: 2800 mg
  — during pregnancy: 2800 mg
  — during lactation: 3200 mg
* men: 3800 mg

Sodium

Nobody living on a typical Western diet has a sodium deficiency. In fact, we are all drastically overloaded with this essential (but, in excess, damaging) electrolyte mineral. Sodium is found mostly in the fluid surrounding our blood cells (extracellular fluid), and is intimately involved in the regulation of our body fluid. In a nutshell, excess sodium (usually along with insufficient potassium) tends to cause retention of fluid, increased blood volume and increased blood pressure. Our concern should not be with ensuring sufficient supplies of this mineral, but rather with trying to cut down on our intake of it. Most of our dietary sodium comes in the form of sodium chloride (salt) added to processed foods. Minimising your intake of these foods (especially the high-sodium foods such as cheeses, processed meats, snack foods), and avoiding salting at the table or during cooking, will greatly reduce your sodium intake.

Chromium

This essential trace element is needed in tiny amounts for good health, but is difficult to absorb. In countries like New Zealand, soil concentrations of chromium are low. Processing and refining of food further compromises chromium content in our diet. Chromium is poorly absorbed from food, and increasingly so with age. Low dietary chromium intake has been associated with an increased incidence of heart disease (in particular atherosclerosis) and diabetes.

Sugar cane is actually extremely rich in chromium, but by the time it ends up on our table as white (or brown) sugar, it has lost 93% of its chromium content (don't get me wrong: I'm not advocating that we should increase our sugar intake to get more chromium!). The same applies to whole wheat, which undergoes a 40% loss of chromium during its conversion to white flour. A diet high in fat will also reduce your ability to absorb chromium.

A particularly effective way of boosting your dietary intake of chromium is to include brewer's yeast in your daily diet (as long as you don't suffer from thrush, or find that yeast causes you bloating and digestive problems). Brewer's yeast and torula yeast are both rich in GTF (glucose tolerance factor). GTF is a combination of chromium, niacin (a B-vitamin), and three amino acids. GTF is found in certain foods, and is readily utilised by the body to help regulate carbohydrate metabolism and insulin function. If yeast is not for you, other chromium-rich foods include beef, liver, brown rice, potatoes, wheatgerm, eggs, spinach, bananas and chicken.

Supplementing with chromium

The issue of chromium supplementation has been fraught with controversy in the past few years. Some preliminary animal studies suggest that chromium picolinate may cause cellular changes which could potentially lead to cancer. There is no human evidence of such an effect; more research is needed in this area, and it is too early to make a definitive decision either way about this form of chromium.

Chromium supplements have been heavily pushed in the weight-loss market. In truth, there is little evidence that chromium will increase your rate of fat loss; it will, however, help to regulate your blood-sugar levels and stave off cravings. If you suffer from blood-sugar problems such as diabetes or hypoglycaemia, or have trouble with elevated cholesterol levels, boosting your chromium intake would be of benefit. Pre-formed GTF supplements are not available (other than by using brewer's yeast), but try to use a chromium supplement that also provides niacin.

Chromium has extremely low toxicity, and a safe daily supplementary range is 200–300 mcg. Do not consume your supplement together with milk and other dairy products, red meat or cola drinks (all high in phosphorus), as phosphorus makes chromium less absorbable. Many multivitamins contain chromium, and indeed chromium is absorbed more readily in the presence of vitamin C.

RDI for chromium

* children (1–18 years): 90–150 mcg

* women: 150 mcg
— during pregnancy: 220 mcg
— during lactation: 270 mcg

* men: 150 mcg

Iodine

Iodine is another micromineral needed in only tiny (but crucial) amounts. Iodine is especially vital for normal functioning of the thyroid gland. Iodine enables the thyroid gland to produce the hormones we need to regulate metabolism, and to regulate cellular respiration and energy production.

Iodine deficiency is rarely a problem today, as most table salt is enriched with iodine. Our soil may lack this trace element but iodine is also supplied through seafoods such as fish, shellfish and seaweed. Kelp is the form of iodine most commonly used as an iodine supplement, and sprinkling small amounts of kelp over food is a good way of ensuring adequate iodine intake if you are a vegetarian (that is, don't eat seafoods), and use little or no salt. As with all good things, though, you can overdo it. Excessive iodine intake through ingesting too much kelp over long periods may reduce the thyroid's production of thyroxine and cause sluggish thyroid function, or over-stimulation and hyperthyroidism.

A diet low in iodine can lead to a dramatic enlargement of the thyroid gland, called a goitre. Goitre is rarely seen now in this part of the world, but this problem was especially common in America in the 1930s and 1940s, especially in the Midwestern states where the soil lacked iodine.

A less dramatic manifestation of low iodine intake is a gradual under-functioning of the thyroid gland (*hypothyroidism*). Signs of sluggish thyroid function include: weight gain; lethargy; poor temperature regulation and a tendency to feel cold; dry skin and hair, and mental symptoms such as depression and apathy. There are often also menstrual problems such as irregular or absent periods or excessively heavy periods. (See hypothyroidism in the A–Z section in Part Two.)

RDI for iodine
* children (1–18 years): 90–150 mcg
* women: 150 mcg
    — during pregnancy: 220 mcg
    — during lactation: 270 mcg
* men: 150 mcg

Iron
See anaemia in the A–Z section in Part Two.

RDI for iron
* children (1–18 years): 9–15 mg
* women: 18 mg until menopause, when reduced to 8 mg
    — during pregnancy: 27 mg
    — during lactation: 9 mg
* men: 8 mg

Selenium
Selenium, like chromium and iodine, is a micromineral, needed in small (but essential) amounts. New Zealand is renowned for its low soil concentrations of selenium, and New Zealand farmers routinely supplement their livestock with selenium (while most New Zealanders remain unsupplemented and unaware of the consequences of a selenium deficiency). Worldwide studies show that there is a strong correlation between low soil selenium levels and high rates of cancer, especially of the breast, colon and lung (all cancers prevalent in New Zealand) (see Chapter 6). However, the question of whether or not supplemental selenium can prevent cancer is still controversial, with some studies demonstrating a positive effect, and others showing none.

Common sense nevertheless strongly suggests that adequate selenium levels are vital for long-term good health, as selenium is an essential factor for the enzyme glutathione peroxidase, an important component of the body's antioxidant defence system.

Selenium also plays a vital role in the prevention of cardio-vascular disease, acting as a potent antioxidant to prevent the oxidation of the potentially damaging LDL cholesterol. I say 'potentially' damaging, because while LDL is dubbed 'bad' cholesterol, it only causes its artery-clogging problems when it is oxidised by free-radicals. Selenium prevents or reduces this oxidation, thus protecting arteries.

Where do you find selenium in your diet? Bearing in mind that a food can only be as mineral rich as the soil it is grown in, the following foods are good sources of selenium: brewer's yeast, wheatgerm, liver, fish, lamb, whole grains, brazil nuts, brown rice, garlic and onions.

Supplementing with selenium

Selenium supplementation has become popular, with many multi-vitamin and mineral supplements containing small amounts of selenium. When it comes to supplementing with selenium, it is definitely possible to have too much of a good thing. Excessive supplemental selenium can cause illness and, in extreme cases, even death. However, it is an extremely safe supplement when taken in the recommended amount. RDIs vary from country to country, but it is generally agreed that adults need between 50 mcg and 200 mcg a day, and are able to tolerate long-term upper limits of 400 mcg a day. Vitamin E enhances the utilisation of selenium in the body, while vitamin-C supplements block the absorption of some forms of supplemental selenium.

Taken as a nutritional supplement, selenium comes in two forms — selenomethionine (organically bound) or sodium selenite (inorganic). Generally, the sodium selenite form has the potential to be more toxic than the organic selenomethionine form, and the selenomethionine form is considered to be more absorbable.

Until 1987 the average New Zealander had a very low dietary selenium intake compared with people in many other parts of the world. In 1987 New Zealand deregulated wheat imports, and we began receiving substantial amounts of selenium-rich wheat from Australia. As a result of the widespread consumption of this wheat, the selenium status of the average New Zealander has increased to at least the minimum recommended levels for health.

However, I believe there is enough evidence of the protective benefits of higher levels of selenium to warrant supplementation in many cases. Generally, I recommend selenium supplementation as part of a complex, along with other antioxidant nutrients such as vitamins A, C and E.

RDI for selenium
   ✳ children (1–18 years): 25–60 mcg
   ✳ women: 60 mcg
       — during pregnancy: 65 mcg
       — during lactation: 75 mcg
   ✳ men: 70 mcg

Zinc

After iron, zinc is the trace mineral we need most of . . . and zinc deficiency is also one of the most common nutritional deficiencies, especially in pregnant or lactating women, rapidly growing children, adolescents, and vegetarians!

Zinc is abundant in a wholefood diet rich in whole grains, nuts and seeds (especially pumpkin seeds), some red meat and shellfish. However, vegetarians who are denied the most abundant supples of zinc (animal flesh and seafood), often develop symptoms of zinc deficiency, despite their high intake of wholefoods. This is partly because our soils are lacking in this trace mineral, and consequently so are our grains and vegetables. Processing and cooking of foods also destroys what zinc is present. Zinc is water soluble, and is leached from food during cooking. Vegetarians are more likely to be zinc-deficient for other reasons too — the zinc bound with phytates and oxalates present in grains and vegetables is poorly absorbed compared with that found in animal protein sources. High-fibre foods also tend to inhibit zinc absorption.

Other useful sources of dietary zinc include herrings, oysters, liver, mushrooms, wheatgerm, pumpkin seeds, onions, and good old brewer's yeast. Zinc needs to be a daily component of a healthy diet, as we are unable to store zinc for times of increased need.

Pregnancy and lactation increase zinc requirements dramatically, as do taking the oral contraceptive pill, going on repeated weight-loss diets, and regular alcohol consumption. Stress and injury increase zinc loss through perspiration and urine, and consequently zinc requirements following surgery or injury are greatly increased.

Zinc is needed for nearly all metabolic functions, and is essential for the manufacture of over more than 300 enzymes. It is an integral part of the formation of hormones such as insulin. It is essential for proper growth and development, especially of the reproductive organs. Zinc is needed to heal wounds, and for our immune system to fight infection.

Signs of zinc deficiency include frequent infections, skin problems such as acne or stretch marks, blood-sugar problems, little white flecks on your fingernails, falling hair and a poor sense of taste, reduced appetite, and poor wound healing. Zinc-deficient teenage girls have delayed onset of menstruation and, thereafter, irregular periods.

Zinc and pregnancy

Pregnant women who are lacking in zinc are at increased risk of a range of health problems such as high blood pressure, oedema, toxaemia and eclampsia. They are also more likely to deliver a pre-term, underweight baby. Less serious, but still unpleasant, is the increased likelihood of stretch marks from zinc deficiency.

Taking iron supplements during pregnancy, combined with a low dietary intake of zinc, is a sure-fire recipe for zinc deficiency as iron competes with zinc for absorption. The recommended daily intake of zinc for pregnant women is 20 mg, and since most women studied are found to have intakes of no more than 10 mg a day, a multivitamin containing zinc and other minerals is a good idea during pregnancy.

A note on supplementing with zinc

People who are vegetarian, pregnant, lactating, or growing quickly (early childhood and adolescence) may well need additional supplementary zinc. Remember that zinc competes with iron and calcium for absorption, so if you use large amounts of these supplements, you can actually induce a zinc deficiency!

In terms of supplements, chelated zinc is usually the best tolerated and most efficiently absorbed (as well as the most costly!) form of zinc. You can further enhance your absorption of this mineral by taking your supplement on its own two hours after your meals, or first thing in the morning.

As with all the other nutrients we have discussed, simply taking large amounts of this mineral in isolation can cause deficiency problems with other trace minerals. Whenever possible, use balanced multimineral and multivitamin supplements to ensure a balanced supply of all the associated nutrients needed for utilisation of zinc. Zinc is essential for the absorption and utilisation of vitamin A: taking vitamin-A supplements while you are deficient in zinc will be of little benefit.

RDI for zinc

* children (1–18 years): 3–7 mg

* women: 8 mg
  — during pregnancy: 11 mg
  — during lactation: 12 mg

* men: 14 mg

Chapter **3**

Exercise

You've got to move it, move it . . .

What strange times we live in. Gone are the days of polio, scarlet fever, death during childbirth, and the risk of death through a simple tooth extraction. In their place have come obesity, diabetes, heart disease, cancer, depression, arthritis. These are the modern pandemics responsible for felling Westerners in their prime. Since the advent of antibiotics, acute, infectious disease is no longer as feared. Instead, we are killing ourselves, or devastating our quality of life, with chronic, degenerative, lifestyle-related illnesses. Illnesses which we could virtually eradicate overnight if we could only be persuaded to make different choices. We choose to smoke, drink to excess, stress our minds to breaking point, consume lifeless, denatured food, pollute our environment with toxins . . . and sit on our ever-expanding behinds while we do so!

Most of us are lucky enough to have freedom of choice. Making the right choices gives us the opportunity to create a different future for ourselves and our children. The choices you make today . . . whether to lie on the sofa with the remote control, or put on your walking shoes and take the dog for a walk . . . will gradually, one by one, determine your future health legacy.

While it is human nature to delude ourselves that there's always tomorrow to give up smoking, go on a diet, or start exercising, the truth is there is absolutely no time like the present. And remember, these choices benefit nobody but yourself. You can choose to lose weight or throw the cigarettes out because you know you 'should', or because you value yourself enough to want the very best quality of life in the years ahead. A life filled with opportunities, excitement, meaningful relationships with those you love — and above all, a life filled with good health and contentment.

One of the most significant choices you can make to ensure that you won't be one of the contributors to the depressing chronic disease statistics is to use the miraculous body you were given in the way it was designed. While our culture and technology have evolved at lightning pace, for millennia the human form has undergone little change. We are designed to run, climb, jump, hunt wild animals, roam the plains foraging for food; sprint out of harm's way; and carry the kill home at the end of the day. Today we use these same bodies to climb into the car; sit behind a desk all day; climb back into the car, and collapse exhausted on the sofa in front of the television. Is it any wonder that there is a real risk that our children may not live as long as we do?

Choose wellness

You can spend a fortune on organic foods, follow a myriad of different fad diets, and swallow handfuls of vitamin pills every day. The cold hard truth is that unless you add regular exercise to your regime, you are missing a vital part of your health equation. Despite what the advertisers may tell us, health does not come bottled in a supplement jar, or even in an organic apple, and sound nutrition is but one of the building blocks of optimum health.

Those who think they have not time for bodily exercise
will sooner or later have to find time for illness.

Edward Stanley

Why exercise?

Exercise enhances the efficiency of every function in the body,
as well as making us stronger and fitter. When we are active we
breathe more, our heart beats faster and stronger, and blood is
pumped more efficiently through the thousands of kilometres of
blood vessels in our body. More life-giving oxygen and nutrients
are delivered to every single cell in the body, and, at the same
time, exercise allows us to move the waste products from cells to
our eliminative organs for elimination. Increased cellular nutrition and oxygenation, coupled with a cleaner, less-toxic system,
translates into feeling fantastic!

The ultimate heart medicine

There is no controversy or debate over the fact that regular
exercise strengthens the heart and keeps the whole cardiovascular
system in condition. Stated simply, regular exercise reduces your
risk of heart disease, high blood pressure, clogged arteries, angina
and heart failure.

Regular aerobic exercise also changes blood fats (lipids) in a
positive way, lowering potentially troublesome LDL cholesterol
and triglycerides, and increasing cardiovascular-protective HDL
fats. HDLs help to prevent the build-up of fatty plaques in the
arteries (arteriosclerosis), which in turn cause high blood pressure
and heart disease. Added together, these cardiovascular benefits
translate into a fit person reducing their risk of heart attack or
stroke by approximately eight times, compared with their unfit
peers.

While all types of exercise benefit the human body in some
way, when the aim is to increase the health of the cardiovascular

system, it is *aerobic exercise* which offers the greatest benefits. Aerobic literally means 'using oxygen', and that's exactly what this form of exercise makes you do. Aerobic exercise is sustained, repetitive and strenuous movement which boosts your heart rate and oxygen uptake and gives your heart and lungs a serious workout. 'Stop/start' exercise such as tenpin bowling is not aerobic. Aerobic activities to choose from include: running or jogging, walking, swimming, cycling and dancing, and using exercise machines such as rowing machines or exercycles.

Because aerobic activity places a stress on the heart and lungs (albeit a good one in the long term), it's important that you build up to peak activity gradually. So many people have the totally unrealistic expectation of transformation from slothdom to athletic prowess within a matter of days, having made their decision to become fit. If you attempt such a rapid transformation, not only will the physical pain deter you from further efforts, but such heroic feats may place you at risk of injury or even a heart attack.

Taking your pulse regularly during aerobic activity allows you to moderate your efforts to keep heart rate in a safe range. How do you work out the intensity of exercise needed to increase your cardiovascular fitness? By taking your pulse and doing some maths. Subtract your age from 220. For example, if you are 40 years old, your maximum heart rate would be 180 beats per minute (bpm). To work at 65% of your maximum heart rate, multiply 180 by 0.65 (which equals 117 bpm). To take your pulse, simply count your heartbeat for 10 seconds, and then multiply this figure by 6 to give you your pulse rate per minute. When you first start exercising, keep cardiovascular rate within 50–60% of maximum heart rate until you are finding this level of exertion easy and comfortable. At this point you can increase your heart rate to a higher level of around 65–80% of maximum. Exercising within this band will increase your fitness and your cardiovascular health. Of course, it's not a matter of one or two sporadic bouts of activity, but building regular exercise into your

Tips for maximum benefit
from your exercise programme

An effective programme should include:

* Aerobic exercise involving continuous repetitive action of large muscle groups to increase heart rate and respiration. Examples of such exercise include walking, cycling, swimming.

* Strength training, working with weights or resistance equipment at the gym, to increase muscle tissue.

* Flexibility training, through regular stretching, to prevent injury, increase physical performance, increase the delivery of nutrients and the blood flow to joints, and to improve balance.

How to set about it

* Choose an exercise that you enjoy, and alternate new activities with old ones regularly to prevent boredom.

* To improve cardiovascular fitness, exercise 3–5 times weekly, with a training heart rate 60–85% of your maximum, for 20–60 minutes per session. Start by exercising at 50–60% of maximum heart rate, increasing the rate only when you are fitter and more comfortable.

* Be patient, start slowly. If it hurts too much, not only could it be dangerous for your health, but it's also likely to work as a form of 'aversion' therapy, quickly putting you off exercising.

* Find a fitness partner for companionship and encouragement.

* Schedule your workouts in your diary, and stick to the appointment you have made with yourself!

* Use an iPod™ to entertain yourself if exercising alone.

life that will pay long-term health dividends. For maximum heart benefit, aim to exercise within your target band for 30 minutes on most days (although this can be performed in three 10-minute exercise 'snacks'). Don't worry if you can't sustain the upper end of your target range for long, as you will reap more benefits from longer periods of lower-intensity exercise (as long as it's still within your target range) than from short bursts of the higher-intensity exercise.

While this may all sound completely overwhelming if your current lifestyle is devoid of physical activity, take your reformation in small, bite-sized and manageable steps. Trick yourself into exercising by playing little games with yourself, such as parking the car further from the office, or getting off the bus a few stops early on the way home from work. Make a commitment to use stairs instead of lifts whenever possible, and always walk to close destinations such as the local dairy, instead of getting the car out of the garage. Invest in a pedometer and work up to a goal of 10,000 steps a day. Find a friend to buddy you — someone of similar fitness level to support you on your journey. Choose your form of exercise wisely and find something that stimulates and excites you. Sitting on a sweaty exercycle staring at the concrete wall in the gym may not set your soul on fire. On the other hand, brisk weekend walks along the cliff tops with the sea wind blowing in your hair will leave you feeling spiritually recharged — as well as sweaty and fit.

Not all exercise costs money. Simple brisk walking is free, and has the benefit of being one of the best forms of exercise for weight loss. If you need some additional motivation besides feeling fitter and looking fabulous, why not invoke a personal reward system. Draw up some realistic exercise goals. Whenever you meet a goal, stash some money away in the exercise account, to be used specifically for nurturing or pleasuring you in some way. How about treating yourself to a massage or facial without feeling guilty or self-indulgent? Remember, you earned it with sweat (but hopefully no blood or tears).

While you may feel boundless enthusiasm at the start of your fitness venture, it's realistic to expect that your enthusiasm and commitment will wane from time to time. When you feel boredom setting in, use it as an opportunity to discover new and enjoyable forms of exercise, rather than as an excuse to take up residence on the sofa again. Just as with dieting, if you skip a couple of your regular workouts, remember that tomorrow is a new day, and simply pick up where you left off.

Whatever form of exercise you choose to embark upon, there are a few essential guidelines.

You may now be burning with enthusiasm and ready to race out the door, but please resist the urge if you are seriously unfit, very overweight, over the age of 40, or have any medical conditions including heart disease, obesity, high blood pressure or cholesterol, or if you're a cigarette smoker. If this is you, it's very important to visit your doctor for a thorough check-up before starting your exercise programme.

For everyone else, there's no time like the present to start exercising. Always make time for a pre-exercise warm-up and stretch routine, and a post-exercise cool-down (gradually slowing down the pace of activity) and stretch. Most important of all, remember to start out slowly and listen to what your body is telling you.

More great reasons to sweat regularly

Weight regulation

Everyone knows that aerobic exercise benefits the heart and lungs, but there are a multitude of other great reasons for getting active. We live in an era of the 'telly-tubbies'. Take a good look next time you're walking through the mall, or dining in the food hall, and you'll be amazed at how many seriously overweight New Zealanders you see. While the typical Western diet leaves a great deal to be desired, one of the most significant reasons for the obesity epidemic is our resistance to exercise and the sedentary ways that have become the modern norm.

Some degree of weight gain with ageing has always been common, but the phenomenon of childhood obesity is a modern one. Studies indicate that childhood obesity is more a result of lack of exercise than of overeating, and a high percentage of adult obesity tracks back to weight gain starting in childhood. If you are a parent, there is no greater motivation to begin a personal exercise programme than the awareness that your children take their lead from watching your habits and behaviour. If you live with 'telly-tubby' ways, you encourage your children to do the same, and the health consequences for them can be enormous. In addition to the social difficulties and emotional impact of living as an overweight child, obese children also face a hugely increased risk of developing type-two diabetes.

Maintaining a healthy weight, or losing weight if needed, is not really rocket science. It's simply a case of balancing energy in with energy out. If you eat more kilojoules than you burn, the excess will gradually build up into a spare tyre slung around your once svelte waistline.

Not only does aerobic exercise burn up kilojoules, it also does a great deal more to aid weight regulation. Cutting back on your kilojoule intake without exercising may lead to some initial rapid weight loss, but it quickly leads to a decline in your basal metabolic rate (BMR) (that is, how efficiently your body burns energy). That means that you need fewer and fewer kilojoules for your body to perform its basic housekeeping duties, and therefore you can maintain your weight on a lower kilojoule intake. This phenomenon accounts for the plateaus that occur when you're on a weight-loss diet. Regular aerobic and weight-bearing exercise helps to prevent this diet-induced decline in BMR, and thus helps to maintain weight loss. In fact, exercise actually boosts the BMR, not just during the exercise itself, but for an hour or two afterwards. Doing aerobic exercise along with strength training while dieting also helps to improve the composition of your body by reducing body fat and simultaneously increasing muscle mass — and muscles burn more energy than fat.

When it comes to keeping off excess kilos, weight-bearing exercise is as important as regular aerobic activity. Resistance training such as working out on the weight machines at the gym also boosts BMR, during the workout and for up to two hours afterwards (compared with an average of one hour after an aerobic workout). Resistance training is especially important for women over the age of 45, as it's not unusual to lose up to 250 g of muscle mass every year after this age . . . and with the loss of muscle comes a decline in BMR. Working with resistance training two or three times a week can lead to an increase in muscle mass of around a kilogram in four to six months. While the scales may say you weigh more, this extra kilogram of muscle will help you burn an extra 400 kilojoules a day. Lifting weights or using resistance machines at the gym is also a vital part of maintaining bone density as we age.

Exercise tips

* Best exercise for weight loss is moderate aerobic activity of long duration, rather than high-intensity aerobics.

* Minimal aerobic activity to induce fat loss consists of at least 30 minutes (and preferably 45 minutes) of continuous moderate-intensity activity, 4–6 times weekly.

* Optimum heart rate level for fat burning is 40–55% of your maximum heart rate.

* Perform 20–30 minutes of weights or resistance training before beginning your low-intensity aerobics to maximise fat burning.

* Most effective time for fat-burning exercise is in the morning before breakfast.

Walk away the blues

Depression is predicted to be the next great Western pandemic; and one of the most effective self-help tools for improving mood, banishing anxiety and calming the mind is regular aerobic exercise. Studies show that people who exercise regularly have higher self-esteem and are happier than non-exercisers, regardless of their body shape. Aerobic activity stimulates natural mood-elevating substances in the brain, called endorphins. The January 2005 *American Journal of Preventative Medicine* looked at adults aged 20–45 suffering from mild to moderate depression. They found that those who exercised aerobically for 30 minutes, three to five times a week, reduced their symptoms by half.

Studies published in the *Archives of Internal Medicine* in 1999 and 2000 compared the effects of regular exercise with those of using antidepressants in older adults suffering from major depression. Patients were divided into three groups. One group simply exercised aerobically for 30 minutes, three times a week. Another group received the antidepressant Zoloft and exercised, and the third group received the antidepressant but did not exercise. Surprisingly, the group which did exercise without taking an antidepressant showed the greatest decrease in symptoms of depression! There are many other studies demonstrating the same antidepressant effect of aerobic exercise. Resistance training, while beneficial in other ways, does not demonstrate the same mood-boosting benefits as aerobic activity.

For women only

As a woman, no matter what your age, condition, or state of fitness, exercise is an important part of your self-help health care. You can safely exercise throughout pregnancy, during the postnatal period, throughout the menopausal years and at any other stage of your life cycle. Regular exercise helps to balance female hormones; decrease PMS symptoms such as irritability, anxiety and depression; relieve period pain; decrease or eliminate many of the common minor health problems of pregnancy including constipation, varicose veins, haemorrhoids, excessive weight gain, and backache; reduce the severity of hot flushes during menopause; and prevent the chronic bone degeneration of osteoporosis.

If you are playing a vigorous sport like tennis or squash, or jogging, invest in a good-quality sports bra, designed to provide additional breast support. This will help prevent sagging or stretching of the delicate breast tissue during exercise. Cotton underpants are also a good idea to help prevent any proliferation of vaginal yeast which thrives in hot, damp environments.

Pregnancy and fitness

The days of being cosseted and fussed over during pregnancy are long gone. Those days of strict instructions to 'rest and take it easy' have been replaced with a general acknowledgment that exercise during pregnancy is as important as at any other time of life.

Some research suggests that women who exercise regularly throughout pregnancy have easier deliveries, with fewer complications and shorter labours. The incidence of problems during the actual pregnancy, in particular toxaemia, is also considerably lower for fit women. While pregnancy is a perfectly normal and healthy state, there are considerable extra demands placed upon you — demands that will be more easily met by a fit and supple body. Even a healthy pregnancy results in considerable weight gain, which itself places added strain on the lower back and abdomen. Ligaments soften and stretch under the influence of pregnancy hormones, contributing to the problem of backache. The volume of blood coursing through the veins is also greatly increased, causing your heart to work harder and beat faster, even at rest. On the birth day itself, there will be some real work to do (it's not called labour for nothing), and fitness may really come into play.

When it comes to exercising during pregnancy, common sense

is important. Choose a form of exercise appropriate to your new body shape and changed condition. Contact sports are absolutely out, as are any other forms of exercise which increase the risk of falling or hurting the abdomen. High-impact sports such as jogging are also not a good idea unless you are already an avid runner prior to pregnancy, in which case you can continue to run for as long as you can comfortably manage it. If you were unfit prior to pregnancy and want to change your ways, by all means start exercising gently and slowly, but listen to your body at all times. If you get excessively breathless, faint, or notice an

The 'do's' and 'don'ts' of exercising during pregnancy

Don'ts

* Avoid any exercise which causes excessive heating, since the increase in your core temperature could potentially cause foetal harm. During the summer, avoid exercising during the heat of the day. Instead get active in the early morning and evening. When exercising indoors, use a fan to keep your temperature down.

* Never use a sauna during pregnancy.

* Never perform aerobic activity to the point where you are unable to talk comfortably while exercising. If you can't carry on a normal conversation, you are placing an excessive load on your cardiovascular system.

* Avoid contact sports or any activity in which there is a risk of falling.

* Avoid exercise which places a strain on the lower back, or overstretches the abdominal muscles. An example of this type of exercise is sit-ups with legs straight out in front

increase in contractions it's a clear sign to slow down and take things more easily.

As the pregnant abdomen begins to swell significantly, it is often more comfortable to do non-weight-bearing exercise (such as swimming, water aerobics or stationary cycling).

Precious pelvic floors

The pelvic floor muscles are out of sight, and consequently out of mind. That's why pelvic floor repair in middle-aged women is one of the most frequently performed gynaecological surgeries.

of you (in fact, don't do these at any time, not just during pregnancy).

* After 3 months of pregnancy, avoid exercises where you lie flat on your back for lengthy periods, as the growing weight of the uterus can interfere with blood circulation.

Do's

* Design an exercise programme which involves aerobic activity to increase or maintain your fitness level, cardiovascular health and oxygen uptake. Also include some stretching exercises to increase flexibility and reduce backache in the lower back.

* Start every exercise session with a 10-minute warm-up such as gentle walking, followed by gentle stretches.

* End every exercise session with a gentle cool-down (such as slow walking) followed by 5–10 minutes of stretching.

This sheath of muscle supports all of the lower abdominal organs (especially the uterus and bladder), and keeps them firmly where they belong. When these rarely exercised muscles begin to weaken and sag, uterine and bladder prolapses occur.

Stress incontinence is an early sign of pelvic floor weakness. If you wet your pants when you sneeze, cough or laugh hard, then you are suffering from stress incontinence . . . and you need to start exercising your pelvic floor muscles today!

The specific exercises designed to strengthen and tone these muscles are named after a Los Angeles surgeon by the name of Kegel. Before you can start to exercise these hidden muscles, you first need to find them. The easiest way to do this is when you're urinating. The next time you pass water, try stopping the flow in mid-stream by tightening your pelvic muscles. By the way, if you can't completely stop the flow, it's another sign of lax pelvic floor muscles.

So now that you know where the muscles are, how do you do the exercises? Imagine that your pelvic floor is like the lift in a tall building. Start with the lift at the bottom floor (pelvic floor muscles are totally relaxed) and then gradually draw the elevator up through the building by gradually tightening the pelvic floor muscles. Move the lift slowly, floor by floor, by increasing the muscle contraction gradually. Between each incremental increase in tension, hold the current contraction for 5 seconds, before increasing it to the next 'floor', where you once again hold the contraction for 5 seconds.

Once you have tightened your muscles to their maximum, repeat the whole process in reverse, gradually relaxing the pelvic floor muscles floor by floor, until they are completely relaxed again. Try to repeat these exercises in sets of 5, with about 10 repetitions a day (making a total of 50 exercises a day). As in the case of any other muscles in the body, it will take time and patience to strengthen the pelvic floor and gradually work up to comfortably performing these 50 repetitions a day.

Unlike other forms of exercise which are easy to make excuses

Benefits of regular exercise

Heart

- Strengthens heart function and lowers resting pulse rate.
- Lowers blood pressure.
- Decreases 'bad' LDL cholesterol and triglycerides while increasing heart-friendly HDL cholesterol.
- Increases oxygenation of every cell in the body.

Mind

- Elevates mood and helps prevent or treat depression.
- Reduces anxiety and raises self-esteem.
- Induces feelings of relaxation and well-being.
- Helps regulate sleep patterns and prevent insomnia.
- Relieves symptoms of pre-menstrual syndrome.

Weight

- Burns kilojoules during and after exercise.
- Increases basal metabolic rate.
- Reduces fat and increases muscle mass.

Other

- Builds strength, flexibility and bone density.
- Improves immune function.
- Reduces risk of some cancers, including breast and colon cancer.
- Normalises blood-sugar levels and reduces risk of hypoglycaemia or diabetes.

to get out of . . . for this type of exercise there are none! You don't need to find extra time in an already busy schedule, because they can be done any time, anywhere. Try linking this exercise time to something you do every day such as driving the car, watching television, or peeling the vegetables. Exercise away, and no one will be any the wiser.

Chapter 4

Body/mind connection

This thing called stress

> Stress is basically a disconnection from the earth, a forgetting of the breath.
>
> Stress is an ignorant state. It believes that everything is an emergency. Nothing is that important. Just lie down.
>
> Natalie Goldberg

Missing the bus in the morning; locking the keys in the car; having a fight with your partner; worrying about the unpaid bills . . . these are a few of the many potentially stressful situations we face in a typical day. Humans have always had some form of stress to deal with, but modern living has changed our stress parameters substantially from the days of prehistoric living. Back then most of our stresses were short, sharp, sudden and life-threatening. Faced with the prospect of becoming the prey of some carnivore, and the consequent grizzly death, prehistoric man relied on the life-saving heightened awareness and speed conferred by the body's stress response. Primed for action by the body's 'fight-or-flight' response, he or she was able to act out the final resolution of the stress response by either fighting the threat, or running away from it. Either action allowed the body to break down the potent cocktail of stress hormones circulating through the bloodstream, thus shutting down the myriad of physiological changes triggered by stress. Recovery, and a return to a state of balance or homoeostasis, then quickly followed.

Fast-forward to the twenty-first century and the once positive, potentially life-saving benefits of the 'fight-or-flight' response have turned against us and are now an underlying cause of stress-related illness. Constrained by the behavioural expectations of our society, it is often impossible to either fight or flee a perceived threat. For example, in the workplace we may be pushed to the brink as a result of unreasonable deadlines, overwork, excessive responsibility and unsympathetic superiors, and yet the opportunity to either punch someone on the nose (fight), or storm out of the office never to return (flee) is usually denied. Add to this common scenario relationship issues, or financial and time stresses, and it's easy to see how we can be left in a state of almost constant stress arousal by a succession of ongoing 'threats', with little or no opportunity to restore our internal balance before the next onslaught.

Acute bursts of stress trigger the well-known 'fight-or-flight' response, with an outpouring of the stress hormones adrenalin and noradrenalin from the adrenal medulla. In preparation for fighting the sabre-toothed tiger (or, more sensibly, running away from it), blood vessels constrict, heart rate and blood pressure increase, cholesterol and blood-sugar levels rise, and blood becomes stickier in preparation for rapid clotting in the case of an imminent injury or wound. Once the danger has passed, all these changes rapidly revert to normal.

These body changes are perfect for giving us the best possible chance to survive isolated, acute, life-threatening stresses. They are not so perfect for the more common modern-day scenarios. Today our stress is more likely to be chronic, low-grade psychological stress, leading to very different physiological consequences. Unlike our ancestors, we cannot fight back by running from or fighting with the source of our stress. Instead, we live constrained, frustrated lives marked by emotional and physical suppression, with nervous and cardiovascular systems left in a chronic state of over-preparedness for attack. In these chronically stressful situations the adrenal cortex (the outer part of the adrenal glands) pours cortisol into the bloodstream. Over time, elevated cortisol levels cause the arteries to harden and clog. Living with a constantly heightened sense of vigilance increases our likelihood of heart attack, arrhythmia (irregular heart beat) and sudden death.

The heightened state of sensory arousal which characterises the stress response only occurs at the onset of stress. When we live with chronic stress, the state of hyperarousal gradually shifts into a condition of chronic exhaustion. At its extreme, the exhaustion becomes 'burnout' and is accompanied by a multitude of seemingly unrelated symptoms — including depression, insomnia, mood swings, irritability, poor libido, back pain, and digestive and cardiovascular problems.

Workplace stress is an issue for many people and is implicated as a root cause of many mental, emotional and physical ailments. Employees who have a high degree of responsibility, but little control over their work, are at a significantly increased risk of heart disease and hypertension. Stress is known to increase the risk of developing back and upper-body muscular-skeletal disorders including carpal tunnel syndrome. Several studies suggest that differences in rates of burnout, depression, suicide and other mental disorders for various occupations are partly due to different levels of job stress. Some studies suggest there may be a relationship between stressful working conditions and reduced immune-system resistance to infections and to viral-linked disorders like cancer.

If workplace stress (or any other kind of stress) is an issue for you, how do you protect yourself from the inevitable destructive effects of long-term or intense stress? There are no simple answers, and a truly effective strategy is complex, involving a combination of attitudinal change, environmental change, and lifestyle management to increase your physical and emotional resilience.

Of course it makes sense to modify as many external stressors as possible. However, what is often overlooked by focusing on the external stressors is that stress is an 'inside job' — an internal response to an external cue. Stress is not what happens to someone: these outside forces are the stressors. The stress is generated by how a person perceives and reacts to those outside forces. Given that the pace of modern life is inherently stressful, simply putting in place strategies of avoidance is not the answer. The secret to reducing the impact of stressors is to shift the focus from the outside chaos and turmoil to the inner world, dwelling instead on altering the perceptions of the mind, and thus altering the biology of your body. Stressors will always be present. By focusing on understanding the way in which our body reacts to these outside stressors, and on learning new psychological skills, it is possible to enhance our body's ability to stay in a state of homoeostasis, or balance, despite the outside turmoil. The mind and body are inextricably linked, and their second-by-second interaction literally creates our internal biological soup. Our thoughts and the resulting physical responses support good health or lead to physical breakdown, depending on their nature. Our attitudes, beliefs, and emotional states — be they love and compassion or fear and anger — trigger biochemical chain reactions that affect our blood chemistry, heart rate, and the activity of every cell and organ system in our body.

Our psychology influences our stress response. There are some psychological characteristics which increase stress hardiness and reduce the development of physical illness associated with stress. Studies looking at executives running top companies have identified several personality characteristics in those executives who remained healthy in the face of ongoing stress. One trait is the ability to respond to challenge with excitement and energy.

Such people look at new situations as opportunities to learn, grow, and develop personally. Another characteristic is having a commitment to something they feel is meaningful, be it their work, their community, their family, a charity, and so on. The third, and critical characteristic, is a sense of being in control, of being able to make decisions that make a difference and make things happen.

Conversely, there are other mental traits which increase vulnerability to stress. Remember that stress lies in the eye of the beholder, rather than in an external event itself, and that what we think and feel causes immediate biological changes that increase the sensation of 'being stressed'. Mental characteristics which aggravate our tendency to feel stressed include: negative mental processes such as 'deficiency focusing' — the habit of always focusing on the negative instead of on the positive. Usually this is accompanied by a mindset which anticipates and expects difficulties and problems. Another mental characteristic which exacerbates stress is the habit of negative self-talk. People with this characteristic bombard themselves with internal messages of failure and low self-esteem, such as 'I always mess up'; 'I'm not good enough to do that'; 'they won't pick me, of course'. When these negative records play endlessly in your brain, they actually have the power to trigger a stress response, causing a release of adrenalin and cortisol, and eventually leading to the development of stress-related illness. Negative self-talkers often have an associated tendency of low skill recognition. They have low perception of their own abilities, and underplay the role of their abilities in their success — instead attributing everything positive to an external factor such as luck or another person.

> Nobody can go back and start a new beginning, but anyone can start today and make a new ending.
>
> Maria Robinson

It's time to relax

The body/mind connection is now indisputable and we no longer believe the autonomic nervous system to be an 'automatic' nervous system. In the late 1960s, researchers at the Harvard Medical School discovered a phenomenon they labelled the 'relaxation response'. By studying Transcendental Meditation (TM) meditators, they found that the simple act of sitting quietly and giving the mind a focus decreased the metabolic rate, slowed the heart rate, decreased the breathing rate, and produced significant changes in brain waves. Since that time, more than 100 studies have verified that relaxation and meditation can lower blood pressure. Biofeedback studies have demonstrated numerous ways in which the mind can be used to influence the working of the autonomic nervous system. Through relaxation and mental focus, subjects have been able to perform very specific tasks such as raising the temperature of one finger, or the temperature of one small square of skin on the back by imagining a candle flame at the spot. People who regularly induce the relaxation response through meditation reduce their body's responsiveness to stress hormones at all times, not just while meditating. In meditators it takes a stronger stress reaction to bring about an increase in blood pressure and heart rate.

Learning the relaxation response

You don't have to learn a complicated or difficult meditation technique to teach your body how to readily slip into a state of deep relaxation. There are a number of simple methods for perfecting the relaxation response if you're willing to practise daily (and ideally twice daily) for at least 20 minutes. Once you can induce your own relaxation response regularly you will notice a number of benefits, including: increased body awareness; an ability to relax even in the midst of high-stress situations; a generalised feeling of being more relaxed most of the time; improved concentration; and a generally greater sense of well-being.

✳ Pick a focus word or short phrase, which has personal meaning to you. For example, a non-religious person may pick a word like 'peace', or 'love', while a Christian may pick a short Bible verse.

✳ Sit quietly in a comfortable position. Don't lie down, as it is too easy to fall asleep.

✳ Close your eyes and relax your muscles.

✳ Breathe slowly and naturally, repeating your focus word or phrase silently as you exhale.

✳ Throughout the process, try to stay passive and 'non-attached' to the outcome. Don't focus or worry about how well you're doing. Simply observe any distracting thoughts you have, and gently return your attention to your focus word.

✳ Continue the process for 10–20 minutes. When you have finished, sit quietly for a couple of minutes before returning to full consciousness.

To maximise your results, it is important to practise regularly, setting aside time at the same time each day. Setting the alarm clock 20 minutes earlier than usual and starting the day with a relaxation exercise will improve your ability to cope with stressful situations in the day ahead. Pay attention to some basic comforts. Don't try to practise your relaxation when you are either excessively full, or hungry. Keep the room well ventilated and heated to a comfortable temperature. Make sure you won't be disturbed by a telephone.

The breath of life

It is impossible to perfect the art of relaxation without first learning how to breathe properly. Most people who are chronically stressed inadvertently develop a very poor breathing technique, which itself contributes to further feelings of anxiety, stress and panic. When we are stressed, our breathing tends to become rapid and shallow, and we utilise only the upper part of the chest, rather than breathing deeply into the diaphragm. Often, stressed breathers begin to gulp air through their mouth instead of breathing through the nose. This type of 'over-breathing' or hyperventilation increases blood-histamine levels, causing sweaty palms and a red, flushed face. Chronic hyperventilators can develop a wide range of debilitating symptoms which can easily be mistaken for serious diseases. Common symptoms include: body aches, pains and stiffness; cardiovascular and respiratory symptoms such as a racing heart, chest pain or tightness, feelings of 'air hunger' and an inability to take a full, deep breath; palpitations; poor sleep; dreaming; chronic exhaustion.

If you recognise yourself in this description, I would advise you to consult a breathing specialist to get help. Serious hyperventilators need assistance in retraining their breathing mechanism. For less-serious breathing problems, self-help is often effective. I recommend you read Dinah Bradley's book, *Hyperventilation Syndrome*, and practise the exercises regularly.

So just how do we breathe properly? It's easier to learn how to breath properly lying down. Lie on the floor with a pillow under your head, and another under your knees. Place your hand lightly over your diaphragm (the area in the centre of the abdomen just below your breastbone). With your lips lightly together, breathe in slowly through your nose, imagining the air going down to your stomach, not your lungs. Once your lungs are comfortably filled, let go straight away and allow the air to be expelled, gently and naturally. You should feel your hand gently dropping back down towards your spine. Focus on natural breaths, rather than large gulping inhales and forceful exhales. The ideal breathing rate is around 12 breaths per minute.

And it's back to exercise . . .

One of the most effective and beneficial ways of managing stress in the long term is to exercise daily. Regular exercise — whether it's a brisk walk around the block, a visit to the gym, or vigorous gardening — will reduce anxiety, improve your mood, and increase your resistance to depression, as well as strengthening your cardiovascular health. Exercise helps improve self-esteem, as well as releasing endorphins, brain chemicals that trigger positive feelings of well-being. Aerobic exercise also allows the body to rid itself of 'fight-or-flight' hormones, such as adrenalin and cortisol, more quickly, reducing the physical and emotional repercussions of chronic stress.

Is your glass half full or half empty?

The optimist sees the rose and not its thorns;
the pessimist stares at the thorns,
oblivious to the rose.

Kahlil Gibran

One of our most powerful self-help tools for staying well is as simple (and as difficult) as attitudinal change. Life will always find ways of challenging us, but how we view those difficulties has a direct influence on our emotional and physical well-being. Positive, optimistic and cheerful people are not only more pleasant to be around, they are unwittingly practising their own powerful form of preventative medicine.

Studies show that having a positive attitude to life pays off. Optimists do better in school, in their careers, and in their personal lives than do pessimists. They suffer from fewer depression and anxiety disorders, and are more likely to take care of themselves by eating healthy diets, exercising and getting regular physical check-ups, compared with their more pessimistic peers. A positive attitude is also kind to our cardiovascular health, with optimists experiencing a 50% reduction in cardiovascular disease risk irrespective of age, race or sex (thought to be a result of their reduced production of stress hormones).

When an optimist does get sick, he or she recovers more quickly than a pessimist. A study found that heart-bypass patients who were more upbeat recovered faster from surgery and felt better at a five-year follow-up than pessimists who had had the same operation. A 2001 report in the *Canadian Medical Association Journal* reported on a review of 16 studies published between 1966 and 1998 that addressed the relationship between patient expectation after surgery, and their recovery. Fifteen of the studies showed that when patients had a positive expectation about their recovery from surgery, they recovered more quickly, even when psychological and social factors were taken into consideration.

Those with a gloomy or hostile outlook on life, who are constantly fretting, waiting for the 'inevitable' disaster to happen, have an increased risk of developing depression and anxiety. They also are more likely to perform poorly at school or work. Pessimism not only makes life a misery, but it may directly contribute to early death. A negative outlook can shorten life expectancy, and when accompanied by feelings of hostility (especially aggression and cynicism towards others), it increases the risk of developing heart disease.

The link between mind and body has long been contemplated but few long-term studies have closely examined the association. An exception is a study carried out at the Mayo Clinic, during which the medical histories of 839 people were tracked for 30 years. Each participant had completed standard personality tests as adults between 1962 and 1965. Of the participants, 124 were classified as optimists, 197 as pessimists, and 518 fell somewhere in between. Results showed that the participants whose test scores reflected high degrees of pessimism were significantly associated with a higher-than-expected mortality rate compared with the optimists or 'middle-of-the-road' types.

Paradoxically, some of the greatest optimists are people who seemingly have the most to feel depressed about. Conversely, those who appear to 'have it all', focus on what they perceive to be lacking in their lives. Whether we see the glass as half full or half empty is not simply determined by our life circumstances. Genes play a role too. In 1996 scientists announced that they had located genes linked to anxiety, addiction, happiness and pessimism. None of us can use genetic inheritance as an excuse for an unappealing character, for while part of your personality may be inherited, genetic disposition is estimated to account for only 50% of our pessimistic or optimistic make-up.

Life constantly bombards us with challenges, but how we see our world in the face of such challenges partly comes down to choice. Genetics aside, through applying some simple mental techniques it is possible to gradually change your outlook to one of increased positivity and optimism, and to reap the rewards of improved physical health and well-being.

Changing thinking patterns first demands of us an increase in consciousness and awareness of the endless self-talk that pervades our every waking moment. For most of us, the constant chatter of the undisciplined mind rolls on like a stuck CD, much of it in the realm of the subconscious. If we want to change our thinking, we first need to become aware of just what we are thinking. It can help to use a notebook as a 'thought log', and start recording what you are thinking and feeling when faced with a challenge. After a while, clear patterns emerge. In particular, look for recurring negative themes such as blame, guilt, anger, pessimism or despair.

After a few weeks of logging your reactions, apply some cold, hard logic to your observations. Challenge the validity of your own thoughts. Ask yourself if your reactions are true and reasonable, and what proof exists to support the validity of your thoughts.

When your constant self-chatter becomes conscious you may well be surprised at how much self-condemnation you indulge in . . . 'I should have known I'd get it wrong, I always do.' 'Of course I didn't get the job, who would bother with me?' That being the case, make a conscious decision to treat yourself with the same patience and support that you would offer to a close friend in times of trouble.

'Reframing' means looking for the silver lining in any situation which initially appears to be negative. Reframing means learning a new way of looking at things. When a friend doesn't return your call for days on end, entertain the possibility that he or she didn't get your message, or has been working back-to-back shifts, or is out of town, instead of assuming that you are being snubbed. Look at criticism as feedback which will afford you the opportunity of improving something.

Try looking at life's inevitable and inescapable challenges as opportunities to find out something new and positive about yourself. Researchers at the University of California asked 2000 people about the worst times in their lives (divorce, job loss, combat, and so on). Surprisingly, they found that even through these times of maximum adversity most people were able to salvage something positive from their experience. It may have been a realisation of how much strength they had; what wonderful friends and human resources they had; even of a renewed and strengthened faith in God. Most thought, in retrospect, that their harrowing experiences had made them better able to cope with other problems and challenges in life. In other words, they 'reframed' trauma into a more positive experience.

There are some simple ways of changing your attitude to challenges, almost immediately. Start by shifting the focus of your attention. It is always easier to pay more attention to the annoying, difficult or challenging aspects of your life. It's amazing how profoundly your experience of life can change by consciously focusing instead on those areas that bring you happiness. Make a list of all the positive, joyful things in your life, and when optimism has deserted you, read and reread your list. Another powerful way of 'reframing' is to end each day by recording five different events, moments or observations of the day which have brought you happiness.

Set some boundaries and carve out regular time just for yourself. In our frantic-paced world of 24-hour-a-day demands, it is easy to lose touch with who you are and what is important in your life. Give yourself the gift of a half-hour several times a week, spent totally alone with your thoughts. Resist the temptation to worry about work or the bills, and instead practise some kind of relaxation which allows you to step back from the annoying minutiae and contemplate the bigger picture. Constant busyness takes away the opportunity to assess where you're going and where you've come from . . . and to feel grateful for where you are right here and now.

> Your living is determined not so much by what life brings to you, as by the attitude you bring to life; not so much by what happens to you as by the way your mind looks at what happens to you.
>
> Kahlil Gibran

Body/mind and a healthy heart

Numerous studies now substantiate the long-held holistic belief that mental, emotional and spiritual well-being are vital components of physical health. While Western medical practice remains slow to integrate this perspective of well-being, traditional healing methods such as Chinese and ayurvedic medicine have observed this profound body/mind connection for millennia. Traditional Chinese medicine speaks of the heart as the home of the 'shen' or spirit. A disturbed shen often leads to physical manifestations of heart problems such as palpitations and chest pain. Similarly, physical heart problems can disturb the shen (mind or spirit). What disturbs the shen in the first place? In a word, emotion — especially excessive sadness, joy (mania), and anger.

Nearly 3000 years after the advent of traditional Chinese medicine, science is verifying the link between psychosocial imbalances and heart disease. According to a comprehensive international study reported in the *Lancet* in 2004, psychosocial factors (such as mental and emotional disharmony, chronic stress and a lack of social support) are just as important cardiovascular risk factors as smoking, high blood pressure, obesity and cholesterol problems.

So how do feelings of chronic anger, sadness, depression, or anxiety adversely affect our heart health? The body and mind are inextricably linked, and 'negative' emotions, thoughts and feelings, literally change the chemistry of the physical body. Such emotions increase blood pressure and levels of LDL (bad) cholesterol; constrict the arteries; and increase the stickiness of the blood.

Tests on accountants show that they experience significant elevations in cholesterol levels during tax time. Tertiary students told that they had failed an exam experience the same immediate

Self-help heart healing

* Be honest about your emotional state, and address any unresolved emotional issues such as anger, resentment and lack of forgiveness for past grievances.

* Remember that forgiveness is a gift to yourself, not to the person you are forgiving, and that holding on to old hurts simply gives more power to the perpetrator.

* Use journaling, visualisation, meditation and psychotherapy (if needed) to help resolve and release emotional baggage.

* Become more assertive and express your emotions freely. Speak out when you feel wronged or hurt by someone . . . but not in an angry or blaming way!

* Cry, cry and cry again to release 'stuck' emotion. Take an afternoon in front of the television and watch sad movies to get the tears flowing if you can't do it any other way.

* When all the crying is done, try laughter therapy. Laughter is a profoundly powerful medicine, which produces

changes in cholesterol levels. The good news is that feelings of love and connectedness produce similarly significant changes in blood cholesterol, only this time in a positive direction.

It's not just stress which increases the risk of heart disease. Specific emotional states such as anger, anxiety, sadness and depression also produce biochemical changes with potentially damaging effect. Researchers from the HeartMath Institute in California have shown that feelings of anger, frustration or insecurity change the rhythms of our heartbeat, making them more chaotic and erratic. Conversely, positive, heartfelt emotions such as love, compassion, care and appreciation all produce a smoother, more harmonious heart rhythm.

biochemical changes beneficial to the heart and immune system. This time watch some funny movies.

* Make love lovingly and often. Feelings of love, compassion and nurturing lower blood pressure, regulate the heartbeat and burn up stress hormones in the bloodstream.

* Love your pets and stroke and cuddle them frequently, to diffuse stress hormones and lower blood pressure.

* Change your focus of attention to one of gratitude. Instead of moaning about all the things that are wrong in your world, make a conscious effort to dwell on all the blessings instead. Start a gratitude diary and take a moment each night to write down five different things that you are grateful for in the day that has passed.

* Reach out to others who need help. Whether you do charity work, or simply help out a neighbour or friend in need, living a life of compassionate caring produces significant health benefits for the heart.

There is little evidence that anger can cause heart disease by itself, but once there is existing heart disease, having an angry disposition can hasten your demise. Hot-headed personalities who regularly 'blow their top' increase their cardiovascular risk profile — but so, too, do those angry individuals who seemingly effectively suppress and bottle up their anger. Anger-suppressors who have had a previous heart attack are 30% more likely to die

Fight or flight

Whenever your mind interprets a situation as stressful and potentially dangerous, a powerful physiological process, called the 'fight-or-flight' response, is triggered.

* The stress hormone adrenalin is pumped into the blood from the adrenal glands, to sharpen senses and give you 'super-hero' qualities of speed or strength.

* Unnecessary physiological processes are slowed or stopped. These include digestion, growth, tissue repair and healing.

* Cardiovascular changes give you strength to run or to fight. Heart rate increases; blood pressure increases; blood flow is redirected away from extremities; blood thickens to shorten clotting time in the event of an injury.

* Pupils dilate and hearing becomes more acute.

These adaptations are all designed to help you survive in situations of acute stress such as when you are in life-threatening danger. In the modern world of chronic, ongoing stress, these fight-or-flight responses can become chronic, and contribute to the development of stress-related cardiovascular disease, diabetes, and mental and emotional illness.

of a heart attack in the following 6–10 years, compared with non-suppressors, regardless of other biological factors. Hot-headed explosions and tight-lipped repression both cause biochemical changes detrimental to the cardiovascular system. The only way to mitigate the detrimental effects of anger is to address the underlying core issues feeding the anger.

Depression is one of the most serious and rapidly escalating epidemics of modern time. Prescriptions for antidepressants continue to soar year after year, with increasingly younger sufferers. While depression is itself a debilitating illness, it may also be

Some common symptoms of excessive stress

Anxiety

Hostility and anger

Irritability and resentment

Irrational fears or phobias

Obsessive, repetitive thoughts

Muscle tension, especially in shoulders, neck, chest and jaws

Headaches, backaches and neck aches

High blood pressure, chest pain or palpitations

Indigestion, excessive gas, abnormally large or small appetite

Chronic constipation or diarrhoea

Tics or tremors

Difficulty getting to sleep, restless sleeping and early waking

Physical weakness and exhaustion

Low or no interest in sex

Menstrual irregularities

Dependence on caffeine, cigarettes or alcohol to help you cope with life.

playing a significant role in feeding the cardiovascular epidemic. Depressed people are more prone to coronary artery disease and heart attacks. If they have a heart attack, people suffering from depression tend to have worse outcomes, and are more likely to die in the aftermath than are their happy peers under similar circumstances. A study by the Duke University Medical Centre followed a group of 700 Danish men and women for a 27-year

Traditional Chinese medicine and the body/mind connection

Two-and-a-half thousand years ago, practitioners of traditional Chinese medicine understood the profound connection between our emotional state and our physical well-being. Emotions are a normal, natural part of the human life experience and they only become a cause of disease when they are very intense, or when they are experienced 'chronically' over a long period of time . . . especially when they are suppressed or driven inwards instead of being expressed in a healthy way. Traditional Chinese medicine views the body/mind connection as working in both directions. While emotion can cause physical imbalance, a physical disharmony can also lead to emotional problems.

The seven emotions of traditional Chinese medicine
Anger — repressed emotion, frustration, resentment, irritability
Chronic anger detrimentally affects the liver organ and meridian, leading to hormonal imbalance, fatigue, headaches, digestive disorders, eye problems, and muscle and tendon problems.

Joy — mania and hyper-excitability
Chronic excitability and mania detrimentally affect the heart organ and meridian, leading to palpitations, insomnia, dream-disturbed sleep, restlessness, and agitation.

period. All the subjects performed a psychological test at the start of the study and again after 10 years. Those whose scores reflected despair, low self-esteem, difficulties in concentrating and low motivation had a 70% greater risk of heart attack and a 60% higher risk of dying than those who did not describe themselves in these terms.

Living a heart-healthy life involves much more than eating a

Sadness — grief, sadness, depression
Chronic sadness detrimentally affects the lungs and the heart. Sadness leads to a deficiency of lung qi (vital force) and results in asthma, breathlessness, a tendency to bronchitis, fatigue, depression and crying.

Worry and pensiveness — anxiety, excessive thinking or studying
Chronic worry weakens the spleen organ and meridian and leads to fatigue, poor appetite, abdominal bloating, loose stools, prolapses, and varicose veins.

Fear — terror, chronic anxiety
Chronic fear weakens the kidney organ and meridian leading to bladder problems, fatigue, dark rings under the eyes, premature ageing, palpitations, night sweats.

Shock
A severe and sudden shock detrimentally affects both the kidney and heart organs and meridians and leads to palpitations, breathlessness and insomnia.

Note that sadness and grief are sometimes considered separate emotions, thus making seven emotions.

great diet, exercising regularly and throwing away the cigarettes. Emotional and spiritual well-being is the third, vital, element for cardiovascular health. Unresolved emotional issues such as anger, resentment and lack of forgiveness will exact a silent but profound toll on your heart.

The power of forgiveness

The weak can never forgive, forgiveness
is the attribute of the strong.

Mahatma Gandhi

Holding on to bitterness, anger and resentment resulting from memories of a wrongdoing against you not only makes you miserable and exhausted, but also translates into biochemical changes within your body that adversely affect your physical health. Negative feelings about the past smother our ability to feel peace, contentment and happiness in the present. Forgetting or suppressing painful memories is virtually impossible, and so the only way to regain inner peace is through a process of genuine forgiveness. Many people struggle with the concept of forgiveness, especially when they are left living permanently with the consequences of wrong action by another. They feel that to forgive the perpetrator is in some way tantamount to sanctioning those actions, and giving the perpetrator a gift that they don't deserve. They may feel that forgiveness is, in a sense, unjust and unwarranted. In truth, refusing to forgive someone simply gives that person the power to continue to hurt you in your daily life, long after the actual event of wrongdoing has faded into the past. Choosing to hold on to your anger and unforgiveness (and yes, it is actually a choice) bequeaths to another power and control over your peace of mind and positive experience of life. Not forgiving does not hurt the offender . . . but to you, the legacy is one of a life lived in the shadow of sadness and bitterness. In such a life there is little opportunity for gratitude, joy and inner peace to grow.

Even if you genuinely come to a place of readiness to forgive, moving to your final emotional destination of surrender and peacefulness can be a lengthy and turbulent journey. Sometimes, professional help in the form of psychotherapy or counselling may be needed to guide you along your path. Hold on to the knowledge that the final joyful destination of release from the heavy burden of unforgiveness makes the temporary challenges of the journey worth all the effort required.

Be the change you want to see in the world.

Gandhi

Chapter 5

Menopause

From the time of a woman's first menstruation until her final bleed, she is ruled by the powerful hormonal cascades which ebb and flow through her monthly cycle. Even before her first period, from the age of seven or eight, minute amounts of the powerful hormone oestrogen begin imperceptibly to orchestrate subtle body changes in preparation for menstruation. By the age of 15 most teenage girls are menstruating regularly. From menarche to menopause, the cyclical interplay of progesterone and oestrogen (and a variety of other female hormones) is a defining characteristic of female health and well-being.

After approximately 35 years of riding the cyclical hormonal roller coaster, there comes a new hormonal 'blip' to deal with — the perimenopause. The perimenopausal years encompass the five or more years leading up to the last menstrual period. This is often a time of hormonal volatility and unpredictability, and for many women these years are more symptomatic and troublesome than the true menopausal years following the last menstruation.

A baby girl is born with ovaries already filled with all the egg follicles she will ever produce. From the time of puberty until the time of menopause, around 400 of these egg follicles will ripen with the potential of fertilisation. At the same time, many thousands of other eggs are partly ripened only to be degenerated and resorbed by the body. By the age of 45 there are very few egg follicles remaining in the ovaries. Around this age, the ovaries begin to produce less and less oestrogen and progesterone. Ovulation becomes more sporadic and some months the ovaries fail to release a ripened egg, and no progesterone is produced. This leads to the common perimenopausal experience of erratic menstrual cycles with shortened, lengthened or missed periods.

Along with the obvious changes in monthly bleeding, common perimenopausal symptoms include:

* vaginal dryness or irritation
* bladder irritability
* insomnia
* fatigue
* muscle pains
* breast tenderness
* mood swings
* depression
* palpitations
* hot sweats and flushes
* night sweats
* poor memory and concentration
* dry skin.

While these symptoms have a very real physiological basis, the passage to menopause is made no easier by the general negativity surrounding ageing in our youth- and beauty-obsessed Western culture.

Everywhere we look we absorb the message that women are only desirable when they are young, 'flawless', and perfect. Our sexuality is displayed and discussed with more intensity and frankness than ever before. Periods, contraception, PMS, STDs — all get constant in-depth coverage and attention. With the advent of pharmaceutical 'solutions' to the 'problem' of menopause, this once taboo aspect of female sexuality has also become a hot topic, albeit often a distinctly negative one!

There is no denying that the menopausal years are a time of great physical and emotional change. Our mindset and attitudes towards ageing and menopause can partly influence our experience of the transition. As with every other challenge in life, we always have the power of choice and free will in determining the way forward. We can choose to accept menopause as just another life transition, and move through it with a focus on the positive . . . or we can get caught up in the media con job, and believe the ageist propaganda. The choice is ours! If you're currently going through menopausal challenges, you may be wondering what there is to find positive about menopause. What about an end to the mess, pain, inconvenience and expense of monthly periods; an end to years of worrying about unplanned pregnancies and contraceptives. What about seeing menopause as the beginning of a new era of freedom and opportunity with the years of child-rearing responsibility behind you?

Indigenous cultures around the world generally have a very different attitude to menopause and ageing of women. Cultures such as the Native American Indians, or the Chinese, see menopause in a far more positive light. Native American lore saw mid-life women as the gatherers (of wisdom), blessed with an inner ripening and maturing, along with their outer ageing. The menopausal years were seen as the time during which outer energy is redirected deep within to nurture the seeds of the heart and soul. Similarly, traditional Chinese culture (and traditional Chinese medicine today) see the menopausal years as the time during which the physical muscles may weaken, but the inner muscles of the soul (perception, wisdom and inner knowing) are strengthened.

Understanding the connection between our cultural heritage and our experience of ageing and menopause is important. Scientific research tells us that the cultural milieu in which we are 'bathed' as we go through the menopausal years actually influences our experience of menopause. In cultures such as our own, in which menopause is seen in a negative light, women are more likely to experience troublesome symptoms, compared with those cultures in which menopause is considered a gathering of life experience and wisdom.

After years of being the nurturers and carers in roles as mothers, wives and partners, we can experience menopause as a time of rebirth; a time when women finally have the time and space and freedom to pause, breathe deeply, survey all that has been, and set a course of rediscovery of themselves in the years to come. This mid-life transition may become a time to travel, take up new hobbies, focus on strengthening or forming new love relationships, study, contemplate and grow.

The mechanics of menopause

To understand the biology of menopause, it's best to start by understanding the mechanics of the menstrual cycle (see Chapter 1). The official definition of menopause is limited, referring to just the time of the last menstrual period. The months and years after the last period are officially termed the 'postmenopausal' years. While this is a working definition, in reality the changes of menopause stretch from up to 10 years before the last period to several years after the last period. These are the menopausal years.

At the time of her birth, a baby girl already has tiny ovaries, filled with the full quotient of eggs she will ever have — enough to last through the monthly ovulation cycle until some time in her forties or fifties. Besides secreting eggs every month, the ovaries produce most of the oestrogen in a premenopausal woman's body. When there are few remaining eggs left in the ovaries, the ovarian production of both oestrogen and progesterone hormone begins to decline noticeably.

Contrary to the belief of many women, menopause does

not mean a complete shut-down of oestrogen production. Post-menopausally, the ovaries and adrenal glands produce hormones which are converted into oestrogen in the fat cells on the hips and abdomen . . . yes, there is a therapeutic reason to have some fat here . . . just not too much! This is one of the reasons that plumper women often find the menopausal changes less traumatic than very thin or lean women.

As oestrogen levels decline, the body goes into overdrive in an attempt to 'kick-start' normal ovulation and menstruation. The hormone involved in stimulating the production of an egg follicle — follicle stimulating hormone, or FSH — is superboosted. By measuring FSH levels, it is possible to determine whether or not you are going through the perimenopausal years.

A traditional Chinese medicine perspective of menopause

The Chinese believe that the transition from regular menstruation to menopause is a time of strain on all the resources of the body, especially the 'qi' or life force which circulates through the energy meridians. However, this strain will only manifest as symptoms of ill health and imbalance if a woman fails to keep balance in her life, through adequate rest, contemplation, sleep, exercise and sound nutrition.

It is the kidney energy that is most vulnerable to depletion during the transition of menopause. In traditional Chinese medicine, the kidneys store the 'jing' (a type of inherited vital force) which governs the entire life cycle of birth, maturation and decline. By the age of 35–40 the prenatal jing with which a woman is born is completely depleted, and the kidney energy requires continuous replenishing and support, through 'right living'. For many Western women, this is where the problems start! Rather than acknowledging menopause as a time of energetic vulnerability, we continue to push ourselves through barriers of exhaustion, overcommitment, emotional turmoil and stress. Coupled with the fragility of kidney energy at mid-life, the typical Western lifestyle of overactivity and stress commonly leads to symptoms of kidney qi deficiency. Typically these include fatigue, hot flushes, irritability, mood swings and poor libido — all typical symptoms of menopause.

Before we get down to the nitty gritty . . .

Yes, menopause may be challenging, and there may well be uncomfortable or annoying symptoms to contend with. This is a time of profound physiological, emotional and spiritual change in your life. Staying well through the flux is possible, with some proactive steps.

Stillness without for stillness within

With annoying symptoms of perimenopause such as hot flushes, night sweats and disturbed sleep, mood disturbances are fairly common. Taking stock of life, and letting go of extraneous responsibilities or commitments, or letting go of friendships which feel more like a burden than a gift, will help to release you from externally draining circumstances.

Balance in all things

Look closely at the balance in your life. If you are exhausted, overcommited, and suffering from an overabundance of work and an undersupply of relaxation and recreation — do something about it! Make some changes to bring more balance between the energy you expend versus the nurturing, restorative pleasures you have in life. Take up a new hobby or revisit old passions which you may have let slip by the way through the years of family responsibilities. Rediscover your passions, your creativity and your artistic talents.

Let food be your medicine

Perimenopause is a time when years of poor nutrition and unwise food choices may come home to roost! Feeling blue, exhausted or regularly self-combusting is a great motivation for improving your nutrition. Balancing blood-sugar swings will also help restore mental and emotional balance (see Chapter 2). Focusing on low-GI carbohydrates, combined with protein, in small, frequent meals will prevent blood-sugar dips.

Avoid sugars and processed foods containing sugar, which will cause blood sugar to escalate rapidly, followed by just as rapid a drop. Try to include plenty of foods that are sources of phyto-oestrogens. Asian women who traditionally consume diets higher in phyto-oestrogens suffer from fewer menopausal problems such as hot flushes, sweats and vaginal thinning. Useful phyto-oestrogen-rich foods include soya products, nuts, beans, lentils, linseed, alfalfa sprouts, soya and linseed bread. (See Chapter 6 for full list.)

Joy jive

Where does your joy come from? Do you remember how it feels to be deeply and profoundly touched by life? What makes your heart sing? What are you passionate about? When was the last time you really laughed until it hurt? Menopause is a time of reawakening, rather than a decline. Find some new pleasures to explore — express yourself, maybe take up singing, dancing, acting or painting. Get in touch with unexplored creativity.

Exercise therapy

One of the most effective self-help strategies for managing your menopausal change is a regular exercise programme. If you've been a lounge lizard until now, be assured that regular sweat sessions will help to minimise a number of common menopausal health challenges, such as those listed below.

* *Increase in cholesterol levels*
With the decline in oestrogen, total cholesterol levels sometimes increase. Regular aerobic exercise elevates the level of HDL (good cholesterol), lowers triglycerides and improves total cholesterol to HDL ratio, and lowers LDL (bad cholesterol).

* *Weight gain*
On average, woman gain 5–6 kg during the menopausal years. Regular exercise will help prevent or minimise this potentially unhealthy weight gain. Strength training will boost muscle mass, thus increasing your metabolic rate and fat burning, and is important, along with aerobic exercise, for weight regulation.

* *Aerobic exercise*
Some women find that regular aerobic exercise reduces the frequency and severity of hot flushes.

* *Insomnia*
Regular exercise deepens sleep, and makes it easier to fall asleep. Fit people have fewer awakenings, and experience more delta sleep (non-dreaming sleep that promotes the greatest body recovery).

* *Mood disorders*
Exercising aerobically for 40 minutes, 4–5 times a week will help relieve mild to moderate anxiety and depression.

* *Bone loss*
Up to 20% of bone mass can be lost in the eight years following menopause. Weight-bearing activities and resistance exercise can help build and maintain bone density. The US Surgeon General states 'physical activity, through its load-bearing effect on the skeleton, is likely the single most important influence on bone density and architecture'.

Is there a fire in here?

Around 80% of menopausal women experience the joys of intense surges of sweat-inducing heat, commonly called 'hot flushes'. The first heat surge can occur during the perimenopausal years when periods may still be regular, and there may be no other signs of impending menopause. The last heat surge usually pays a visit within the two years after the last period. Women experience hot flushes differently. For some they are an almost pleasant, mild sensation of warmth which passes over the body quickly. For others they are earth-shaking torrents of fire which burn up through the body to the face, and result in drenching rivers of sweat. Sometimes they are accompanied by anxiety, nausea, or palpitations.

There is much we do not know about the cause of hot flushes. Generally it is believed they have something to do with the tiny gland in the brain known as the hypothalamus. Falling oestrogen levels irritate the neuroreceptors in the hypothalamus, which in turn sends messages to blood vessels in the skin, to dilate. As more blood flows through dilated blood vessels, the skin heats up and this is perceived as a flush. Despite the rise in the skin temperature, the body temperature is actually dropping during a flush. Perspiration evaporates from the skin, and the cooling sensation is noticed. The declining body temperature triggers the release of the stress hormone adrenalin. As adrenalin levels increase, the blood vessels constrict and the flush comes to an end. Hot flushes are often extremely severe for women who experience an 'induced' menopause following hysterectomy, with or without the removal of ovaries. Thin women, and those who don't sweat easily, also tend to experience the most severe flushing.

Drenching sweats which occur at night and wake you from your sleep are a similar phenomenon to the daytime hot flushes. Because you are sleeping, the hot flush sensations are often not noticed, and it is only when the drenching cold sweat occurs that you wake from your sleep.

There are a number of basic self-help measures which may help you cope with your hot flushes. First and foremost, stay calm and try not to panic. Although they may feel overwhelming and embarrassing, hot flushes are in no way dangerous or life-threatening. Try a little psychological 'reframing': how about thinking of them as 'power surges' rather than hot flushes. Dress for the occasion! Avoid synthetics such as acrylic and polyester, which simply trap perspiration. Choose materials that breathe, such as wool, cotton and linen, and dress in several layers so that clothing can come off and go back on a hundred times a day if needed. Use cotton sheets on the bed, and a woollen or cotton-filled duvet rather than synthetics. A fan set on 'low' focused on your side of the bed may also help you cope at night. Carry a sipper bottle of water with you at all times. Avoid foods which commonly trigger hot flushes, such as spicy foods, hot drinks (especially tea and coffee), alcohol and sugar. Try eating quality food, in small amounts and often, rather than sitting down to large meals. If you are a smoker, flushes are likely to be worse as the chemicals in cigarettes tend to constrict blood vessels and intensify flushes.

Nutritional therapy

Many women find that vitamin E and selenium reduce the frequency and intensity of flushes, as do bioflavonoids. While some women's flushes improve if they take 400 iu of vitamin E a day, others need up to 1200 iu to notice a significant improvement. Persevere, as it can take four to six weeks of consistent use of vitamin E before you notice a change in flushes. Preferably use a mixed tocopherol vitamin-E supplement (rather than simply alpha-tocopherol), starting with a dose of 400 iu a day. This is best taken after a meal containing a fat source, and not at the same time or soon before or after any iron supplement you may be taking. Gradually increase dosage to 800 iu a day over a week (you'll need to get some 200 iu capsules to increase the dose gradually). Take this dose for four weeks before deciding whether you need to increase dosage again, up to 1200 iu a day. If you do need to increase again, once your flushes have been under control for several weeks, try experimenting with cutting down on your intake to find the minimum dose of vitamin E to effectively keep your flushes at bay. If you are diabetic, taking blood-thinning medication, have a blood-clotting problem or have high blood pressure, consult your health professional before using any supplemental vitamin E in doses higher than 400 iu a day. Small doses of selenium in the range of 100–150 mcg a day will help the body utilise vitamin E, as well as offering a myriad of powerful antioxidant properties (see selenium in Chapter 2 and Chapter 6).

Bioflavonoids occur naturally in a wide variety of fruits and vegetables, especially citrus fruit, apricots, cherries, grapes and plums. Bioflavonoids greatly enhance the absorption and utilisation of vitamin C, as well as strengthening the walls of the blood capillaries. Taken as a supplement (containing hesperidin and other citrus bioflavonoids) in doses of 500–2000 mg a day, along with vitamin C (500–2000 mg a day), bioflavonoids may help control the severity of hot flushes. Taking a high-potency balanced B-complex will help support the nervous system and reduce the impact of the stress of frequent hot flushes.

Green medicine

Herbal medicine has much to offer in the way of time-tested 'green' medicine to effectively reduce the frequency and severity of flushes and night sweats. The most widely used herbal remedies include the following.

If you have a history of oestrogen-positive breast cancer, consult a registered herbalist before self-prescribing any of these herbs.

Black cohosh (*Cimicifuga racemosa*)

Black cohosh has a long history of use in the treatment of a wide range of female health problems, including menopausal symptoms, uterine fibroids, absent or painful periods, pelvic inflammatory disease and PMS. Black cohosh was revered by the Native American Indians who used it to treat painful periods and menopausal problems. When used during the menopausal years, it has the added benefit of antispasmodic and pain-killing effects, and can help to ease the physical aches and pains common during menopause.

Remifemin is a commercial standardised extract of black cohosh used as a herbal alternative to HRT (hormone replacement therapy). Widely tested, this product effectively reduces hot flushes and sweats, as well as vaginal thinning and drying, and menopausal depression. Remifemin is also safe to use in women who have experienced or who have oestrogen-sensitive breast cancer.

Chaste tree (*Vitex agnus castus*)

One of the ultimate female herbs, with a long history of use, *Vitex* is a female hormonal regulator which can be safely taken for lengthy periods of time with few, if any, side effects. Very occasionally, a woman may experience headaches or breast tenderness while taking *Vitex*. Traditionally, *Vitex* is used to treat a wide range of female hormonal problems resulting in irregular or absent menses, period pain, PMS, infertility, fibroids, endometriosis, etc. *Vitex* has an effect on the pituitary gland in the brain, helping to normalise levels of the hormones FSH, LH and prolactin (see Chapter 1). As a menopausal herb, *Vitex* reduces symptoms of flushing, fluid retention, anxiety, depression and nervousness.

Sage (*Salvia officinalis*)

This common culinary herb is renowned for its ability to reduce sweating. It is an oestrogenic herb which has traditionally been used to regulate the menstrual cycle, treat period pain and reduce menopausal hot flushes and sweats. It can be taken as a simple herbal tea with one heaped teaspoon of fresh herb or ¾ teaspoon of dried herb added to one cup of hot water, two to three times a day. Make in a teapot and leave to steep for 10 minutes.

Dong quai (*Angelica sinensis*)

This ancient herb is one of the most popular and widely prescribed female tonics in Chinese herbal medicine. Dong quai has a powerful effect on the heart, liver and spleen meridian, and is a 'blood-building' tonic. It is prescribed for a range of 'women's problems' including painful, irregular or absent periods, and menopausal hot flushes.

Dong quai is especially useful for menopausal women suffering from weakness, dizziness and palpitations along with their flushes. Dong quai also helps 'moisten the intestines' and so is useful for gently restoring normal bowel function to lazy or sluggish bowels. This herb should not be used by women who have heavy menstrual periods or any kind of blood-clotting problems.

Fennel (*Foeniculum vulgare*)

This is another popular culinary herb which, like sage, has oestrogenic properties. Along with its ability to reduce flushing, fennel is an excellent digestive carminative in cases of indigestion, bloating, or flatulence.

Make a herbal tea with one teaspoon of fresh herb added to a cup of hot water, three times daily.

Homoeopathic help

Belladonna

Indicated for intense hot flushes with reddening and burning of the face, accompanied by restlessness and irritability. There may also be palpitations, and all symptoms are made worse by any kind of movement, touch or jarring.

Lachesis

A very important remedy for hot flushes that are accompanied by sweating and severe headaches centred on the top of the scalp. The flushes and headaches are worse in the morning and worse after sleep. Lachesis patients cannot stand any kind of pressure on their bodies, such as a tight waistband.

Pulsatilla

For the very emotional woman who is prone to fits of crying and bothered by mild hot flushes that come and go quickly. Symptoms are made worse by any kind of heat.

Vaginal dryness

It is common to notice vaginal and vulval changes during the menopausal years, caused by the declining levels of oestrogen. The vagina becomes shorter, thinner and less elastic and the once plump outer lips of the vulva begin to thin noticeably. Blood supply to the vagina decreases, and the mucous membranes lining it become more fragile and prone to infection. Vaginal secretions diminish, reducing the acidity of the vagina and increasing the propensity to vaginal infections and thrush. Vaginal lubrication during sexual arousal can also decrease, leading to dryness and difficulty with intercourse. Minimise the likelihood of vaginal thrush and cystitis by always using a quality personal lubricant during sexual intercourse. In New Zealand, Sylk (made from kiwifruit vines) is a gentle, effective lubricant containing no parabens or petrochemicals.

Oestrogen creams are frequently prescribed for vaginal thinning and discomfort, and they effectively thicken the vaginal walls (and may, or may not, improve lubrication). While they rapidly produce an improvement in vaginal health, they are not without drawbacks. The mucous membranes of the vagina are extremely porous, and small amounts of the oestrogen applied to the vagina rapidly cross the membranes into the bloodstream. However, the resulting increase in blood oestrogen levels is small, compared with the levels resulting from use of systemic hormone replacement therapy (HRT). The use of these creams in women who have had breast cancer is still controversial.

Some women find that regular use of a natural wild yam cream improves the tone and lubrication of the vagina effectively. There are a number of herbs which can be taken orally to improve vaginal health at menopause. Motherwort (*Leonarus cardiaca*) is a beautiful and gentle ally for all things menopausal. Twenty drops of tincture added to a little water and taken three to four times a

Keeping the vagina healthy at menopause and beyond

* Avoid using soap, bubble baths, douches and personal hygiene products in and around the vagina. They all tend to dry the vaginal area and may cause irritation. If you are still menstruating, avoid tampons, and use pads (preferably 100% unbleached cotton) instead.

* Avoid tight-fitting underwear and wear only cotton underpants. If you wear pantyhose, buy those with a cotton panty or no panty. Ventilate the vaginal area as much as possible by going without underwear (at home!) whenever possible.

* Use a personal lubricant during intercourse and take time with plenty of foreplay to ensure you are well aroused before penetration. Vitamin E oil is useful for treating vaginal dryness symptoms. Pierce a capsule containing vitamin E oil, and apply to a finger. Rub the oil up into the vagina, onto the vaginal walls. Repeat 2–3 times daily if needed. Vitamin E taken orally can also help ease vaginal dryness and thinning.

* Regular douching with unsweetened *Lactobacillus acidophilus* yoghurt may help prevent thrush problems. The same effect can be obtained, but with decidedly less mess, by inserting a *Lactobacillus* capsule high into the vagina at night.

day will help restore vaginal thickness as well as soothing nerves, insomnia and palpitations. Chaste tree (*Vitex agnus castus*) may also improve vaginal health as well as easing problems with heavy menstrual bleeding, PMS and irregular cycles, hot flushes, anxiety, depression and nervousness.

You've heard the old adage 'use it or lose it'? When it comes to keeping a strong, vibrant sexuality into old age, never a truer word was spoken. Regular sexual stimulation to orgasm is one of the most effective (and enjoyable) forms of self-help for keeping the vagina healthy through menopause and beyond. If you don't have a sexual partner, all is not lost: research shows the same vaginal health benefits result from masturbation to orgasm. For more information on preventing and treating vaginal infections, see Thrush in the A–Z section in Part Two. All the advice given there is also relevant for coping with vaginal difficulties during menopause.

Insomnia

Bleary-eyed exhaustion is synonymous with menopause for many women. Regular drenching night sweats are hardly conducive to deep sleep, and even if you're lucky enough to escape them, hormonal changes alone often disrupt the ability to fall into a deep and peaceful sleep. If life has become a battle with drooping eyelids and hours of tossing and turning in the dark, resist the temptation of a 'quick fix' with sleeping tablets, and instead try some simple self-help remedies. Not only can sleeping tablets rapidly create a dependency, they also cause abnormal sleep cycles, and suppress valuable REM (rapid eye movement) sleep. Each night we go through different phases or cycles of sleep, each of which is essential for our health. It is during the REM sleep that most of our dreaming occurs. Using pharmaceutical sleeping tablets suppresses this vital REM sleep. When the tablets are withdrawn, there is frequently a rebound effect during which sleeping is light, or disturbed by vivid dreams. However, there are some instances when the short-term use of medication (when all else has failed) may be needed to re-establish a normal sleep pattern.

A study published in the *Journal of the American Medical Association* (July 2001) showed that sleeping tablets are not the most effective long-term way of overcoming insomnia. The six-month study compared methods of dealing with insomnia, amongst a group of 75 chronic insomniacs. At the end of the six-month study, participants who had simply taken sleeping tablets reported a 16% reduction in the amount of time spent awake at night. The placebo group reported a 12% reduction. The group that improved the most was the one educated about better sleep habits and put on a consistent sleep schedule, but who had taken no sleeping tablets. This group got over 50% more sleep through the night than those who did not have the therapy.

Take a good look at your evening routine. It's important to get into the right frame of mind for falling asleep. This means going to bed in a relaxed state, not stewing over the dramas of the day. Try not to work up until bedtime; instead, indulge in at least an hour of quality relaxation time before hitting the pillow.

Combined with hormonal fluctuations, one of the most common causes of insomnia is an overactive autonomic nervous system (the part of the nervous system which controls the stress-related 'fight-or-flight' reaction). Days filled with constant stress, tight deadlines and endless demands cause the primitive autonomic nervous system to remain stimulated and active long after you switch off the lights at night. If you run on adrenalin all day, don't be surprised if your body continues to run on adrenalin all night. Many chronic insomniacs have found that following a programme of regular relaxation and stress management provides a permanent solution to sleeplessness. Yoga, meditation, or progressive relaxation techniques, practised as little as three times a week, gradually bring the autonomic nervous system back into balance, allowing you to switch off your brain and bedside light simultaneously.

Try a warm bath with candles, soft music and essential oils. Invest in some quality aromatherapy oils and add two or three drops of oil to the bathwater — lavender and sweet marjoram are especially useful. Other useful sleep inducers include: bergamot, roman chamomile, lemon, neroli and sandalwood. Alternatively, make a herbal bath by adding half a pint of your favourite herbal tea to your bathwater. Use a china or pottery teapot to steep the herbs. Pour boiling water over 3–4 teaspoons of fresh herbs or 1–2 teaspoons of dried. Cover the pot and leave to infuse for at least 10 minutes. Strain, and add to bathwater. A beautifully scented and relaxing combination includes lavender flowers, lemon balm, elder flowers and rosemary leaves. Or why not try a chamomile or hops bath.

Chamomile or relaxing teas can be sipped as a nightcap, and are useful to drink through the evening in place of stimulating caffeine drinks such as coffee, tea or hot chocolate. Beware the trap of drinking yourself to sleep with an alcoholic nightcap. You may fall asleep more easily, but chances are that you won't sleep through the night. Herbal teas are more reliable and longer-lasting relaxants.

If you're struggling with daytime sleepiness, try to resist, as much as possible, the urge to nap. A daytime nap of as little as half an hour can take the edge off night-time sleepiness. Instead, force yourself outside for fresh air and exercise — try a brisk walk along the beach or in a local park. Half an hour to an hour of aerobic activity each day will usually see your nocturnal habits improve immensely. A sedentary lifestyle, coupled with stress, stimulates a build-up of adrenalin which is simply not dissipated by physical activity through the day. Regular walking is one of the most sleep-inducing forms of exercise, as it is rhythmic, non-competitive and allows the mind to be stilled. After studying the sleep patterns of 43 sedentary adults suffering from insomnia, researchers at Stanford University in California found that exercising for 20–30 minutes every other afternoon decreased the time the insomniacs needed to fall asleep by 50%. Avoid vigorous exercise in the three hours before bedtime as it may boost your alertness. Studies suggest that doing exercise more than three to six hours before bedtime has the most effect on falling and staying asleep.

Not all sleep is equally beneficial. Slow wave sleep (SWS) is a very deep and restorative phase of sleep. The amount of time you spend in this beneficial phase of sleep can be increased by regular exercise. The best time of day for exercising to induce more SWS sleep is between 4 and 8 p.m. Interestingly, this particular benefit of exercise appears to be most pronounced in people who are already fit.

Low blood sugar is a common cause of frequent night waking. If you eat dinner at 6 p.m. and don't eat again through the evening, your blood sugar may be low by bedtime. Symptoms of this include yawning, sighing, tension, anxiety and an inability to relax enough to get off to sleep. A small complex-carbohydrate snack such as a little oatmeal, a slice of wholegrain bread or a banana will boost your blood sugar before bedtime.

Tryptophan is a naturally occurring amino acid (a building block of protein) found in a number of foods, including bananas, milk, yoghurt, dates, tuna and peanut butter. In theory, snacking on these foods in the evening gives your body the raw materials it needs to create serotonin, which is essential for sleeping well. In practice, however, tryptophan-rich foods don't always lead to increased serotonin as the other amino acids in these foods block the brain's uptake of tryptophan. In fact, it is carbohydrate-rich foods such as cereal, wholemeal crackers, rice or oats which result in the biggest serotonin increase. Tryptophan can also be taken as a supplement in tablet form before bedtime, in order to boost serotonin levels, and a calcium and magnesium supplement taken an hour before bedtime helps to relax body and mind, and induce a deep sleep.

Dietary patterns can influence both our ability to fall asleep and the quality of our sleep. Heading the list of dietary 'sleep wreckers' comes caffeine, in the form of coffee, tea, chocolate and energy drinks. Limit your total intake of caffeine, and try not to have caffeinated products for at least four to six hours before bedtime. Alcohol can also spoil a good night's sleep. Many people respond to alcohol as a stimulant. Some studies show that even as little as one glass of wine can disturb sleep, and reduce REM sleep in much the same way as do sleeping tablets. Other factors which may make it difficult to fall asleep include an excessively salty diet, eating your evening meal too close to bedtime, and, if you are a smoker, having a cigarette in the four to six hours before bedtime.

Take a close look at the environment of your bedroom. Is it a sleep sanctuary, or just another room used for working, eating, telephone calls, studying and ironing your shirts? Try to re-establish the bond between sleep and your bedroom by using the bedroom solely for sleep and sex. Make the environment conducive to sleep by keeping the room as cool as possible to encourage your body's natural drop in temperature through the night. Sensory stimulation by noise or light will disrupt your production of melatonin, a hormone directly related to the sleep cycle. If you wake for a toilet trip, resist the urge to turn on any lights, as even brief exposure to bright light will disrupt melatonin levels and make it more difficult to get back to sleep.

The prescription hormone Melantonin is gaining popularity as a seemingly safe and effective means of re-establishing normal sleep patterns. Produced by the tiny pineal gland in the brain, melatonin influences circadian rhythms which affect sleep patterns. With age, melatonin production declines, especially between the ages of 50 and 60. Quality of sleep appears to be directly influenced by melatonin levels circulating in the body. Melatonin levels can be negatively affected by prescription drugs such as beta blockers, which are used to treat high blood pressure. Excessive consumption of alcohol and caffeine will also disrupt normal melatonin levels, as will sleep deprivation due to overwork or shift work. (See Chapter 6 for melatonin and the breast cancer link.)

Riding the emotional roller coaster

Many previously balanced women undergo an unsettling personality transformation at the time of menopause, something akin to a Jekyll-and-Hyde experience. Many of my patients describe their emotional changes as resembling a severe and ongoing case of PMS. Irritability, inexplicable anxiety, depression and almost phobic fears are not uncommon, and can be partially explained by the profound hormonal fluctuations of perimenopause and menopause. While hormones are definitely part of the equation, I believe that some of our mid-life emotional strife has a psychosocial basis related to the negative connotations associated with female ageing and fading physical beauty.

The menopausal years may also be the first time in your life that you have absolutely no excuse for not getting on with the things that you have always talked about, but never quite managed to do such as furthering your education, getting a better job, or leaving an unhappy marriage. Children are grown and independent and for the first time in 20 or 30 years you have the time and the space to sit back and do some serious stocktaking. New insights (both happy and disturbing) may seep to the surface of your consciousness. Being faced with choices, potential new directions, and the chance to express your independence and freedom can be both exhilarating and daunting and unsettling.

Issues of sexuality often arise around the mid-life transition. Sexual difficulties or a feeling of insecurity and uncertainty around your own sexuality, waning libido and perceived loss of physical attractiveness may surface. Physical difficulties such as vaginal dryness, loss of libido and bladder infections may put a damper on the fiery sex goddess you may once have been!

Putting it all together, hormonal changes aside, it's hardly surprising many women experience some emotional upheavals as they pass through the transition into mid-life liberation.

How do you take this opportunity for reinventing yourself and turn it into the gift that it is, rather than buying into the cultural conditioning that would have us believe that life is all but over once the 'big M' arrives? Start by defining your own personal parameters of self-worth. Seek out and dwell on the many positive qualities and strengths which make you the special woman you are. List them, dwell on them, affirm them and be proud of them. Maybe you value your creativity, passion, compassion, wisdom, humour, intuition, patience, exuberance . . . focus on them and enhance them. Look within for your positive reinforcement and worry less about the opinions of others. The ability to feel good in your own skin and proud of who you are can be one of the greatest blessings of ageing. Focusing on your new-found freedom from child rearing, mid-life prosperity (hopefully), and the opportunity to develop friendships and personal relationships with other women and men, can turn the menopausal years into an exciting journey.

If anxiety, depression or mood swings are still a problem, don't be afraid to turn to others for help. Talk to other women who may be experiencing similar changes, or older female friends who have already weathered the mid-life experience. Talk to your partner, sharing books about the menopause and encouraging greater understanding and emotional support. Seek professional help in the form of counselling, acupuncture, homoeopathy or herbal medicine. In the case of severe depression, see your doctor.

Self-help and natural therapies

Nutrition

Sound nutrition is a vital precursor to a healthy nervous system and balanced mood. Are you fuelling your precious body with a nutrient-rich feast of wholefoods, or are you consuming a diet of worthless and disease-promoting junk food, refined carbohydrates and sugar? If it is the latter, don't be surprised by your erratic moods.

What you put into your mouth can make a tremendous difference to your emotional balance. As well as lacking in nutrients, junk food diets also supply an abundance of simple carbohydrates (high-GI carbs) and sugar that play havoc with blood-sugar regulation. (See Chapter 2 to understand the relationship between carbohydrates and your blood-sugar levels and mood regulation.)

Depression or emotional volatility may be a cry for help from your body for more nutritional input. Although the standard 'balanced diet' will usually supply enough nutrients to keep you alive and relatively healthy, it may not meet the increased nutritional requirements that result from the emotional and physical stress of menopause. During mid-life transition, nervous system nutrients such as B-complex vitamins, vitamin C, calcium,

Nutritional supplements that may help reduce depression and anxiety during menopause

✳ A high-potency B-complex supplying 50 mg of the key B-vitamins. This should be taken twice daily with breakfast and mid-afternoon snack.

✳ Vitamin C, mixed ascorbate powder. Take 1000 mg of vitamin C, 2–3 times a day, mixed in a little juice or water.

✳ Fish oil — take between two and five 1000 mg capsules daily with food. Consult your medical practitioner if you are taking blood-thinning medication.

✳ Calcium and magnesium — quality calcium supplements always contain magnesium. A formula containing calcium hydroxyapatate or citrate is most useful. Follow instructions on the product and take with a little fruit juice to enhance absorption. If you are using a combined calcium/magnesium formula, you can take additional magnesium separately to further boost magnesium levels, if anxiety, tension and insomnia are a problem.

magnesium and essential fatty acids are all needed in greater amounts.

Herbal help

Herbal help for the nervous system falls into three main groups:

* nervine tonics to strengthen the nervous system

* nervine relaxants to ease nervous tension

* nervine stimulants to stimulate the nervous system.

In cases of anxiety, depression and tension, both tonics and

* 5-HTP — a natural derivative of an amino acid (a building block of protein), 5-HTP is a metabolic precursor to the brain chemical serotonin (thought to be low in most depression sufferers). Common prescription antidepressants SSRIs (including Prozac and Aropax) help to boost serotonin levels in the brain by delaying the body's breakdown of the chemical. Some studies have shown 5-HTP to be as effective as SSRIs in the treatment of depression and anxiety, with no side effects. Dose range is 50–150 mg per day. Take 100 mg for two weeks or until symptoms improve, and then change to a maintenance dose of 50 mg a day. Do not use with antidepressants before consulting your GP.

* SAM-e — S-adenosyl-methionine is an antioxidant supplement which has been found to be as effective as some pharmaceutical antidepressants. To date there have been more than 40 clinical trials using SAM-e in the treatment of depression. In some people, symptoms of depression begin to improve in as few as seven days.

relaxants may be used. One of the best herbs for nourishing and strengthening the nervous system is the humble oat, which can be taken as a herbal remedy, food or tea. Oats are rich in calcium and silica, and traditionally the herb has been used if there is nervous debility and exhaustion along with depression. A tea made from oat straw was a traditional remedy to relieve fatigue and weakness, especially when emotional imbalance was a root cause.

Relaxant herbs help ease nervous tension and anxiety. Certain herbs have earned a reputation as being particularly effective to ease anxiety and tension associated with the hormonal shifts of menopause. Passion flower is a beautiful, gentle but effective nervine herb used to relax the nervous system and ease anxiety symptoms. Black cohosh effectively eases hot flushes and night sweats and has the additional benefit of being slightly sedative and calming to the nervous system. Motherwort is the herb of choice when menopause-related anxiety is causing heart symptoms such as palpitations and a racing heartbeat. Hyssop, lady's slipper, lime blossom, rosemary and skullcap each have a nervine relaxant effect.

These herbs are most effective when taken in appropriate combinations, and for this reason I recommend a consultation with a registered medical herbalist, rather than self-prescribing. However you can go right ahead and self-administer calming herbal teas such as lemon balm, oatstraw tea and chamomile.

Giving your menopausal body the right fuel, and supporting good nutrition with supplements and herbal medicine (if needed), will help restore your mental and emotional equilibrium. Just as important is a commitment to regular aerobic exercise. Going for a brisk walk, jog, swim or cycle every day stimulates the production of your body's own mood-enhancing brain chemicals (endorphins). As endorphin levels rise, nervousness, anxiety, depression and mood swings will abate. A number of clinical trials have shown regular aerobic exercise to be as effective as antidepressants in the treatment of some types of depression.

Diet tips for menopause

* Drink plenty of water and herbal tea for good hydration despite hot flushes and sweats.

* Follow the healthy eating recommendations for blood-sugar regulation in Chapter 2. Blood-sugar swings will aggravate menopausal fatigue and mood swings.

* Avoid 'heating' food and drinks which aggravate hot flushes. These include: spicy foods, tea, coffee, alcohol, chocolate, and sugar in general.

* Include plentiful dietary sources of calcium such as calcium-enriched soya milk, leafy green vegetables, nuts and seeds, bony fish (salmon, sardines, herrings), tahini, peas, beans and lentils, and low-fat dairy products. Avoid 'calcium leechers' such as soft drinks, salt, caffeine, sugar and too much red meat.

* Boost antioxidant levels to protect cells from age-related free-radical damage. Antioxidant-rich foods to have in your daily diet include: berries, fresh fruits and vegetables — including generous servings of onions and garlic — green tea, dark chocolate 70% cocoa mass (in moderation!). (For more information on antioxidants, see Chapter 2 and Chapter 6.)

* Avoid refined grains and high-GI carbohydrates. Not only will they cause blood-sugar fluctuations, but the resulting high insulin levels will encourage weight gain and potentially increase the risk of breast cancer. Rid the cupboards of white flour, white bread, sweetened, refined and processed foods. In their place put whole grains, wholemeal bread, basmati or brown rice, fruits and vegetables, nuts and seeds.

✳ Avoid the 'fat-free' trap. Fats are vital for staying healthy, and are especially important during menopausal years when there is a generalised drying of skin, hair, and mucous membranes. Boost your intake of healthy omega-3 and omega-9 fats to support skin, hair, connective tissue, bone, immune, cardiovascular and nervous system health.

Choose from flax oil (mix with balsamic vinegar to make an easy salad dressing); extra virgin olive oil; avocado oil; rice bran oil; nuts and seeds (especially almonds, macadamias and walnuts); avocado; LSA (ground linseeds, sunflower and almonds); oily fish (salmon, sardines, herrings, tuna).

✳ Increase dietary phyto-oestrogens (plant compounds with a weak oestrogenic effect). Women with a high dietary phyto-oestrogen intake tend to have fewer problems with hot flushes and night sweats. There is also strong evidence that a phyto-oestrogen-rich diet reduces risk of cardiovascular disease, cancer and osteoporosis.

Choose from soya milk, tofu, miso, linseed, fruits and vegetables, lentils, beans and legumes. (See phyto-oestrogen list in Chapter 6.)

✳ Increase dietary fibre to keep your gut and digestion healthy. A high-fibre intake along with balanced gut microflora is important for optimum oestrogen detoxification, and breast health.

Fibre-rich foods to choose from include: fresh fruits and vegetables; whole grains, brown rice, nuts, seeds, lentils and beans; linseed (take 10 g a day soaked in water overnight). Cultured products such as *acidophilus* yoghurt will help to maintain a healthy population of friendly gut bacteria.

It's also important to make time for regular relaxation or meditation (see Chapter 4). This may take the form of walking somewhere beautiful and relaxing, gardening, having a hot bath or listening to music. Whatever calms you . . . make the time to do it regularly.

Move it or lose it

While optimum nutrition and a balanced lifestyle are vital measures to peacefully navigate the sometimes turbulent waters of the menopausal years, regular exercise is equally important. That means that no matter how great your diet is, staying healthy through menopause simply cannot be achieved by obsessing about your diet while settling into a comfortable state of slothdom! Regular exercise minimises many of the symptoms of menopause such as flushes and night sweats, mood swings, depression and insomnia. The increased risk of osteoporosis, heart disease and breast cancer in the postmenopausal years is also reduced by regular exercise.

For many women, the menopausal years are the first time they notice something amiss in the pelvic area. It may be slight stress incontinence; more trouble with vaginal or bladder infections, or an uncomfortable feeling of dragging in the lower abdomen. Triggered by declining oestrogen levels, these problems are aggravated by lack of physical activity and the resulting poor muscle tone and lack of blood circulation in the lower abdomen. What encourages blood circulation? — exercise of course. Aerobic exercise such as brisk walking, swimming, jogging or even bike riding will help improve blood circulation through the abdominal and pelvic area.

Lovemaking and sexual arousal do wonders for pelvic blood circulation. When it comes to vaginal health and menopause, the old adage 'use it or lose it' definitely applies. Regular lovemaking or masturbation helps keep the vagina strong and lubricated. Pelvic floor exercises (see Chapter 3) are specifically designed to exercise the sling-like pelvic floor muscles which support all the pelvic organs and keep them sitting in their rightful places. These exercises are easy to do and can be done discreetly, anywhere and at any time . . . whether you are washing the dishes, driving the car, or even standing in line at the supermarket!

Up to the menopausal years, women have a significantly lower incidence of cardiovascular disease than do men, due to the cardioprotective effects of oestrogen. After menopause, as a result of declining oestrogen levels, our risk of cardiovascular disease sharply increases. Regular aerobic exercise is one significant lifestyle choice proven to minimise this increase in cardiovascular risk. Not only will it protect you against coronary artery disease, high blood pressure and high blood fats, but aerobic activity will also reduce your risk of weight gain, diabetes, breast cancer, depression, and osteoporosis! If you can find just 30 minutes a day, 5 days a week, for a brisk walk or a bike ride, you'll reap all of these many health benefits, and you will also have increased energy and positive self-esteem.

In the last decade of HRT hype (see below), osteoporosis has become almost synonymous with menopause. So much so that many women believe it is almost inevitable they will end their days as a stooped, frail and osteoporotic shadow of their former selves. This is simply not true, and if you're serious about keeping your skeleton strong throughout the postmenopausal years, it's probably not a drug you need but a pair of good walking shoes and a set of hand weights. It is impossible to slow down bone loss with good diet alone. An adequate dietary intake of calcium and other mineral cofactors is important for bone health, but without weight-bearing exercise calcium cannot be 'fixed' into the bones. We lose the most calcium from our bones during times of inactivity, including sleep. Increased amounts of calcium leach from the bones of people who are immobilised due to illness (or who choose to spend most of their life on the sofa), or astronauts living in an environment of weightlessness. Weight-bearing exercise, during which your body exercises against some kind of resistance, is essential for bone strengthening. For the bones of the lower body this type of exercise could be walking, running, dancing, golfing, or racquet sports; and for your upper body, racquet sports, weight lifting or using resistance machines at the gym.

Hormone replacement therapy (HRT) — a spectacular fall from grace

July 2002 will go down in history as the time when the massively lucrative HRT bubble burst. This was the month in which the largest-ever study into the long-term risks and benefits of HRT (the Woman's Health Initiative (WHI) study) was prematurely terminated. This American study came to an end three years early, when it became abundantly clear that risks of long-term combined HRT use outweighed any benefits it might have.

Throughout its 40-year history, HRT has been shrouded by a complicated and confusing mythology largely created by aggressive and somewhat creative pharmaceutical marketing campaigns, and a resulting medical practice based on a dearth of clear scientific evidence. Since its inception, HRT has been touted as a panacea for the mid-life woman, claiming to restore ageing women to their former glory, complete with sharper minds, stronger sex drives, healthier hearts and stronger bones, not to mention being devoid of annoying flushes, sweats, mood swings and wrinkling skin.

Until 2002, HRT had been a phenomenal marketing success. Wyeth, manufacturers of the once popular Prempro and Premarin, boasted pre-2002 worldwide sales totalling US\$3 billion per annum. The marketing of HRT involved redefining the natural condition of menopause as a medical condition resulting from 'oestrogen deficiency'. It was a condition which, of course, could be miraculously 'cured' by taking supplemental oestrogen, or oestrogen combined with progestogen (also known as progestin, a synthetic progesterone). Because every single woman who lives past mid-life is guaranteed to develop the 'condition' of menopause, the potential market for HRT was enormous. From 1992 to 1999, the oestrogen drug Premarin was the most prescribed drug in America.

Until the Woman's Health Initiative study, there were two main categories of HRT use. It was prescribed either for relief of acute menopausal symptoms such as hot flushes and sweats, or with the intention of long-term use for the supposed prevention of osteoporosis, heart disease and Alzheimer's disease.

The federally funded WHI trial of HRT begun in 2001 was due to end in 2005. It involved more than 16,000 women aged 50–79 years. The study was prematurely aborted when data revealed that women who use combined HRT for more than five years face a 26% increased risk of breast cancer, and a 29% increased risk of heart attacks or other coronary events. Equally alarming was the realisation that the greatest risk of coronary events occurs in the first year of HRT use. It wasn't all bad news though, and along with these increased risks came a one-third decreased risk of hip fractures, and a slightly decreased risk of bowel cancer.

These percentage increases translated into the following changes in disease incidence per 10,000 women taking combined HRT for five or more years:

* 7 more coronary heart disease cases
* 8 more invasive breast cancer cases
* 8 more stroke cases
* 8 more cases of blood clots on the lungs
* 6 fewer cases of bowel cancer
* 5 fewer hip fracture cases.

In 2004, another arm of the WHI trial was prematurely aborted. This arm of the study was examining oestrogen-only hormone replacement, and was terminated early when it became evident that ERT (oestrogen-only replacement therapy) also carries an increased risk of stroke, blood clots and dementia, as well as increasing the risk of endometrial cancer (cancer of the lining of the uterus).

The WHI study caught the attention of the world, but in truth it was only one of a series of (smaller) studies casting doubt on the safety and efficacy of long-term HRT use.

New Zealand author Gill Sanson, in her book *The Osteoporosis 'Epidemic'*, provides an informative roundup of reputable HRT studies presaging the WHI results. As far back as 1997, the esteemed journal *Lancet* published the results of an analysis of 51 studies showing that women who used HRT for 11 years had a 35% increased risk of breast cancer compared with non-users. The risk was shown to increase with age and length of use. Three years later the *Journal of the American Medical Association* published the results of a study involving 46,000 women, followed for 10 years to assess the effects of combined HRT. The study concluded that combined HRT use significantly increased a woman's risk of developing breast cancer by age 70. The authors concluded that each year of HRT use increased the risk of breast cancer by 8%. The results of a large study published in the August 2003 *Lancet* estimated that, in Britain alone, an additional 20,000 breast cancer cases in the past decade resulted directly from HRT use.

Until recently, common medical practice saw vast numbers of mid-life women placed on HRT at the onset of hot flushes, with the expectation of indefinite use as a safeguard against heart disease and osteoporosis. The WHI study has changed this practice by showing that not only will combined HRT not protect cardiovascular health, it may in fact have the opposite effect and precipitate a heart attack, stroke or blood clot. Once again the findings had been previously indicated by other studies.

The HERS study conducted in the mid-1990s is considered to be a landmark study on the use of HRT and heart disease. Nearly 3000 women with known heart disease were given either a placebo or a combined HRT drug. Women receiving HRT showed a decline in their 'bad' (LDL) cholesterol and an increase in 'protective' (HDL) cholesterol. Despite these favourable changes there was no reduction in heart disease, and their heart attack rate actually increased. Triglyceride levels and blood clots also increased.

The terminated WHI trial produced the same findings of increased cardiovascular risk in the first year of HRT use, but this time amongst a population of women with *no* established risk factors for heart disease.

Historically, the other main rationale for long-term HRT use was to prevent thinning of the bones and osteoporosis. The WHI bombshell effectively removed osteoporosis prevention as an indication for long-term use . . . but the question of whether it was ever an appropriate indication has been the source of international controversy for some time.

The June 2001 *Journal of the American Medical Association* published a paper on the subject. An editorial accompanying the paper states, 'Why take it? If it's for hot flushes, it's clear it works. If it's for the prevention of anything else, it's not clear yet.' The study, an analysis of 22 HRT trials, found a reduction in bone fracture risk only in women who started treatment before age 60. The accompanying editorial questions whether HRT even prevents fractures in women who start taking it before the age of 60, because the studies in the analysis weren't designed to look at osteoporosis. It says, 'the study highlights the fact that evidence about the efficacy of postmenopausal oestrogen for prevention of fractures is weak'.

Natural progesterone therapy

In the past few years, increasing numbers of New Zealand women have turned to natural progesterone therapy to solve a myriad of hormonally related health issues. Well-known long-term champions of natural hormone replacement include Dr Mike

Lee (a passionate advocate of natural progesterone therapy for more than 20 years); English doctor Katrina Dalton (long-term advocate of natural progesterone therapy in the treatment of PMS); and closer to home, Dr Sandra Cabot, who has used the therapy extensively for nearly a decade. Natural progesterone cream (or oil) is prescribed not only to ease a multitude of menopausal ills, but it is also widely used in the treatment of fibroids, endometriosis, PMS, heavy menses, ovarian cysts and osteoporosis.

Many female health issues result from a relative excess of oestrogen in relation to the amount of progesterone in the body. From the perimenopausal years (mid-forties) on, it is not uncommon for women to experience cycles in which there is no ovulation. Without ovulation, production of progesterone is greatly reduced, leading to an excessively oestrogenic environment in the body. Oestrogen excess is also a common phenomenon amongst women of all ages, as a result of the highly oestrogenic environment in which we live (see Chapter 6). Oestrogen dominance is implicated in the development of menstrual problems including irregular cycles, heavy periods and PMS; hormonal migraine; fibroids; endometriosis; fibrocystic breasts; and even breast cancer. By using bio-identical natural progesterone therapy to rebalance the progesterone/oestrogen ratio, many of these health problems are significantly improved or eliminated.

Natural progesterone is not the same as the progestogen (synthetic progesterone) used in pharmaceutical hormonal compounds such as HRT or the oral contraceptive pill. Natural progesterone is 'bio-identical'; in other words, it precisely matches the molecular configuration of the progesterone produced by the body itself. Synthetic progestogen, on the other hand, is a chemical alteration of the progesterone molecule, and is not the same as the progesterone produced in the body. For this reason, natural progesterone therapy rarely produces unpleasant side effects, and certainly none of the dangerous side effects associated with progestogen use.

HRT — the facts

Heart disease

✻ Combined HRT use increases the risk of coronary artery disease, stroke and blood clots on the lung.

✻ Combined HRT use may favourably affect cholesterol levels but this does not translate into decreased mortality.

✻ Risk of heart attacks increases within the first 3 years of combined HRT use.

✻ Combined HRT increases the incidence of blood clots. One out of every 263 women treated with HRT will experience a drug-related blood clot.

✻ Prevention of cardiovascular disease is no longer a rationale for HRT use.

Breast cancer

✻ Most observational studies show that women using combined HRT or oestrogen-only replacement therapy (ERT) have more cases of breast cancer than do women not on these drugs. The increase in risk translates into 1% per year for women on ERT and 8% per year for those on combined HRT.

✻ Increased risk of breast cancer becomes apparent within 1–2 years of commencing HRT use, and increases with duration of use.

✻ All forms of HRT, including continuous and sequential regimes, oestrogen-only therapy, HRT patches and implants, are associated with increased breast-cancer risk.

* The risk of breast cancer significantly decreases after stopping HRT, and within 5 years the residual risk is not significantly different from that observed for those who have never used HRT.

* HRT use also increases breast density, making it more difficult to obtain accurate mammograms.

Ovarian cancer

* Postmenopausal women using combined HRT for 10 years or more have been shown to have an increased risk of dying from ovarian cancer.

Dementia

* The WHI study showed that combined HRT use doubles the risk of dementia (predominantly of the Alzheimer's form) in women aged 65 and above. The increased risk becomes apparent after 1 year of HRT use. The increased risk translates into an extra 23 cases of dementia per 10,000 women per year.

If HRT or ERT is used, it should be prescribed in the lowest possible effective dose and for the shortest possible period of time, for the management of acute menopausal symptoms (and preferably only after drug-free options have been exhausted). It should never be taken long-term as a preventative for any kind of health condition.

Reported benefits of using natural progesterone therapy

* Prevention of bone loss, and in some cases increase in bone density.

* Reduction of hot flushes, vaginal thinning and dryness.

* Cardiovascular benefits including reduced risk of heart disease, stroke and abnormal cholesterol.

* Reduction in fluid retention.

* Reduction in, or elimination of, hormonal migraines.

* Improvement in sleep, moods, memory and concentration.

* Improvement of libido.

* Reduction of PMS.

* Protective role against breast cancer.

* Reduction in postnatal depression.

Another significant difference between oral progestogen therapy and transdermal (through the skin) natural progesterone therapy is the dose required to achieve a therapeutic effect. Oral progestogen may be administered in doses of as much as 200–400 mg a day, compared with the usual transdermal progesterone dose of 15–20 mg a day. When hormones are taken orally, they enter the bloodstream from the small intestine and go directly to the liver, where they are rapidly broken down, leaving only small amounts in circulation and available to cells. By administering hormones through highly porous skin, natural progesterone cream circumvents the digestive system, thus allowing cells to absorb hormones efficiently — hence the much smaller doses required.

Signs and symptoms that respond to natural progesterone therapy

* PMS — abdominal bloating, acne, mood swings, anger, fluid retention, breast tenderness, migraine.
* Irregular periods.
* Palpitations, high blood pressure.
* Arthritis.
* Asthma.
* Spontaneous bruising.
* Cold hands and feet.
* Endometriosis.
* Cervical dysplasia.
* Bone and joint pain.
* Bleeding gums.
* Allergies.
* Fibroids.
* Vaginal thinning and dryness.
* Headaches.
* Hypoglycaemia.
* Insomnia.
* Menopause.
* Panic, anxiety, tearfulness.

Replacing progesterone in the body simultaneously impacts on a number of other vital hormones such as DHEA, oestrogen, testosterone and thyroid hormones. Natural progesterone is the precursor of adrenal corticol hormones (coricosteroids) and the entire group of oestrogen hormones (bear in mind that oestrogen is a generic name given to several different hormones), and testosterone. Frequently, when natural progesterone cream is used for a period of time, low levels of these other hormones also increase to normal.

Signs and symptoms of oestrogen dominance

* Fluid retention.
* Breast swelling and lumpiness.
* Uterine fibroids.
* Endometrial cancer.
* Endometriosis.
* Breast cancer.
* Weight gain and fat deposition at thighs and hips.
* Low libido.
* Heavy or irregular menses.
* PMS, mood swings and depression.
* Migraines.

Chapter **6**

Breast-cancer prevention

It's hard to find anyone who doesn't know someone whose life has been personally touched by breast cancer, such is the prevalence of this most feared of female cancers. Women in every corner of the globe are affected by breast cancer, but it is Western women in particular who face the greatest risk of developing the disease. Prior to 1940, breast cancer was a rare occurrence, but in the past 65 years the incidence of breast cancer in the Western world has doubled, rising by approximately 1% annually. Globally, approximately 1.1 million new cases of breast cancer are diagnosed every year.

In New Zealand, breast cancer is the most common form of cancer affecting women, with 1 in 10 women (around 2300 new cases annually) receiving a breast-cancer diagnosis in her life, and 650 women a year dying from breast cancer. This equates to a breast-cancer incidence of around 117 cases per 100,000 person-years in New Zealand, in contrast to only 22 cases per 100,000 person-years in Africa and Asia. In the past 50 years there has been an alarming increase in breast cancer amongst New Zealand women. Between 1956 and 1997, the number of cases in New Zealand has almost quadrupled — from 488 to 1936 per annum. The 'face' of breast cancer has also changed in the past few decades. Once considered a disease of 'older women', breast cancer is increasingly found in ever-younger women. Almost 30% of new cases in New Zealand are diagnosed in women under 50. The one small glimmer of statistical light in an otherwise gloomy picture is a decrease in breast-cancer mortality of more than 16% between 1991 and 2000.

The figures speak for themselves. No woman can consider herself immune from the possibility of one day developing breast cancer. In October each year, New Zealanders and Australians dig deep into their pockets to give generously to the annual breast-cancer appeal. The media blitzes us with their annual campaign of breast-cancer awareness, centred on the importance of early detection through regular mammograms. Indeed, it is true that the earlier a breast cancer is detected, the less likelihood there is that it has spread to other parts of the body. Early, small, localised cancers are much less likely to be lethal. Despite the ongoing emphasis on early detection, it is hard not to be disheartened by the ever-increasing numbers of new cases detected . . . albeit early.

While early detection is vital, if we are serious about reducing the terrible loss of life as a result of breast cancer, what is even more vital is a major paradigm shift. Instead of focusing our attention predominantly on screening and early detection (in other words finding cancer once it is present), greater emphasis must be given to educating women about *prevention* of breast cancer. We need to ask the hard questions about the causes of cancer — even if the answers are disquieting, politically incorrect and threatening to powerful industries.

In truth there is much we still don't know about the causes of breast cancer, but there is already much that we do understand, and a great deal of research suggestive of likely (but still not fully proven) causative factors. Around the globe, vocal groups of women (such as our own New Zealand-based Breast Cancer Network) are calling for a precautionary approach to breast-cancer prevention, using the evidence of harm rather than the proof of harm to be the impetus for action. In other words, why wait until a possible causative factor has undergone many years of research and pronounced a thoroughly proven cause of breast cancer, when we can begin to change our lifestyles and nutrition *now*, based on existing evidence of harm?

What causes breast cancer?

In short: we still don't know, with the causes of more than 50% of breast cancers still unexplained. That said, there are already some clearly defined breast-cancer risk factors. We do know that breast-cancer risk is complex and that many factors play a role, and that simply having one or two of the established risk factors is unlikely to significantly increase your risk of developing breast cancer. There is also much for us to learn in the realm of diet and nutrition, as well as about exposure to environmental pollutants and their impact on breast health.

Risk factors can be broadly divided into two groups. The first group includes those factors that are simply the 'luck of the draw' and which we can do little about, such as ageing; our genetic heritage; the age at which we had our first menstrual period (although this is partially modifiable through dietary choice and avoiding obesity); age of menopause. The second group of variables are those which present us with choices and an opportunity to do things differently; to be proactive in an attempt to minimise our breast-cancer risk. These are the 'lifestyle' variables — such as diet, nutrition, exercise, stress management, and so on. Then there is a third group of risk factors which are 'partly' modifiable. These include our exposure to environmental pollutants which are either directly carcinogenic, or which have a hormonal effect in our body, potentially stimulating the development of hormonally linked cancers such as breast cancer. I call these factors 'partly modifiable' as we can partly limit our exposure to such toxins by choosing organic diets and safety-conscious personal care and cleaning products. However, even if we make such conscious choices, there are numerous avenues of exposure which we are largely powerless to prevent, living as we do in our polluted petro-chemical-laden modern world.

Before you read on, I need to emphasise once again that there are many factors involved in breast cancer, and that there is still much we do not understand about its causes.

If you already have breast cancer, spare yourself the agony of self-recrimination, guilt and the common experience of feeling you have in some way caused your own illness. Even if you have practised little of the preventative medicine discussed below, it is still impossible to definitively state the cause of your breast cancer. Environmental, genetic, and probably other factors, as yet undiscovered, combine in little-understood ways with lifestyle choices to create a complex picture of causality. However, it is never too late to adopt the precautionary principle, and to make as many proactive changes as possible to optimise your health from this point forward.

Breast-cancer risk factors you cannot change

Being a woman over the age of 50

Eighty per cent of all female breast cancers occur in women over the age of 50. Growing older is a risk factor which you simply cannot change!

Family history of breast cancer

Just because another woman in your family has had breast cancer does not mean that your risk is automatically increased. For example, having a grandmother who is diagnosed with breast cancer at the age of 75 does not increase your risk. There are, however, some familial patterns of breast cancer which suggest that you may have inherited a gene which increases your risk of breast cancer (see below). Suspect a possible genetic involvement if:

∗ you have a mother, sister or daughter with breast cancer

* multiple generations of your family have been affected by breast or ovarian cancer

* you have female relatives who were diagnosed with breast cancer before the age of 50

* you have female relatives who have had breast cancer in both breasts.

Genetic predisposition to breast cancer

Purely hereditary breast cancer accounts for only 5–10% of all breast cancers. True genetic breast-cancer risk is the result of a woman carrying the BRCA1 or BRCA2 gene. Women who carry the BRCA1 gene have an increased incidence of breast cancer, often at a young age, as well as an increased risk of ovarian cancer. The BRCA2 gene is less common, and while an increased risk of breast cancer comes with it, the increased risk of ovarian cancer is smaller than with the BRCA1 gene.

Age at onset of menstruation and menopause

Girls who begin menstruating at an early age are considered to have a higher risk of breast cancer, as do women who cease menstruating at an older age. Both these scenarios prolong a woman's exposure to oestrogen during the reproductive years. Menstruating for 40 years or more especially accentuates this risk.

Size, shape and growth patterns

A 2004 study in the *New England Journal of Medicine* looked into any possible connection between patterns of childhood growth and subsequent breast-cancer risk. The study involved over 117,000 Danish women. The findings suggest that high birth weight, early age at peak growth, high stature at 14 years of age, low body mass index at 14 years of age, and high growth rate during childhood, especially around puberty, were all independent risk factors for breast cancer.

Risk factors you can do something about

Age and frequency of pregnancy

If you have never had a pregnancy, breast-cancer risk is increased compared with that of a woman who has had a child before the age of 30. However, leaving a first pregnancy until after the age of 30 increases the risk to levels greater than that of a woman who has never had a pregnancy. This apparent anomaly appears to be linked to the time that elapses from the first period until the first pregnancy. During this time, breast tissue seems to be especially prone to damage by poor diet, radiation exposure and alcohol consumption.

Never having breastfed

Cumulative time of six years or more spent breastfeeding decreases breast-cancer risk. Women who have pregnancies at a young age appear to reap a breast-protective benefit from breastfeeding, regardless of how long they breastfeed for.

Exposure to radiation

In our modern world of high-tech medicine, exposure to ionising radiation in the course of medical diagnosis is increasingly common. X-rays, mammograms, and CT scans are routinely used to peer into the body. Despite their routine use, all these procedures expose our cells to ionising radiation, for which a safe exposure level has never been established. Even the lowest doses of radiation can damage the genetic material within a cell, increasing the risk of abnormal cell replication and the development of cancer. In fact, exposure to ionising radiation is one of the few irrefutable causes of cancer. Prominent researchers such as Dr John Gofman and well-known breast specialist Dr Susan Love go as far as to suggest that some of the modern escalation in breast-cancer incidence can be accounted for by previous exposure to medical radiation. Between 1950 and 1990, breast-cancer incidence soared by 90% in the USA, with similar increases seen in other Western countries. How much of this rapid increase is related to radiation exposure will never be certain.

In 1993 the *Journal of the National Cancer Institute* concluded that 'total dose, age at first exposure, and time since first exposure are all determinants of the incidence rate ratio of breast cancer after exposure of the breast to ionising radiation'. Time of exposure to radiation influences how great a negative impact there will be on breast tissue. Radiation exposure during childhood is thought to impart the greatest cancer risk, with exposure after the age of 40 having much less of an impact. Adolescent girls undergoing rapid breast tissue development are at the most risk of radiation damage to breast tissue.

A fact sheet from Cornell University states that 'age at exposure is one of the most important determinants of future risk of developing breast cancer due to radiation later in life. Young girls are at highest risk and women irradiated around the menopausal ages are at low risk.' Before menopause, breast tissue has an increased sensitivity to radiation, possibly due to higher oestrogen levels, so cumulative exposure to radiation prior to menopause poses a greater risk than the same cumulative exposure after menopause.

While one exposure to radiation may not significantly increase our risk of breast cancer, cumulative exposures almost certainly do. Modern X-rays and mammograms deliver about 10 times fewer rads than did earlier models, but their cumulative impact is still of concern. When it comes to X-rays, it is X-rays of the chest and coronary X-rays which pose the greatest risk to the breasts. However, radiation can scatter from X-rays anywhere in the body — including from dental X-rays — to affect the breasts. (Always request that a lead apron be used for dental X-rays.)

CT scans are now widely used in medical diagnosis, despite the fact that the radiation exposure from a CT scan is many times greater than that from an X-ray. The American National Cancer Institute says, 'CT scans comprise about 10% of diagnostic radiological procedures in US hospitals, but contribute an estimated 65% of effective radiation dose to the public from all medical X-ray equipment'. Professor Eric Hall, from Columbia University, New York, says that a modern CT scan will expose a patient to the same amount of radiation as the inhabitants of Hiroshima and Nagasaki were exposed to!

Given what we know about the effects of radiation on breast tissue, it is ironic that the most widely used breast-screening tool, the mammogram, exposes our breasts to ionising radiation! How much of a risk this exposure poses is a question of debate. Dr Samuel Epstein, writing in the *International Journal of Health Services* (2001, 31:3) states that 'each rad of exposure (increased) breast-cancer risk by 1%, resulting in a cumulative 10% increased

Reducing radiation exposure

❋ Question the necessity of X-rays and CT scans on a given occasion. Are they absolutely vital?

❋ Always request that your chest, breasts and abdomen be covered with a lead apron during X-rays — even dental X-rays.

❋ Resist the dentist's suggestion of a dental X-ray at each visit, and save them for when they are absolutely necessary.

❋ Ask what dosage of radiation you will be exposed to. Be very concerned by radiographers who either won't tell you or tell you they don't know. Cancel the procedure and go elsewhere!

❋ Go to specialist radiography centres for procedures involving radiation. They are most likely to have radiation-emitting equipment calibrated regularly and accurately.

risk over ten years of premenopausal screening, usually from the age of 40–50'.

In New Zealand the typical rad exposure during a mammogram is considerably less than that surmised by Epstein, with a typical mammogram (two shots per breast) exposing a woman to a cumulative total of just over 0.2 cGy (rads). Two-yearly mammograms over a decade would give a cumulative exposure of 3.6 cGy per decade. New Zealand code of practice states that a dose of 0.15 cGy per single view should not be exceeded in a mammogram. The more your breasts are squashed between the X-ray plates, the lower will be the dose of radiation!

Taking all the factors into consideration, experts still conclude that the low risk of radiation exposure from mammograms is outweighed by the increased likelihood of early cancer detection. However, common sense suggests that this equation is altered by age, with premenopausal women being at greatest relative risk from radiation exposure, and also having the lowest projected

Measuring radiation

1 Seivert = 100 rads
1 milliSeivert (mSv) = 0.1 rad
1 Grey = 1 Seivert
1 centriGrey (cGy) = 1 rad

Background radiation 0.5 cGy/year (depending on location)
Chest X-ray (1 view) 0.025 cGy
Mammogram (4 views) 0.5 cGy
Full-body CT — breasts 6+ cGy exposure
In terms of breast tissue exposure from mammograms,
    1 Grey equals 1 Seivert

Reproduced with permission from Breast Cancer Network.
Source: Breast Cancer Network NZ (2005) *Upfront* 62, p. 5.

benefit from mammograms (due to their lower absolute risk of developing breast cancer, combined with the increased rate of false-negative results due to denser breast tissue). The combined effect of these two variables is a significant reason for women to seriously consider questioning the widespread recommendation of beginning mammograms at the age of 40. (See discussion under 'The mammogram debate' below.)

Cigarette smoking

We know that cigarettes are packed full of toxic chemicals and carcinogens. We know that these chemicals cause lung cancer, and contribute to our shocking cardiovascular mortality statistics. We also know that these toxic chemicals reach breast tissue and are found in breast milk. Amazingly, we are not so sure about their effect on our breast-cancer risk. A number of significant studies have failed to find any link between active cigarette smoking and increased risk of breast cancer. (Critics suggest that this failure is based more on a lack of high-intensity, long-duration smokers in studies, rather than a true absence of correlation between smoking and breast cancer.) There is compelling evidence, however, that women who are consistently exposed to second-hand smoke ('passive smokers') are at increased risk of breast cancer. So much so that the American EPA concluded that the evidence regarding second-hand smoke and breast cancer is consistent with a 'causal relationship'. The US Surgeon General, in 2006, was slightly less definitive in his findings, concluding that, at this point, 'there is a suggestive but not sufficient' evidence of a link.

In women with a family history of breast or ovarian cancer, cigarette smoking appears to be a major risk factor for breast cancer. In these families, breast-cancer patients' sisters and daughters who smoke are twice as likely to develop breast cancer when compared with the non-smoking sisters or daughters.

Given that we already know about so many devastating health consequences of cigarette smoking, the fact that the correlation between breast cancer and cigarette smoking is still being debated is hardly a reason to start or continue smoking. If you are a smoker, the single most powerful thing you can do to gift yourself a healthier and probably longer life is to give up your habit — *now*.

Use of synthetic hormones

HRT

Do synthetic hormones, such as the oral contraceptive pill and hormone replacement therapy, increase your risk of breast cancer? This question has stimulated controversy and debate for decades. A number of studies have suggested a connection between synthetic hormone use and breast cancer, while others have refuted any such link. Partly this is because both 'the pill' and HRT come in a wide variety of different formulations containing varying amounts of synthetic oestrogen and progestogen; progestogen alone (as the contraceptive mini-pill), or oestrogen alone as oestrogen replacement therapy.

Hormone replacement therapy (HRT) or oestrogen-only replacement therapy (ERT) came quietly onto the pharmaceutical scene during the 1940s. During the 1990s, with the glut of baby-boomers reaching mid-life, the pharmaceutical industry recognised the potential for HRT to become a bestseller.

Marketing campaigns transformed our perception of the mid-life woman into one of a 'diseased' person (suffering from oestrogen deficiency!) and HRT was promoted as a virtual panacea for her hormonal ills. Not only would HRT stop your hot flushes and keep you calm, but it would also keep you slim, wrinkle free and sexually primed . . . according to the glossy pharmaceutical ads. Wyeth, the manufacturers of Prempro and Premarin, was experiencing annual sales of US$3 billion per year until the HRT bubble burst overnight in July 2002.

One arm of the Women's Health Initiative (WHI) trial (see Chapter 5) was stopped prematurely when it became apparent that the risks of HRT use (more heart attacks, strokes, thrombosis and breast cancer) outweighed the benefits (fewer cases of fractures and colon cancer). Panic swept the globe as millions of women the world over abruptly stopped using HRT. The data showed that women who use combined HRT for more than five years face a 26% increased risk of breast cancer, and a 29% increased risk of heart attacks or other coronary events. Equally alarming was the realisation that the greatest risk of coronary events occurred in the first year of HRT use.

The other arm of the study into unopposed oestrogen (instead of combined oestrogen and progestogen HRT) is continuing and has not yet detected an increased risk of breast cancer with oestrogen-only HRT. Only women who have had a hysterectomy can use unopposed oestrogen therapy because of the dramatic increase in the risk of endometrial cancer with HRT.

A follow-up study to the WHI study, published in June 2003, concluded that:

> . . . relatively short-term combined oestrogen plus progestogen use increases incident breast cancers, which are diagnosed at a more advanced stage compared with placebo use, and also substantially increases the percentage of women with abnormal mammograms.

These results suggest oestrogen plus progestogen HRT may stimulate breast-cancer growth and hinder breast-cancer diagnosis. Putting all the stats in perspective, a paper in the *Journal of the American Medical Association* states that:

> the increased risk of oestrogen/progestogen combination means that in 10,000 women taking the drug for a year, there will be 7 more coronary heart disease events, 8 more invasive breast cancers, 8 more strokes and 8 more pulmonary emboli, but 6 fewer colorectal cancers and 5 fewer hip fractures.

Women who go through the menopause at an older age have an increased risk of breast cancer compared with women experiencing menopause when younger.

For every year over the age of 50 that a woman continues menstruating, her breast-cancer risk increases by 1% — which equates to the increased risk associated with HRT. Most of the studies to date have shown that the most significant increase in breast-cancer risk is seen in women who have used hormone replacement therapy for 10 or more years. Using HRT for 5–10 years increases breast-cancer risk by 50%, and 20 years of use doubles your risk of breast cancer (that is, it increases risk by 100%).

Synthetic hormones affect different breasts in different ways. Approximately 3 in 10 women using HRT will have a noticeable increase in the density of their breast tissue. This makes accurate mammographic screening more difficult. It is clear that drinking too much alcohol will increase breast-cancer risk, but the combination of HRT and alcohol may increase risk even more. Two studies have found that if you're on HRT, that delicious little tipple will send your blood oestrogen levels soaring to three times their usual level, suggesting that HRT and alcohol are a risky combination for breast health.

One of the 'gold standard' studies examining the relationship between HRT use and breast health was the 'one million women' study. This English study involved over a million women (average age of 56 at onset of study) registered through National Health Service breast-screening centres. They were each given a comprehensive questionnaire covering a multitude of factors, including HRT use and menstrual history.

The study found that current use, but not past use, of HRT was associated with an increased breast-cancer incidence, and with deaths from breast cancer. Women taking combined HRT over the duration of the study were twice as likely to develop breast cancer compared with women who had never used HRT. Women taking oestrogen-only replacement therapy (ERT) were 30%

more likely to develop cancer. Over a 10-year period, the risk of breast cancer is four times greater in those taking combined HRT compared with those taking the oestrogen-only forms of HRT.

The study also showed that HRT increased the risk of breast cancer much earlier than previously thought, with increased risk evident after only two years of use. However, once women stopped using HRT, their increased risk dropped back to a normal level within 1–5 years. The risk of breast cancer was also seen to increase in direct proportion to the length of time that combined HRT was used. Also worrying was the discovery that women who develop breast cancer while using HRT were more likely to die of their cancer than non-users.

In summary, the researchers stated that the use of HRT (whether oestrogen-only or combined) for 5–10 years from the age of 50 resulted in 1–19 extra cases of breast cancer per 100,000 women. The huge variation in risk reflects the differences in preparations and duration of use of the drug.

Extrapolating the study results to reflect risk to the whole of the United Kingdom population gives a sobering insight into the link between HRT and breast cancer. Study author Valerie Beral points out that '20,000 extra breast-cancer cases in the last decade in the United Kingdom are likely to be attributable to the use of HRT. Of these 15,000 are likely to be linked to the oestrogen–progestogen combination.' Putting this increased risk into perspective, it is interesting to note that during the same time frame, obesity was probably responsible for 50,000 extra breast cancers, and alcohol consumption responsible for at least 16,000 breast cancers in the United Kingdom.

Oral contraceptive pill (OCP)

Do birth-control pills increase a woman's risk of developing breast cancer? There, it's a nice straightforward question . . . with a complicated answer. For a start, when you talk about 'the pill' you're actually referring to a multitude of different drugs containing various combinations and potencies of synthetic hormones. This is part of the reason for the incredible variations in the findings of studies trying to answer this very question. Some studies give a definitive 'yes', while others argue, just as definitively, 'no'.

In 2002 one of the largest studies on oral contraceptive use, the Woman's Lifestyle and Health study, looked at the relationship between the pill and breast cancer. Following a group of more than 100,000 women between the ages of 30 and 49 for eight years, they found that women who had used the pill at any time had an increased risk of 26% compared with women who had never used it. Women who were currently using the oral contraceptive pill had an increased risk of 58% compared with women who had never used the pill. The news was even worse for women over the age of 45 still using the pill. For them, the risk of developing breast cancer rose to 144% that of the risk of never-users. For women under the age of 20 using the pill, or those using the pill before their first pregnancy, there was no increased risk of breast cancer. The increased risk of breast cancer was reduced back to the level of a woman who had never used the pill 10 years after stopping the pill.

Similarly, a National Cancer Institute-sponsored study in 2003 found that the risk of breast cancer was significantly increased for women aged 20 to 34 who had used the pill for at least six months. In women aged over 35, the risk of breast cancer was still elevated, but smaller than for the younger women. A 1996 analysis of 54 different studies, performed by the Collaborative Group on Hormonal Factors in Breast Cancer, found that women currently using the OCP had a slightly higher than usual breast-cancer risk — a risk which remained elevated for 10 years after cessation of the pill. However, in women who had started using the pill before the age of 20, the risk remained permanently elevated.

In direct (and confusing) contrast to these findings, the Women's CARE study suggested that current or former use of the OCP did not elevate breast-cancer risk, regardless of length of use and dose of oestrogen, and whether or not they began using the pill before the age of 20.

Are you confused? You should be. The bottom line is that researchers still can't agree on whether or not the pill increases breast-cancer risk. What we do know is that the OCP contains synthetic oestrogen, and exposure to any kind of synthetic oestrogen (within the body or in the environment) has the potential to act as a carcinogen. If you choose to use the OCP, try to use it for the minimum time possible; have regular pill-free breaks (between relationships, for example); and use another form of contraception over the age of 45.

Fertility drugs

The trend towards delaying pregnancy until later in life is one of the most pronounced sociological phenomena of our time. Once upon a time a woman's *raison d'être* was to marry young and start a family. In contrast, modern Western women often want it all: an education, career, travel, and then eventually a family. While there is nothing intrinsically wrong with this desire to fulfil themselves in ways other than childbirth, the stark reality is that later in life pregnancy can be more difficult to come by. After the age of 30 there is a significant decline in female fertility, with an even more significant decline after the age of 35. Consequently, infertility has become a modern plague, and along with it there is an increasing reliance on high-tech intervention to achieve conception.

Invariably this intervention involves the use of synthetic hormonal drugs. What impact do these hormonal drugs have on a woman's breast-cancer risk? It's a valid and worrying question, but one to which we still don't have a definite answer. As is so often the case with these big hormonal questions, despite the existence of a number of well-designed studies looking into the link between fertility drugs and breast-cancer risk, results are conflicting, and we are as yet unable to confirm that fertility drugs will not increase your risk of breast cancer.

Antibiotics and breast cancer

Is it possible that using antibiotics could increase our risk of breast cancer? Shockingly, a study published in the *Journal of the American Medical Association* suggests the answer is 'yes'. The significant study involved 10,000 women observed for 17 years. Women who used antibiotics 25 times or more in that 17-year period doubled their risk of breast cancer compared with women who had never used the drugs. The greater the use of antibiotics, the greater the risk of breast cancer.

The most probable explanation for this correlation involves the detrimental effect that antibiotics have on the friendly bacteria living in the gut. Broad-spectrum antibiotics decimate the populations of these vital bacteria, which are involved in the breakdown of oestrogens and carcinogens passing through the gut. Low populations of these friendly bacteria in theory lead to higher levels of oestrogen passing back into the bloodstream and circulating through the body. These same bacteria are also essential for the utilisation of beneficial phyto-oestrogens consumed in the diet.

If you are taking a course of antibiotics, it is always advisable also to take a high-potency probiotic formula for a period of 4–6 weeks. This is to replace friendly gut bacteria and hopefully reduce the possibility of antibiotic use increasing breast-cancer risk.

Light exposure and melatonin

Is it possible that sleeping at night in a room that is poorly darkened could increase your risk of breast cancer? Strange as it sounds, there is evidence to suggest that women who sleep in a room in which there is even low-level light (from curtains not closed properly, or a hall light seeping under the bedroom door) are at increased risk of breast cancer. The hormone melatonin, made by the pineal gland deep inside the brain, is the link. Melatonin is only secreted at night and is important for regulating our body clock, as well as influencing the regulation of several hormones — including oestrogen. Laboratory studies have also revealed that melatonin suppresses the growth of human breast-cancer cells. These effects could explain the phenomenon of significantly increased breast-cancer rates amongst female night-shift workers. The light/melatonin connection has been suggested as being partly responsible for the fact that industrialised nations, with their widespread use of electric light both day and night, have breast-cancer rates approximately five times higher than those of underdeveloped countries. While more research is warranted, the precautionary principle would suggest it best to:

* ensure you sleep in a very dark room at night

* sleep for at least seven hours a night.

Xeno-oestrogens and environmental pollutants

Until we have a more complete understanding of pesticide toxicity, the benefit of the doubt should be awarded to protecting the environment, the worker and the consumer — this precautionary approach is necessary because the data on risk to human health from exposure to pesticides are incomplete.

British Medical Association

In a world so strongly focused on early detection of breast cancer through screening, the contribution of our toxic environment to the development of this disease is shockingly under-emphasised. Billions of dollars of research money are poured into drug development and increasingly sophisticated diagnostic and treatment technology in an attempt to achieve earlier and earlier detection of breast cancers — rather than being spent on measures aimed at preventing the development of breast cancer itself. Governments the planet over appear loath to instigate legislation to protect women from the myriad of chemicals which many suspect play a significant role in the development of breast cancer. This despite a large body of evidence which strongly suggests that exposure to a wide range of synthetic chemicals must be considered a powerful contributing factor in the rapid and widespread increase in breast-cancer incidence in the past 60 years — a time frame closely aligned with the explosive growth in the petrochemical and agrochemical industries.

Organisations pressing for tighter controls and legislation banning such chemicals are rebuffed with the standard argument that the toxicology of the chemicals must first be proven beyond reasonable doubt. As you read on, you'll see why this is a nearly impossible requirement. Instead, many women's advocacy groups are now promoting the adoption of the precautionary principle. Invoking the 'precautionary principle' means that chemicals would be restricted or banned based on *evidence* of harm rather than on *proof* of harm. Because of the complex interaction between multiple chemical exposures, time of exposure and genetic heritage, absolute proof of harm by a chemical is nearly impossible to establish.

We live, eat, breathe and reproduce in a planet soaked in a toxic soup of synthetic chemicals. In the USA alone, an estimated 85,000 of these chemicals are registered for use, with an additional 2000 new compounds coming into use each year. The vast majority of these chemicals have never been tested for their effect on human beings. Once we ingest, inhale or absorb them, most of these chemicals remain in our bodies, stored in our fat cells (of which breast tissue is largely composed). This is one of the most worrying aspects of exposure to endocrine-disrupting chemicals — that once we take them into our body, our body cannot break them down readily, and they are stored in our fat cells (such as those of breast tissue) for many years. Thus we are exposed to low-level, long-term exposure. The resulting chronic hormone exposure is unprecedented in human history. The potency of these chemicals to produce an oestrogenic effect in the human body is huge. Bisphenol-A is a by-product of polycarbonate plastic production. As little as two parts per billion of this oestrogenic chemical has been shown to produce an oestrogenic effect in laboratory animals.

The American National Toxicology Program has identified 42 different synthetic chemicals that are known to cause breast cancer in rats. Other research groups have added another 160 chemicals to this list of 'known mammary carcinogens'. These are chemicals to which we are regularly exposed. Add to this list of known carcinogens the 500-plus chemicals which have been shown to exert an oestrogenic effect in the human body, and it's not hard to see the potentially destructive effect of environmental toxins in the development of breast cancer.

Synthetic chemicals have the potential to increase breast-cancer risk in a number of different ways. First, they may mimic the effects of oestrogens in the human body. They may also act as a direct carcinogen, stimulating the development of cancerous cells in the breast. Depending on time of exposure, many of these chemicals are also thought to adversely affect the development of breasts, and increase long-term susceptibility to breast cancer.

Even those chemicals which have been tested and declared not to be a hazard to human health cannot be declared benign with certainty. Chemical compounds are tested in isolation, usually in high doses over short periods. However, in the real world we are exposed to multiple compounds over long periods. This method of testing completely ignores the fact that the combinations of multiple chemicals we endure in the real world can and do produce completely different toxic effects from those encountered in the arbitrary, isolated testing of the laboratory. We now know that multiple oestrogenic chemicals can act together to produce an effect even when each individual component of the mixture is below a threshold for effect.

In-vitro studies (test-tube studies rather than studies in the human body) demonstrate this phenomenon clearly. Oestrogen-sensitive breast cells individually exposed to small amounts of 10 different oestrogenic chemicals show no significant cell growth. However, when the breast cells are exposed to the same chemicals, this time in combination, the cells show a pronounced increase in growth, and therefore cancer risk. There is also the danger inherent in extrapolating the results of animal or test-tube toxicity studies to human beings. Testing a chemical on an animal or in a test tube does not necessarily reflect the effect it will have on a human being. Chemical toxicity testing also fails to take into account individual differences in our susceptibility to harm from chemicals, based on our unique genetic heritage.

So-called 'body burden' studies test blood, urine, body fat or breast milk to determine the number and type of chemical residues we carry in our body. USA studies show that Americans of all ages now carry an average of 116 different synthetic chemicals in their body . . . some of which have been banned for more than 20 years because of their acknowledged toxicity. Closer to home, Australian research has demonstrated that babies are born already toxified by a veritable witches' brew of potential endocrine-disrupting chemicals. In 2000 an Australian study (Townsville) tested the first bowel discharges of infants in the area. The researchers found lindane in 78% of samples, PCP in 43%, chlorpyrifos in 59%, malathion in 34%, chlordane in 16%, DDT in 52% and PCB in 27% of samples.

Every one of these chemicals, passed on from the mother to her unborn infant, has been associated with promoting cancers, or affecting the endocrine, brain, and immune systems of the unborn. These are the same chemicals that are routinely found in the food analysis performed on the diet of New Zealanders. While proof of the effects of exposure to these endocrine-disrupting chemicals *in utero* is limited, we have enough evidence to suggest we should be very worried. Studies have shown that dioxin, atrazine and bisphenol-A (found in plastic food containers, baby bottles and tin can linings) all affect the development of the breasts, and exposure to a mixture of common organochlorines such as DDT and PCBs has been shown to increase the susceptibility to chemically induced breast cancers.

In New Zealand we continue to use some agrochemicals that

have long been banned in other countries. Endosulfan is one such, banned in 20 countries because of its link with breast cancer, its persistence in the environment, and its ability to act as an endocrine disruptor.

While simply detecting the presence of a chemical does not necessarily prove a link between that chemical and breast cancer, combined with the evidence we already have it should give us a major wake-up call. Mary Wolf PhD from the Mount Sinai School of Medicine, New York, discovered a strong link between blood levels of DDT and PCBs and the likelihood that a woman would go on to develop breast cancer. Using a sample of 14,000 women, she found that the women with high blood levels of DDE (a breakdown product of DDT) had four times the risk of developing breast cancer of women with low levels of the chemical.

A 2003 study reported in the *Occupational Environmental Medicine Journal* found that women with breast cancer are more than five times as likely as their healthy peers to have measurable serum levels of DDT and HCB. By analysing a group of 159 women with breast cancer and 200 healthy women, Belgian researchers found that breast-cancer patients were 5.6 times and 9.14 times more likely to have measurable levels of DDT and HCB, respectively. In New Zealand, a study sponsored by the New Zealand Department of Health in the late 1980s found significant levels of DDE (the breakdown product of DDT) in the breast milk of New Zealand women.

Israeli experience also demonstrates a link between two common organochlorine pesticides (lindane and benzene hexachloride, BHC) and breast cancer. In the 1970s, the Israeli breast-cancer rate was double that of other countries with comparable diets and lifestyle, and was rising. Israeli women were also found to have incredibly high levels of the organochlorine pesticide BHC in their breast milk — levels that were 800 times those detected in the breast milk of women in the USA. In 1978, as a result of public outcry, the organochlorines DDT, BHC and lindane were banned from use in Israel. Over the following 20 years, the Israeli breast-cancer anomaly disappeared, and Israel became the only industrialised nation with a falling rate of breast cancer.

It is widely acknowledged that synthetic hormones such as HRT and the oral contraceptive pill, and even naturally occurring phytochemicals such as phyto-oestrogens, can alter a woman's breast-cancer risk. Despite this acknowledgement, controversy still exists over the part played by exposure to environmental chemicals with an oestrogenic effect (known as *xeno-oestrogens,* meaning 'foreign oestrogens').

Xeno-oestrogens can cause havoc in the human body in a variety of ways. They can plug into the oestrogen receptors on cells, allowing them to mimic the stimulatory effect of oestrogens, prompting breast cells to multiply and grow. Just like oestrogens, xeno-oestrogens can also prompt the body to release tumour growth factor, again stimulating the growth of cancer cells. Lastly, these synthetic oestrogens can actually increase the number of oestrogen receptors in the body, making cells more susceptible to stimulation by oestrogen. As if that's not alarming enough, we also know that these potentially cancer-causing effects are compounded when we are exposed to xeno-oestrogens in combination, such as occurs in everyday living.

Xeno-oestrogens are everywhere. Common sources of exposure include:

* pesticides such as dieldrin (discontinued but still in our environment), and atrazine (the most widely used pesticide in the USA)

* plastic additives such as bisphenol-A (BPA), polyvinyl chloride (PVC)

* benzene (a petrol additive)

* phthalates (found in plastics, cosmetics, personal care products, deodorants and fragrances)

* parabens (preservatives used in food, personal care products and make-up)

* petrol additives

* chlorine compounds used to bleach paper

* solvents such as methylene chloride (used in spray paint and paint removers)

* insecticides such as methoxychlor, endosulfan and lindane (widely used in nit treatments)

* sunscreen lotions — many contain chemicals with an oestrogenic activity

* non-stick coatings in cookware.

Organochlorines including DDT, DDE and PBCs stand out as especially troublesome environmental contaminants when it comes to breast-cancer development. Each of these chemicals is an endocrine disruptor, with the ability to cause female hormonal imbalance. Organochlorines mimic oestrogen and produce an oestrogenic effect in the human body. Chemicals belonging to the organochlorines group include pesticides such as DDT and dieldrin, triazine herbicides and industrial chemicals such as PCBs and dioxin. Many of these chemicals have been proven to cause breast cancers in rats.

While the use of some of these organochlorines was discontinued years ago, they are still present in our environment and in the fat and breast milk in our bodies. If you eat fish, dairy products and meat, you can guarantee that you are exposed to organochlorines at your own dinner table.

Proving definitively that there is a cause-and-effect relationship between our exposure to these chemicals and subsequent breast-cancer risk continues to be difficult, with numerous studies suggesting that such a relationship does exist . . . and numerous others failing to find evidence of any such relationship. Often these studies measure the degree of contaminants in a woman's body at the time of her breast-cancer diagnosis, and fail to consider effects of the mixture of chemicals she has been exposed to, or the degree of exposure to chemicals in the years preceding diagnosis.

The difficulty in establishing the degree of risk with exposure to environmental pollutants is partly due to the fact that not everyone who is exposed to a carcinogen or endocrine disruptor will go on to develop cancer. More usually, cancer develops with multiple exposures over time. Where once the dose of exposure was considered to be of greatest significance, it is now apparent that the timing of those exposures is a major determinant in their potential for negative impact. For example, exposure *in utero* may have a greater impact than exposure during postmenopausal years. It has been repeatedly shown that when a foetus is exposed to endocrine-disrupting chemicals (such as those mentioned above) *in utero*, the hormonal 'soup' he or she is growing in is altered, affecting the development of reproductive organs and potentially increasing predisposition to cancer development in adulthood.

Critics argue that the hormonal potency of endocrine-disrupting chemicals is much lower than the potency of the oestrogen we produce in our own body. Increasingly though, there is evidence that when exposure to these chemicals occurs at times when our own endogenous oestrogen production is low and our tissue sensitivity to oestrogen is very high (*in utero*, during pre-puberty and following menopause), the chemicals' potential for causing hormonal havoc is greatly increased. Mice studies in which foetuses were exposed to the common chemical bisphenol-A (found in many plastics) found that breast development was changed in ways that are associated with the development of breast cancer in rodents and humans. Along with timing, the other important variables include the duration and pattern of exposure. Maximum vulnerability to endocrine-disrupting chemicals appears to occur with exposure before birth (*in utero*), in the pre-pubertal and adolescent years, and the years through to a woman's first full-term pregnancy.

New Zealand prides itself on its international reputation as a 'clean, green haven', but living on our idyllic shores is certainly no guarantee of protection from cancer-causing environmental toxins. There is little research performed here to gauge the exact exposure of the average New Zealander to organochlorines and endocrine-disrupting chemicals. The New Zealand environment is poisoned with a multitude of these chemicals, and based on overseas studies we can be certain that they have found their way into the body of virtually every man, woman and child living here. In much the same way that we see a star burning in the

Chemicals with carcinogenic potential

We are exposed to chemicals with the potential to increase the incidence of breast cancer through:

* cigarette smoke

* pesticides

* industrial emissions

* car fumes

* pesticides

* plastics in the home, including food containers, baby bottles

* household cleaners and detergents

* personal care products

* soft furnishings

* building materials

* dry-cleaning chemicals

* solvents.

night sky long after its death, the potentially devastating legacy of chemical contamination lingers long after a chemical ceases to be used. Thus, the generation of New Zealanders alive today still reaps the sinister repercussions of banned chemicals such as DDT, dieldrin and PCBs.

We are also continually exposed to a wide range of known carcinogens and endocrine-disruptors that are still freely used today in New Zealand. The herbicide atrazine, banned in Europe, is still used in New Zealand crop production despite its known effects as a breast-cancer causing carcinogen and endocrine disruptor. 2,4-D is another commonly used herbicide and endocrine disruptor, and it is often applied through aerial spraying (which means uncontrollable spray drift).

> Because total oestrogen exposure is the single most important risk factor for breast cancer, oestrogenic chemicals, which would add to lifelong exposure, are an obvious suspect when searching for the cause of rising rates (of breast cancer) over the past half century.
>
> Dr Theo Colburn,
> Endocrine Disruptor Exchange (USA)

> The most alarming of all man's assaults upon the environment is the contamination of air, earth, rivers and sea with dangerous and even lethal materials. This pollution is for the most part irrecoverable; the chain of evil it initiates not only in the world that must support life but in living tissues is for the most part irreversible. In this now universal contamination of the environment, chemicals are the sinister and little recognised partners of radiation in changing the very nature of the world — the very nature of life itself.
>
> Rachel Carson, *Silent Spring*

How to minimise your exposure to synthetic chemicals that may increase breast-cancer risk

✳ Choose organic foods whenever possible. If you cannot get organic produce, at least avoid those foods with the highest levels of pesticide residues, including strawberries, bell peppers, spinach, cherries, peaches, celery, apples, apricots, green beans, cucumbers.

✳ If you can only afford to buy limited organic products, ensure that these include dairy products, eggs and meat.

✳ Avoid using pesticides and herbicides in your home and garden.

✳ Avoid organochlorine exposure by using non-bleached sanitary products, toilet paper and coffee filters. Avoid the use of bleach in your home, using hydrogen peroxide instead.

✳ Use safety-conscious personal care products and make-up. Ensure that your products do not contain phthalates or parabens. Don't be fooled by labels with words such as 'organic', 'natural', 'hypoallergenic', 'animal cruelty free' or 'fragrance free'. The products thus labelled may be all of these things, but might nonetheless still contain chemical nasties.

✳ Choose fragrance-free products. Many fragrances contain phthalates which are powerful endocrine disruptors.

✳ Avoid antiperspirants containing aluminium (the majority of commercial formulas). Instead use a deodorant which does not contain aluminium, and will stop odour without preventing perspiration.

* Avoid sunscreen lotions containing chemicals with oestrogenic activity: BP-3; homosalate; 3-(4-methylbenzylidene) camphor; octyl-dimethyl-p-aminobenzoic acid; octyl-methoxycinnamate.

* Dry-clean clothes only if essential, and hang them outside overnight to air before putting them back in your wardrobe.

* Avoid use of plastics in your home whenever possible. Wrap food in brown paper or waxed paper before (or instead of) cling film; store foods in glass, metal or ceramic containers; avoid plastic hot water jugs; never place food in a plastic container to be heated in a microwave oven; never re-use plastic water bottles. Bisphenol-A is found in all polycarbonate plastics (baby bottles, tin can linings, dental sealants, re-usable water bottles and plastic food containers). Bisphenol-A leaches from plastic into food and water, even when the plastic is intact and undamaged.

* Avoid cookware with non-stick coatings. Instead use stainless steel, glass or ceramic cookware.

* Avoid insect sprays in the home unless they are made from natural pyrethrin, derived from chrysanthemums. Fly sprays usually contain synthetic pyrethroids which are fat soluble and a suspected xeno-oestrogen (that is, a synthetic substance having an oestrogenic effect in the body).

Pesticides in New Zealand

The New Zealand Total Diet Survey (NZTDS) periodically analyses pesticide residues in New Zealand foods. In 2000, the survey made the following findings.

* Young New Zealand children are getting approximately five times more pesticide residues in their average diet than equivalent American children.

* Young adolescents around the age of 13 are consuming more pesticide residues than other age groups. This should be of concern, as early puberty is recognised as a time of increased risk from pesticide exposure, in terms of long-term breast-cancer risk.

* The percentage of total samples with pesticide residues is significantly greater than is the case in some other countries, including the United Kingdom and the United States.

* Wine, grains and meat were the food groups most likely to contain pesticide residues.

* Eight endocrine-disrupting chemicals were found in foods tested.

* More than 60% of fruit and vegetable samples were found to contain a fungicide known to have an endocrine-disrupting effect when broken down in the body.

* Organochlorine levels continue to fall but still equate to USA levels found in the late 1980s.

* DDT is the main contaminant found in New Zealand dairy products. New Zealand's rate of contamination is 68% compared with a rate of 3.4% in the USA.

Understanding the paraben debate

Parabens are synthetic preservatives listed on your personal care products as butylparaben, propylparaben, methylparaben and ethylparaben. They are the most commonly used preservative in cosmetics and personal care products, and 90% of personal care products contain them. Traditionally revered for their low allergenicity and effectiveness in preventing the spoiling of products, parabens have come in for a mountain of bad press linked to their potential effects as endocrine disruptors.

Rat and test-tube studies have shown parabens to have a weakly oestrogenic effect. All of the oestrogen-sensitive cells in the human body have 'keyholes' (receptor sites) into which slot oestrogen molecules produced in the body. The problem with parabens is that they are able to slot into these same 'keyholes', stimulating an oestrogenic response in the cell. As yet it is unclear just how much of a problem this is in terms of breast health, and the question of paraben safety remains largely unanswered.

In 2002 the results of a study in which parabens had been administered to rats orally, and by injection, appeared in the *Journal of Steroid Biochemistry and Molecular Biology*. The results showed that oestrogenic effects on cells occurred in a way that could potentially cause problems with the proliferation of cancerous breast cells. The oestrogenic effects of parabens is greatest in butylparaben, and then, in descending order, in propylparaben, ethylparaben, and methylparaben.

More recently, alarm bells have been sounding again with the discovery of unchanged parabens in breast-tumour samples taken from 20 patients. While this sounds disturbing (and may well turn out to be indicative of an association between parabens and breast cancer), all we know at the moment is that parabens can be found in breast tumours. We still do not know whether that is a coincidental finding, or whether there is a correlation between parabens and breast-cancer development.

The American regulatory agency FDA is concerned enough

about the paraben issue to be conducting its own extensive research. With our current knowledge it cannot be definitively proven that parabens are a health hazard, but they certainly are under the microscope and warrant serious investigation. The main problem in stating degree of toxicity (or lack of toxicity) is that there are no studies investigating the effect of exposure to a daily low dose of paraben over a period of years, such as occurs with normal use of cosmetics and personal care products.

Until more is understood about the effect of parabens in the body, it is advisable to use paraben-free personal care products as much as possible.

A sedentary lifestyle

Everyone knows that we need to exercise regularly in order to stay well and avoid the major killers of obesity, heart disease, and diabetes. Not so many people know that this same exercise will help to reduce our risk of a number of common cancers, including breast and prostate cancer. While there have been some conflicting studies, there is enough convincing evidence to suggest strongly that regular aerobic exercise is an important part of any breast-cancer prevention or recovery programme.

Exercise is thought to reduce breast-cancer risk in several different ways. Teenage girls who exercise regularly tend to start menstruating later than their sedentary peers, and age at menarche is an established risk factor for breast cancer. The earlier a girl begins menstruating, the greater is her total lifetime exposure to oestrogen, and consequently her breast-cancer risk. A few studies have also suggested that regular exercise may lower a woman's oestrogen levels, thus reducing her risk of breast cancer. Exercise also helps to minimise weight gain with ageing; and adult weight gain, and being overweight as an adult, are both risk factors for postmenopausal breast cancer. Exercise also stimulates the immune system in ways which may enhance the body's ability to detect and destroy cancer cells.

What remains unclear is whether exercise is more beneficial for breast-cancer prevention, during adolescence, during adulthood or throughout a woman's entire life. That having been said, there is some valid evidence that teenage girls who are physically active have a lower incidence of breast cancer later in life, when compared with their sedentary peers. In 2004 the *European Journal of Cancer Prevention* published a review of research investigating the link between exercise and breast-cancer rates in teenagers and young adults. It found that the most physically active women reduced their breast-cancer risk by 20% compared with their more sedentary peers.

The study authors said that for every hour of exercise performed by an adolescent each week, her risk of breast cancer declined by 3%.

Studies examining the exercise/breast-cancer link in older women have predominantly produced similar results. One such large study involving 74,000 women between the ages of 50 and 79 was published in the *Journal of the American Medical Association* in 2003. In response to their results, study authors concluded that:

> increased physical activity is associated with reduced risk for breast cancer in postmenopausal women, longer duration provides most benefit, and that such activity need not be strenuous.

Similar good news for postmenopausal exercisers came in a large study looking at the association between exercise and breast-cancer risk. It found that women with the greatest leisure time activity had a nearly 40% reduced risk of breast cancer, and that the risk reduction was greatest for premenopausal women, especially under the age of 45. The lowest risk was found in lean women who exercised for more than four hours a week.

So how much exercise do you need for breast health? To reap significant cancer-protective benefits, aim to do four or more hours of aerobic exercise a week. Women who exercise this much during their reproductive years are shown to reduce their risk of breast cancer by up to a massive 58%. Brisk walking, jogging, cycling, playing racquet sports, swimming and working out on the cardio machines at the gym all qualify as aerobic activity.

It's also worth noting that even if you have had breast cancer and are in recovery, the benefits of exercising remain convincing, despite the fact that in reality most women with a breast-cancer diagnosis decrease their level of physical activity by an average of two hours per week. Almost all studies show beneficial effects of exercise in women with breast cancer both during and after cancer treatment. Women with breast cancer who exercise regularly report improved body image and self-esteem, reduced nausea during chemotherapy, and fewer problems with depression, fatigue and insomnia. Postmenopausal women who are overweight increase their breast-cancer risk, partly due to the oestrogen-producing properties of fat. Similarly, women who have had breast cancer increase their chances of survival through weight loss and weight control, a vital component of which is regular exercise.

Obesity

It's no surprise that obesity increases the likelihood that you will one day join the cardiovascular disease or diabetes statistics. The connection between obesity and cancer is less widely discussed, especially the link between overweight and breast or prostate cancer. In the case of breast cancer, there is a connection between obesity, body shape and breast-cancer risk. . . but the connection is changeable depending on your age. If you are a heavy premenopausal woman (weighing more than 79 kg), your risk of breast cancer is reduced compared with that of your slimmer peers! However, once you hit menopause, if the weight comes with you, then your breast-cancer risk escalates compared with slimmer postmenopausal women (those weighing less than 59 kg). Interestingly, not all fat is equal in terms of its cancer-promoting effects in postmenopausal women. Carrying extra kilos on the abdomen, as opposed to having the fat slung around your hips and bottom, is the most dangerous in terms of risk for both breast cancer and heart disease.

The fat which is deposited around the abdomen is almost like an endocrine (hormone-secreting) gland, in the sense that it is 'active' fat, producing a variety of different substances called *cytokines* that have hormone-like functions. At least six of these cytokines promote the process by which cancer cells develop a blood supply of their own, to grow and spread (angiogenesis).

There are several confusing findings in the search to understand the relationship between weight and breast cancer. For example, girls who are heaviest at age 10 appear to have lower breast-cancer rates later in life, compared with thinner girls.

Picture the following common scenario. Beautiful, slim young woman marries, begins producing children and gaining weight, and gaining weight and gaining weight. If she gains 20 kg between the age of 18 and menopause, her breast-cancer risk doubles compared with the slim young woman who manages to stay slim right through to her menopausal years. Time for some more confusion! A woman who gains weight through her thirties and forties (a common scenario) reduces her risk of premenopausal breast cancer, even though her risk of breast cancer after menopause is increased.

The explanation for this seeming anomaly is not clear, although it most probably has something to do with oestrogen and its connection with body fat. We know that the more oestrogen you are exposed to over a lifetime, the greater your risk of both pre- and postmenopausal breast cancer. Before menopause, overweight women have lower levels of oestrogen than their skinnier peers, and consequently also have a lower risk of breast cancer. After menopause, the ovaries radically reduce their production of oestrogen. Oestrogen is, however, produced in the body's fat cells, so postmenopausal women who are overweight tend to have higher oestrogen levels than thinner postmenopausal women, and consequently a greater breast-cancer risk.

Another common female scenario is the never ending 'see-sawing' of weight, with bursts of good-intentioned weight loss followed by a return to the old ways and a gradual creeping back of weight. What's the effect of this on your risk of breast cancer? So far, we don't know the answer. Your weight at the time of a breast-cancer diagnosis also appears to influence survival. Women with a higher body mass index (that is, weight : height ratio) who carry most of their extra fat on the abdomen, have generally been shown to have decreased survival rates.

While common sense suggests that if you are overweight when you are diagnosed with breast cancer, it is a good idea to lose weight, more studies are needed to confirm exactly how weight loss or gain after diagnosis will affect your survival rates.

Diet and breast cancer

Can a poor diet, on its own, cause the development of breast cancer? Almost certainly not. Can a diet aimed at reducing cancer risk be guaranteed to prevent the development of breast cancer? Again, the answer is 'no'. Not even the most ideal of diets can offer an absolute guarantee of protection against breast cancer. While the answer is 'no' in both these extreme scenarios, there is ever-increasing evidence that how we choose to nourish our body can play a significant part in the prevention of breast cancer. As this is a complex disease in which many factors play a role, good nutrition alone will not be a panacea. It is, however, an extremely important part of a multi-faceted approach to preventing breast cancer.

Epidemiological studies which compare rates of breast cancer in different countries around the world consistently show that women consuming a typical Western diet have an increased incidence of breast cancer compared with women consuming an Asian, Mediterranean, or vegetarian diet. When Japanese women (who traditionally have a very low risk of breast cancer) move to Western countries and adopt a Western diet, their breast-cancer risk increases to Western rates, within one generation.

Diets offering protection against breast cancer

Vegetarian, Asian and Mediterranean diets all appear to confer some protection against breast cancer.

Vegetarian diet

* lower levels of animal fats and the endocrine-disrupting chemicals which are stored in animal fat

* high fruit and vegetable intake

* high fibre intake

* vegetarian women have lower levels of toxic oestrogen metabolites compared with meat eaters

Asian diet

* low in fat and largely vegetarian

* high in phyto-oestrogens from soya, beans, kelp

* high in green tea

* low in simple carbohydrates and sugars

* no or low dairy products

Mediterranean

* limited meat and dairy

* high in fruits and vegetables, whole grains, seafood, flax and olive oil

* high in fats, but these are the breast-protective omega-3 and omega-9 fats

* high in fibre

The relationship between nutrition and disease is complex, especially when it comes to understanding how our food affects our risk of chronic illness such as cancer, and there is still much to be understood.

It's true that we don't yet have answers to many of the questions about the relationship between breast cancer and nutrition, and there is a need for ongoing research. Still, there is enough that we do know — or strongly suspect — to create useful dietary guidelines for breast-cancer reduction. Working with the 'precautionary principle' these guidelines are, in some instances, based on evidence of risk or benefit, rather than on absolute proof.

> The more we know about cancer, the more it's clear that diet is related to cancer, but the relationship is complex. Diet and cardiovascular disease is simple compared to diet and cancer because the risk factors differ for different cancers.
>
> Dr Alan Kristal
> Fred Hutchinson Cancer Research Centre

> Diet is one of the most important lifestyle factors and has been estimated to account for up to 80% of cancers of the colon, breast and prostate.
>
> Trevor Smith
> Auckland breast surgeon

The breast health diet

Green for go, go, go

In a word, if it's green and it's a vegetable, it's good for you and your breasts. Vegetables and fruit (organic if possible) are a vital element of a breast-healthy diet. Forget the 'five-plus a day' mantra, striving instead to eat nine delicious servings of a wide range of fruits and vegetables daily. It's really not as daunting as it sounds. Try having fresh fruit on your muesli or porridge in the morning; snack on fruit for morning and afternoon tea; make a huge and varied salad at lunch time; and serve a salad or three different vegetables with dinner every night. Invest in a quality juicer and experiment with different juices as 'pick me ups' throughout the day.

Fruits and vegetables help to keep breasts healthy in a number of ways. They are by far the richest source of dietary antioxidants and phytochemicals, helping to protect breast cells from the damaging effects of unstable molecules called free-radicals. Our own body creates free-radicals as a by-product of the never-ending cellular energy production cycle. Stress increases free-radical production, as does cigarette smoking, consumption of rancid fats, and exposure to environmental pollutants and ultraviolet light. Free-radicals are constantly bombarding the fatty cellular membranes surrounding every cell, and the DNA of every cell in the body. This causes cellular destruction, or alteration of the DNA codes within a cell, and can lead to the development of cancer, premature ageing and chronic disease.

While all fruits and vegetables contain antioxidants, there are some which deserve special accolades. These include all berries (especially blueberries); dark green vegetables (spinach, silverbeet, broccoli, bok choy); and bright red and orange fruits and vegetables (carrots, yams, kumara, pumpkin, red peppers, apricots, plums, tomatoes). Fruits and vegetables supply antioxidant nutrients such as beta-carotene (and a whole range of other carotenes), selenium, and vitamin C, CoQ_{10} and lipoic acid; and a huge array of phytochemicals with powerful antioxidant properties such as lycopene, resveratrol, flavanols and flavones. There is an established link between a high dietary intake of these antioxidants and a reduced risk of breast cancer and a variety of other cancers.

Interestingly, while a high intake of fruits and vegetables correlates with decreased breast-cancer risk in premenopausal women, swallowing handfuls of antioxidant supplements containing vitamins A, C and E, selenium and zinc has not been found to offer the same benefits. Don't delude yourself into thinking that you'll be okay if you're eating a rubbish diet and popping nutritional supplements to compensate! The living 'green foods' contain a complex array of vital phytochemicals, with powerful cancer-fighting properties, which are generally missing from most nutritional supplements. These phytochemicals (the word simply means plant-based chemicals) have powerful antioxidant properties which help safeguard the DNA in our cells from damage by free-radicals. Some also protect the process of methylation which is critical for the activation of cancer-suppressing genes. Yet others stimulate our own immunity and block the growth of abnormal cells which can eventually become a cancer.

Besides supplying essential nutrients and antioxidants, fruits and vegetables offer breast protection in other ways too. They are a rich source of green chlorophyll which helps support the body in the detoxification of the environmental chemicals we are exposed to.

Some phytochemicals help protect us from the acceleration of cell production stimulated by oestrogen. Oestrogen is a vital hormone essential for our health throughout our life. Contrary to common belief, we continue to produce and need oestrogen even after we have passed through menopause. There are several different forms of oestrogen in the female body — some are potentially troublesome in terms of stimulating breast tumours, while others have the ability to actually protect us from breast cancers. The relative balance between 'friendly' and 'unfriendly' oestrogen in our body is partly determined by how our body metabolises, breaks down and excretes oestrogen. Some plant compounds actually help to change potentially harmful oestrogen into beneficial forms of oestrogen.

The brassica family of vegetables (commonly called cruciferous vegetables) are especially useful for enhancing this process. The brassica group includes: broccoli (which is especially beneficial),

Maximising breast protection by eating fruit and vegetables

✳ Buy fruits and vegetables in small amounts regularly, to avoid lengthy storage and loss of vital nutrients.

✳ Eat raw fruits and vegetables as well as cooked ones.

✳ Steam vegetables or stir-fry them lightly to avoid nutrient degradation.

✳ Chop vegetables just before cooking: nutrient break-down is more rapid once vegetables have been chopped.

✳ Aim to eat 9 servings of fruits and vegetables every day.

✳ Eat a generous serving of dark green, leafy vegetables every day.

✳ Eat brassica vegetables such as broccoli, cauliflower, Brussels sprouts and cabbage daily. Cruciferous vegetables should be lightly cooked and thoroughly chewed to maximise their cancer-preventing benefits. Avoid boiling cruciferous vegetables (or any others) as this destroys up to 80% of their cancer-fighting phytochemicals.

✳ Keep the freezer well stocked with free-flow bags of berries such as blueberries, boysenberries, and raspberries. Add a daily serve of berries to breakfast, or mix with *acidophilus* yoghurt for a healthy snack. Frozen berries are delicious on a hot summer day — simply pour out a cupful and crunch while frozen.

✳ Boost chlorophyll intake by drinking barley greens, wheat grass or chlorella and adding a teaspoon of spirulina to smoothies or juices.

Brussels sprouts, cabbage and cauliflower. Of these, broccoli and Brussels sprouts are considered to be cancer-fighting superheroes, closely followed by cabbage. These vegetables (especially broccoli) contain a chemical called indole-3-carbinol or I3C. This chemical helps to convert the potentially troublesome 'strong' oestrogens (known as 4- and 16-oestrogens) into the benign, and even protective, 2-oestrogens. In some ways, I3C could almost

Antioxidant superfoods

Colourful fruits and vegetables are especially rich in antioxidants if they are coloured all the way through, not just on the skin. Examples are berries and tree tomatoes. The following foods are especially rich antioxidant sources:

* dark green leafy vegetables (spinach, silverbeet, broccoli, bok choy)

* dark red or orange fruits and vegetables (peppers, tree tomatoes, apricots, carrots, yams, pumpkin, kumara)

* all berries, but especially blueberries; cherries; black grapes

* fruit juices, especially blackcurrant, grape, cranberry and apricot juice

* prunes and raisins

* garlic and onions

* green tea and black tea

* dark chocolate — 70% cocoa content (while this is a delicious and useful antioxidant source, remember that it packs a significant calorie punch too!)

* herbs and spices, especially turmeric.

be considered to be nature's version of tamoxifen, blocking undesirable oestrogenic effects in breast cells. Women who eat 1 to 1.5 servings of brassica vegetables every day reduce their breast-cancer risk by 25%.

Broccoli is an especially breast-friendly vegetable. Not only is it rich in I3C, but it also contains large amounts of a compound called D-glucorate which supports the detoxification and breakdown of both oestrogen produced in the body and toxic xeno-oestrogens from the environment.

Finally, plants including fruits, vegetables, legumes and grains provide us with dietary fibre. Residues of a high-fibre diet bind with oestrogen in the gut and excrete it from the body, preventing the resorption and recirculation of oestrogen in the bloodstream. A high-fibre diet also helps to feed and support friendly, beneficial bacteria in the gut. These bacteria play a role in oestrogen breakdown and excretion, and so are vital for breast health.

> People are applying the precautionary principle to their own lives by purchasing food that has not been produced by industrial methods. From the simple stance of hazard avoidance, organically produced food is the best option that we have.
>
> Dr Vyvyan Howard
> Toxico-pathologist at the University of Liverpool, UK

Fabulous folate

Not only do fruits and vegetables provide us with a plethora of antioxidant nutrients, they are also our richest natural source of folate. Most women associate the need for this B-vitamin with pregnancy. Taking folic acid supplements prior to conception and during the first trimester of pregnancy is now standard practice, with a resulting proven reduction in the incidence of babies suffering from spina bifida.

This same B-vitamin plays an important part in keeping breast cells healthy. Dietary folate helps us detoxify both oestrogen produced in the body and environmental xeno-oestrogens we absorb or ingest. Folate stimulates the body to produce a powerful natural antioxidant called SAM-e. Women who are lacking in folate have a higher incidence of chromosome breaks in their cells (this is a precursor to the development of an abnormal cell) compared with folate-rich women.

While multivitamin formulas usually contain around 400 mcg of folic acid per tablet, much greater amounts can be obtained by including generous quantities of folate-rich foods in your daily diet.

The following foods are good folate sources:

* leafy green vegetables (spinach, silverbeet, broccoli, bok choy)
* beetroot
* asparagus
* liver
* kidney
* oranges
* pineapples
* bananas
* berries
* brewer's yeast
* bean sprouts
* wheatgerm
* soya beans and soya flour.

Drink up your greens

Next to water, tea is the most popular beverage in the world. Stand in front of the tea section at any supermarket and you are guaranteed to be overwhelmed by the huge range of flavours and colours, many of them with the added therapeutic benefits of herbs. In the West, where black tea has traditionally been the beverage of choice, green tea is rapidly gaining popularity as news of its health-giving properties spreads. Green tea is bursting with polyphenol compounds known as flavonols, or commonly known as catechins. The most impressive of these catechins is called EGCG (epigallocatechin gallate), which has the ability to block cell reproduction in the earliest stages of cancer development. Not all green teas have the same EGCG content, and in general it is the Japanese teas, rather than Chinese teas, which have the greatest concentration of this cancer-fighting compound.

Epidemiological studies looking at Japanese women have suggested that drinking green tea may slow the progression of breast cancer. The Aichi Cancer Centre in Japan has performed much of the research relating to the benefits of green tea. Its studies show that early-stage cancer patients who drink three or more cups of green tea daily have a decreased risk of recurrence of their cancer. Rat studies have compared groups of rats given water or green tea regularly. When primed with a cancer-producing substance, the rats drinking the green tea still developed breast tumours, but their tumours developed later, were less invasive and weighed 70% less than those of the water-fed group.

Most of the studies suggest that a minimum of 3–5 cups of well-

Green tea tips

* Make the green tea in a teapot and steep for 8–10 minutes before drinking.

* Drink at least 3, and preferably 5, cups of green tea daily, spaced out throughout the day.

* For maximum cancer-fighting impact, drink regular caffeinated (not decaffeinated) green tea.

* Choose Japanese green teas.

brewed green tea daily offer the most potent cancer protection, and interestingly it is the green tea still containing its naturally occurring caffeine (albeit four times less than in black tea) which shows the greatest cancer-preventative properties.

Flax (linseed) fantastic

The tiny shiny black seeds of the flax plant are one of my favourite 'superfoods'. Not only do they keep the gut healthy and bowel motions easy and regular, but they also offer powerful protection to breast cells.

Flax belongs to the lignan family, other members of which include sesame seeds, bran, whole grains, and beans. Lignans are a sub-family of phyto-oestrogens. The traditional Western diet is low in lignans and studies show that postmenopausal women with breast cancer tend to have lower dietary lignan intake than healthy women.

Lignans may help to prevent breast cancer in a number of different ways. They are rich in plant-based oestrogen-like substances (called phyto-oestrogens), which lock into and fill the keyhole oestrogen receptors in the breast cells. This prevents the much stronger oestrogen produced in the body from stimulating the oestrogen receptors. In this sense, they function as a natural 'anti-oestrogen' similar in action to tamoxifen. Lignans also bind with oestrogen in the gut, facilitating its excretion, and helping to lower blood levels of oestrogen. Studies have shown that flax seed lignans are protective against breast cancer in the early promotional stages when cancers have not quite formed. (Note: Potentially cancerous cells have damaged DNA. Usually the body kills these cells through programmed cell death — called apoptosis — thus preventing them from passing on their damaged DNA. Sometimes, however, damaged cells regain their ability to replicate and so pass on their potentially cancerous DNA. These cells have undergone 'promotion', and this 'promotional' stage is considered to be the second stage of cancer development.)

It doesn't take much flax to provide rewards. Simply add 10 g of flax seeds (linseed) to your daily diet. Either soak the seeds in a little water overnight and mix into morning porridge or muesli, or grind the seeds to a powder and add to cereal, fruit and yoghurt, smoothies, muffins or soups. Because of its high fat content, linseed quickly goes rancid. Make sure that your flax is fresh, is kept in the fridge in an airtight container, and is used quickly.

The truth about fats

Dietary fat continues to get a bad rap, vilified as the cause of the Western epidemics of obesity, heart disease and diabetes. Women in particular are often slavishly obsessed with reading labels and seeking out fat-free or low-fat products. In reality, the truth about fats is much more complex than the simplistic 'fat is bad' thinking. The relationship between dietary fats and breast cancer is also complex, and still not fully understood.

Our understanding of the relationship between fat and breast cancer has changed over the years. A decade ago, it was believed that a diet high in fats, whatever the type, promoted breast cancer. Comparisons of breast-cancer rates of countries where the population had a high dietary fat intake with those of countries with a low fat intake seemed to confirm the theory that the more dietary fat was consumed, the greater was the incidence of breast cancer. Japanese, with their low dietary fat intake, also have a lower incidence of breast cancer. In comparison, the high dietary fat intake in the USA is accompanied by a much higher incidence of breast cancer. Adding further credence to this hypothesis was the observation that when Japanese women moved to the USA and changed their diets to the American norm, their breast-cancer risk quickly rose to American levels.

Taking the fat hypothesis to the lab and testing the theory on both rats and women failed to definitively confirm the relationship between fat and breast cancer. Some of the rat studies suggested that it was the total caloric intake of the diet, rather than the proportion constituted by dietary fats, which played the most significant role in the increase in breast cancer. The often-quoted Harvard Nurses' Health Study amazingly failed to find an association between fat of any type and breast cancer. (Critics of the study point out that the women with the lowest fat intake in the study still had a relatively high fat intake, comprising 29% of their total daily calorie intake. The breast benefits of low fat consumption are not expected to be seen until calories from dietary fat drop below 20% of total calorie intake.) Since then, other studies have uncovered some connections between dietary fats and breast cancer, but the relationship remains complex and not fully understood.

In trying to uncover the connection between dietary fat and breast cancer, it's not just a case of looking at total fat intake, or what proportions of differing dietary fats a woman consumes. There is also a historical aspect to consider. To what degree do the amount and type of dietary fats eaten during childhood and adolescence affect future breast-cancer risk? For example, children who eat one additional serving of French fries a week from the ages of three to five increase their risk of adult-onset breast cancer by approximately 30%. Is there a different effect when premenopausal as opposed to postmenopausal women eat a high-fat diet? In terms of breast health, is there any point in a 50-year-old woman adhering to a low-fat diet when, as a child, she was raised on a high-fat diet? Has the damage already been done? These are a few of the many questions yet to be answered.

Which type of dietary fat is most likely to contribute to an increased risk of breast cancer — saturated or polyunsatured? The jury is still out, with conflicting information making it impossible to answer this question accurately. In studies using laboratory rats, both saturated and polyunsaturated fats have been shown to increase the growth of breast tumours. In human studies, results have been less conclusive and are confusing.

While some studies have failed to find an increased breast-cancer risk with a higher dietary intake of animal fats, poly-unsaturated fats, saturated fats or trans-fats, there have been several studies indicating that certain types of fat can actually decrease our breast-cancer risk. In particular, monounsaturated olive oil, and omega-3-rich flax seed oil and fish oil show exciting promise. Studies have variably shown a reduced risk of 25–45% with the consumption of at least 2 tablespoons of olive oil a day. Olive oil contains oleic acid, which is highly effective in killing the Her$_2$/neu protein, a factor in the growth of some breast-cancer tumours.

The 1998 *Archives of Internal Medicine* published the results of a study involving nearly 62,000 Swedish women aged between 40 and 76. Examining the relationship between different dietary fats and breast cancer, the researchers found an inverse relationship with the consumption of monounsaturated fats. For example, the more monounsaturated fat there was in the diet, the lower was the incidence of breast cancer. In contrast, the more polyunsaturated fat consumed, the higher the incidence of breast cancer. Interestingly, with all the negative press given to saturated fats, they were found to be completely neutral in terms of influencing breast-cancer incidence!

Greenland Inuit women consume huge amounts of fish-based omega-3 oils in their traditional diet, and also have a strikingly low incidence of breast cancer. (Of course, there are very many other ways in which their diet and lifestyle differ from those of the average Western women, which also contribute to their low breast-cancer risk.)

Epidemiological studies have tended to show that women in those countries where there is the highest dietary intake of omega-3 fats tend to have the lowest incidence of breast cancer. Similarly, there are a number of animal studies showing that omega-3 fatty acids slow the development and decrease the growth of breast tumours. The evidence from human studies is not as clear, with around half showing that a high consumption of fish oil is associated with a decrease in breast-cancer risk.

Omega-3 fats work as inflammatory inhibitors and consequently may prove to be a great deal more breast-friendly than their omega-6 cousins. Eat cold-water fish (salmon, sardines, herrings, tuna) three or four times weekly; make salad dressings using cold-pressed flax oil; sprinkle ground flax seeds on your breakfast cereal; snack on nuts and seeds; add avocados to salads and cook in delicious cold-pressed virgin olive oil . . . then you'll be chockablock full of omega-3 fats!

While there is still a great deal of debate and controversy on the subject of the relationship between fat and breast cancer, it makes sense to apply the 'precautionary' principle, and make some changes based on what we know about fats and their effect on the body in general.

The average Western diet provides an excessive amount of omega-6 fats compared with omega-3 fats. In an optimum diet, the intake of these two types of fatty acid should be approximately equal. The modern diet provides an abundance of polyunsaturated fats in the form of safflower oil, sunflower oil, corn oil, margarine, commercial salad dressings and shop-bought baked goods — even our daily bread is loaded with omega-6 fats. An overabundance of omega-6-rich linoleic acid disturbs the body's ability to absorb and utilise vital omega-3 fatty acids. The skewed omega-6 to omega-3 ratio can act as a potential cause of inflammation in the body, arguably increasing the possible risk of breast cancer. Alpha-linolenic acid (found in flax, pumpkin oil, canola and soya bean oil), on the other hand, appears to reduce the ability of breast-cancer cells to spread out of the breast. A study in the *British Journal of Cancer* found that women who had the highest levels of alpha-linolenic acid in their fat tissues, at the time of their breast-cancer surgery, were five times less likely to go on to experience a metastasis than were women with the lowest level.

Saturated fats are considered by many to be the ultimate 'bad guy' on the fat scene . . . although trans-fats are rapidly picking up the mantle as the most vilified of fats. For years we have been pounded with the 'low-fat, low-saturates' mantra in the name of good health. Standing back and looking at the patterns of disease in the West in the past 50–100 years, we find that there are some noticeable anomalies which prompt questioning of the hypothesis.

The modern epidemics of cancer and heart disease began to emerge in the 1930s (interestingly, this was the era in which the process of hydrogenation of polyunsaturated fats was perfected, and such fats found their way into commercially processed foods). Our ancestors dined on fatty cuts of meat, butter, full-fat cream and milk, and yet many of them lived long and hearty lives free from coronary disease and cancer. Fast-forward to modern times and an obsession with 'heart-tick foods' and low-fat every-thing — and we are dropping like flies from heart attacks, breast and prostate cancer, colon cancer and other cancers. Something seems amiss, doesn't it? In the area of breast cancer and saturated fats specifically, there is similar confusion. While some research has found a link between saturated fats and breast cancer, other research projects have failed to find any such link.

Our supermarkets are filled with processed pseudo-foods which have given us a plethora of new dietary nasties to worry about in the form of colourings, additives, preservatives and 'altered' foods. Hydrogenated fats are one such altered food. These fats never occur in nature, but are the result of a technological process in which hydrogen is bubbled through a polyunsaturated oil, changing it into a solid (saturated fat). Margarine is a hydrogenated fat, as is commercial peanut butter in which the peanut oil is evenly distributed throughout the butter, rather than sitting in an oily pool at the top of the jar. While the process of hydrogenation gives us the convenience and appeal of such processed foods, hydrogenated fats are increasingly implicated in the development of a range of chronic illnesses, including heart disease and breast cancer. These fatty acids, completely foreign to the human body, increase free-radical damage to cells and interfere with our ability to utilise essential fatty acids.

While debate still continues on the subject of dietary fats and breast cancer, the following advice is expedient, based on what we already know about the effect of different dietary fats on the overall health of the human body.

* Ensure that dietary fat is a daily part of your diet.

* Limit dietary intake of saturated fats such as red meat, full-fat dairy products, takeaways, pies, pizza, palm oil.

* Include coconut oil in your diet regularly. Technically it is a saturated fat, but it is rich in long-chain fatty acids, and has been shown to exert a powerful antiviral and antibacterial effect in the body. Coconut oil also works as a powerful immune stimulant.

* Avoid processed foods containing trans-fats, such as margarine, peanut butter, commercially baked goods, French fries, and potato chips.

* Boost omega-3-rich fats by eating cold-water fish (salmon, sardines, herrings, tuna) three to four times a week; adding flax seeds to cereals or porridge at breakfast; using flax oil as a base for making salad oils; eating nuts, seeds and avocados regularly.

* Reduce intake of omega-6-rich polyunsaturated fats and eat monounsaturated fats instead. Polyunsaturates include traditional cooking oils such as safflower, sunflower, soya, corn and sesame oils, along with margarines made from polyunsaturated oils. Instead cook with olive oil and use an olive or avocado spread on your bread.

* Read labels on processed foods to check the relative balance of saturated, polyunsaturated and monounsaturated fats and check for the trans-fat content.

* *Never* use fats which may be rancid. Store all fats in a cool, dark place, and throw them away if they smell or taste unusual. Similarly, ensure that all nuts and seeds are stored in a cool cupboard (or the fridge) in an airtight container. *Rancid fats are extremely carcinogenic.*

The dairy connection

In 2000 Professor Jane Plant published *Your Life is in Your Hands*, in which she outlined her well-researched hypothesis of a connection between dairy-product consumption and breast cancer. Since then, women have come to believe that dairy products cause breast cancer . . . but is this true?

You're getting sick of hearing this by now, but once again, the truth is that the research is contradictory and unclear. Some studies suggest a correlation between consumption of dairy products and breast cancer; while others fail to show any such correlation; and still others demonstrate a protective effect for postmenopausal women who eat dairy products.

One branch of the Harvard Nurses' Health Study, involving 120,000 nurses, found that consumption of dairy products seemed to affect breast-cancer risk differently depending on whether women were premenopausal or postmenopausal. In post-menopausal women, dairy consumption did not appear to have any impact on breast-cancer risk. In premenopausal women, however, those women consuming the most dairy products appeared to also have the lowest incidence of breast cancer. This protective effect seems to disappear after menopause even in women with a high consumption of dairy products.

Pro-dairy product researchers present evidence that the calcium and vitamin D in dairy products may protect against breast cancer. The anti-dairy product faction argues that dairy products are detrimental on three counts: they contain insulin-like growth factors which have been shown to accelerate the growth of breast-cancer cells; they are a source of dietary fat (although there is weak evidence to support a link between saturated fat intake and breast cancer); unless they are organic, they are contaminated with pesticide residues and antibiotic residues which may cause an increase in a woman's oestrogen levels. For now the jury remains out on the dairy/breast-cancer question.

Know your fats

Monounsaturated fats
Heart-friendly, with strong evidence they have a protective effect against breast cancer.

* olives
* olive oil
* canola oil
* peanut oil
* peanuts
* cashew nuts
* almonds
* macadamia nuts
* avocados

Polyunsaturated fats (omega-6 rich)
Omega-6 essential fatty acids are predominant in the following oils. They are rich in linoleic acid. Consumed in excess, they stimulate inflammation.

* corn oil
* soya bean oil
* safflower oil
* cottonseed oil

Rich in gamma-linolenic acid:

* evening primrose oil
* borage oil (natural anti-inflammatories)

Polyunsaturated (omega-3 rich)
Omega-3 essential fatty acids are predominant in the following oils. They are rich in alpha-linolenic acid. They are beneficial for cardiovascular health, and work as a natural anti-inflammatory. There is evidence that they may inhibit cancer development.

* fish and fish oils
* flax seed oil

Be sensible about dairy product intake:

* Moderate intake of dairy products (remember that there are many other dietary sources of calcium).
* Buy organic dairy products.

Trans-fatty acids

Associated with an increase in incidence of cancer and heart disease.

* most margarines (the harder the margarine, the more trans-fats are present)
* hydrogenated peanut butter
* partially hydrogenated vegetable oil
* deep-fried chips
* fast foods
* commercially baked goods
* snack foods — pretzels, some potato chips

Saturated fats

Controversial connection with breast cancer. Link between saturated fats and heart disease (controversial).

* meat, especially red meat
* dairy products — milk, cheese, butter, yoghurt, ice-cream
* vegetable shortening
* palm oil
* coconut oil
* coconut milk

Tofu or not tofu . . . that is the question

If you're feeling a little dizzy after this confusing and contradictory journey through the realms of diet and breast cancer, hold onto your hats — things are about to get even more tricky as we examine the question of soya.

I am frequently asked whether or not soya foods should be added to a 'breast-healthy' diet — and it's a question I dread answering, as the answer is so confusing! Making a broad, sweeping generalised statement, the answer is 'yes' — most probably — but the benefits of doing so may vary depending on your age.

In any discussion of the pros and cons of phyto-oestrogens, it is important to differentiate between phyto-oestrogens occurring naturally in food and dietary supplements containing concentrated extracts of phyto-oestrogens, in particular isoflavones. Some research suggests that taking these supplements for long periods has the potential to stimulate the growth of breast-cancer cells, thus possibly increasing the risk of breast cancer. Test-tube studies have found that isoflavone supplements (usually isolated from soya) encourage the growth of breast-cancer cells. Studies with laboratory mice have similarly found that when isoflavone supplements are used for long periods, in the presence of low oestrogen levels (such as occur during menopause and beyond), breast-cancer development is accelerated. Whether these supplements have the same effect on breast tissue in women is not clear. While there is still so much we are unsure of, it is probably advisable not to use such concentrated phyto-oestrogen supplements in the long term or in high doses. It's worth emphasising here that it is the consumption of isolated, concentrated extracts of isoflavones that has the potential for causing problems, not the consumption of moderate amounts of the wholefood soya bean.

Many plant foods, including soya products, contain molecules known as phyto-oestrogens (meaning oestrogen-like substances that come from plants). The phyto-oestrogens found in soya products belong to a family of polyphenols called isoflavones. The principal isoflavones in soya are genistein and daidzein. These molecules are similar, but not identical, to human oestrogen. Every oestrogen-sensitive cell in the body (such as those in the breast) contains an oestrogen receptor (like a keyhole), into which oestrogen locks in order to stimulate the cell. Phyto-oestrogens are able to lock into these same receptor sites, effectively filling them and making them unavailable to the much stronger oestrogen produced by the body, and potentially toxic environmental oestrogens known as xeno-oestrogens. Stimulation by the much stronger hormonal oestrogen can cause cell replication to speed up out of control, leading to the formation of cancerous tumours. Given that two-thirds of all breast cancers are oestrogen sensitive, in theory filling up lots of receptor sites with phyto-oestrogens thousands of times weaker than estradiol and estrone would seem to be a good thing. Unfortunately, studies have been unable to confirm that these theoretical benefits of phyto-oestrogen consumption always occur. There is still a question regarding the effect of high phyto-oestrogen intake in postmenopausal women. Does filling the oestrogen receptor sites with phyto-oestrogen produce an oestrogenic stimulatory effect on the cells in postmenopausal women who have low circulating oestrogen levels?

There are three main families of phyto-oestrogens:

* *isoflavones* — the richest source of which are soya products

* *lignans* — lentils, beans, flax and grains

* *coumestans* — bean sprouts.

Soya manufacturers have been quick to point out that people in Asian cultures with a naturally high intake of isoflavones (such as those found in soya) have three to six times less breast cancer than those in Western cultures. While this is true, it is highly unlikely that this difference is due to isoflavone intake alone. Whether a high isoflavone intake is beneficial for all women, or only for some subsets of women, and only at certain times of their reproductive life, remains unclear.

Dietary phyto-oestrogens appear to have different effects depending upon the age at which they become a dietary staple. There is strong evidence that regular consumption during childhood and adolescence is strongly protective against breast cancer later in life. Whether eating phyto-oestrogen-rich foods during adulthood or after menopause confers the same benefits is still unknown. What is known is that women who have had a high dietary isoflavone intake since childhood have a clear reduction in breast-cancer risk. Asian American women who ate soya once a week as children demonstrated a 47% lower incidence of breast cancer as adults compared with adults who had had a low consumption of soya in childhood. Phyto-oestrogens consumed in childhood actually change the architecture of a developing breast in a way which makes it more resistant to cancer. Animal studies examining the effect of a diet high in soya have again not been completely conclusive. In many (but not all) of these studies, a high-soya phyto-oestrogen intake has resulted in fewer breast tumours. Interestingly, this reduction in breast-cancer risk amongst animals also seems to be dependent on the age at which they had a high soya intake. When they received the soya diet before the age of sexual maturity, they went on to develop about half the number of breast tumours compared with those animals who were given a high soya diet after maturity.

Studies of breast cells in tissue culture have produced mixed results, suggesting that soya phyto-oestrogens can either encourage or discourage growth within the breast, depending on the amount of isoflavones they were exposed to.

Measuring the amount of phyto-oestrogens in a woman's urine and then looking at whether or not she has breast cancer tells us something about the protective effect of phyto-oestrogens. In just such a study, women in the top 25% of phyto-oestrogen levels had a four times lower incidence of breast cancer compared with the women in the bottom 25% of phyto-oestrogen levels. This applied to both premenopausal and postmenopausal women.

While it is generally agreed that a phyto-oestrogen-rich diet is advantageous to a woman who has never had breast cancer, things aren't quite so clear when it comes to the question of phyto-oestrogens for women who have breast cancer, or who have had it in the past. Such women are generally advised by their medical carers to avoid soya products and other phyto-oestrogen-rich foods for fear that these may exert a mildly oestrogenic effect on the breasts, thus stimulating the return of breast cancer. In truth, there is little clinical evidence to support such a recommendation. What is clear, however, is that any woman who has, or has had, breast cancer should never take supplements containing concentrated extracts of isoflavones.

Despite studies showing that isoflavone supplements cause an increased rate of growth in breast tumours already present, eating the equivalent amount of isoflavones in the form of wholefoods (soya milk, tofu, and so on) has not been demonstrated to have the same negative effect.

Soya experts in general recommend that breast-cancer patients should consume a moderate amount of soya in the diet, consistent with the Asian diet. They caution against the use of high-dose isoflavone supplements, as their safety in breast-cancer patients has not been ascertained. Women on tamoxifen and aromatase inhibitors should avoid soya, since to date the research on the interactions between isoflavones and tamoxifen has been contradictory, with some of it indicating that soya isoflavones can nullify the therapeutic effects of these drugs.

Increasing your dietary phyto-oestrogens in a 'user friendly' way involves more than simply gulping endless glasses of soya milk. By all means make soya milk a dietary addition by using it instead of cows' milk on cereal, in cooking and for making smoothies and coffee. When you get peckish in the middle of the morning or afternoon, why not try a phyto-oestrogen power shake. Mix together soya milk, protein powder, flax seed oil and a teaspoon of ground flax seeds, along with fresh fruit such as berries or banana.

Fermented soya foods such as tofu and miso are especially rich sources of isoflavones. Firm tofu or tempeh can be cut into small cubes and added to stir fries, soups and rice dishes. Miso makes a delicious and filling snack at any time of the day, and studies suggest that daily consumption of miso, as part of a diet

Sources of dietary phyto-oestrogens

These foods are useful sources of dietary phyto-oestrogens:

* soya milk
* soya protein powder
* soya flakes
* soya-based protein bars
* miso
* tofu
* tempeh
* flax seeds (the whole seeds but not the oil)
* soya and linseed bread
* dark rye bread
* alfalfa sprouts
* a wide range of fruits, including berries, apples, bananas, grapefruit, lemons, papaya, peaches, pears, plums, rock melon
* a wide range of vegetables, including asparagus, beetroot, bok choy, broccoli, Brussels sprouts, cabbage, capsicum, carrots, cauliflower, peas, leeks, sprouts, mushrooms, onions, potatoes, spinach, tomatoes, turnip
* baked beans

supplying at least 25 mg a day of isoflavones, is associated with a strong reduction in breast-cancer risk.

Even if you're a soya fan it is a good idea not to overdo the soya products in your attempt to boost phyto-oestrogen levels, as for some women soya can act as a thyroid depressant. It makes more nutritional sense to include a wide and varied range of the phyto-oestrogen-rich foods included in the list above.

* brown rice
* cashew nuts
* chickpeas
* dried apricots
* lentils
* nut butters
* oat bran
* extra virgin olive oil
* prunes
* red kidney beans
* sesame seeds
* stoneground wholemeal or rye flour
* black tea
* green tea
* jasmine tea
* red clover tea
* walnuts
* wheat bran
* wholegrain breakfast cereals.

Fibre to the rescue

If you follow the advice previously given and boost your intake of fresh fruits and vegetables, and phyto-oestrogen-rich beans, grains and flax, you will already have achieved your next aim, that of boosting your fibre intake. Most people think of dietary fibre in the context of regular bowel motions. Certainly, a high-fibre diet is important for preventing constipation, bloating and a range of other digestive problems, but did you know it is also important for your breast health?

A diet high in insoluble fibre (the sort you find in grains, nuts, seeds and beans) decreases the recirculation of oestrogen between the intestines and the liver, thus lowering blood oestrogen levels. A high-fibre diet, whatever the source, also helps to promote a healthy balance of bacteria in the gut, and this in turn helps to reduce the amount of oestrogen recirculated from the gut back to the bloodstream. A strong and flourishing population of 'friendly' gut bacteria is vital for the metabolism of phyto-oestrogens, isoflavones and lignans. Without a healthy bacterial balance, you won't reap the benefits of dietary phyto-oestrogens.

Increase your fibre intake by eating nine or more servings of fresh fruits and vegetables daily; eat wholegrain breads instead of white bread; eat wholegrain muesli or porridge instead of refined breakfast cereals; add extra wheatgerm or oat bran to breakfast cereals and porridge; use brown rice instead of white rice; cook wholemeal pasta instead of white pasta; snack on nuts and seeds; add oat or wheat bran to cereals and baking; add lentils to homemade soups.

The low-down on insulin

Insulin is the blood-sugar-regulating hormone we most often hear about in connection with diabetes. It's true that insulin abnormalities are involved in both type-one and type-two diabetes, and it's looking increasingly likely that this same hormone also has an influence on breast health. In our high-fat, high-carbohydrate society insulin abnormalities are common, and I suspect that in time the role played by long-term elevation of insulin levels in the development of breast cancer will prove to be an important one.

Before an actual diagnosis of diabetes is made, many type-two diabetics have spent years living with a condition known as 'insulin resistance'. Insulin is the hormone responsible for moving sugar from the blood into the cells. Insulin resistance occurs when the body becomes resistant to this sugar-shuttling effect of insulin, prompting the pancreas to pump out ever-increasing volumes of insulin in an attempt to move sugar to where it should go. This leads to increasing levels of insulin in the blood, and it is this abnormally high insulin level which some researchers believe may stimulate the growth of breast-cancer cells. Insulin has growth-promoting properties, and cancer cells are cells which are growth crazy.

Research has consistently linked high insulin levels and insulin-like growth factors with an increased postmenopausal breast-cancer incidence. High insulin levels are often accompanied by a number of other changes in biochemistry, which together have been labelled 'Syndrome X' or metabolic syndrome. This is diagnosed when high insulin levels are accompanied by low levels of HDL (good) cholesterol, high blood pressure, high triglycerides (another type of blood fat), and an increased risk of diabetes. Often metabolic syndrome occurs in obese men and women. Women suffering from metabolic syndrome appear to be at increased risk of breast cancer. While some scientists believe this is due to the effect of high insulin levels stimulating the growth of breast-cancer cells, others believe it is due to high insulin levels increasing levels of the male hormone testosterone.

A number of significant studies have linked high insulin levels with increased mortality for breast-cancer patients. One such study appeared in a 2004 journal and examined whether a woman's insulin levels influenced her risk of dying after having breast cancer. They found that those women who had high blood-insulin levels after their cancer was treated were more likely to go on to die of their breast cancer, especially if they were postmenopausal. In fact, these women were almost twice as likely to die of breast cancer as were their peers who had low insulin levels.

The long-term EPIC study (see below) followed patients who had received standard treatment for their breast cancer, for a period of 10 years. During that time, fasting insulin levels were tested regularly. Researchers found that those women with the highest insulin levels were eight times more likely to die during the study than were the women with the lowest insulin levels. Similarly, those with the highest insulin levels were also four times more likely to suffer from a recurrence of their cancer, with metastases. Some of the women with the high insulin levels were obese, but slim women with high insulin levels were also found to experience the same degree of increased risk.

Women produce the 'male' hormone testosterone, but in much smaller amounts than men. Testosterone replacement therapy is one of the new hormonal therapies being promoted to post-menopausal women to increase energy levels, and specifically to boost flagging sex drive. One of the largest studies ever to look

The European Prospective Investigation into Cancer and Nutrition (EPIC)

The findings of the European Prospective Investigation into Cancer and Nutrition — one of the largest studies ever to investigate the link between diet and nutrition, involving more than half a million Europeans — are as follows:

✳ High oestrogen levels in postmenopausal women increase breast-cancer risk.

✳ High testosterone levels in postmenopausal women increase breast-cancer risk.

✳ Overweight and lack of exercise increase breast-cancer risk in postmenopausal women.

✳ Overweight is not associated with increased breast-cancer risk in premenopausal women.

✳ Consumption of fruits and vegetables is not associated with breast-cancer risk.

into the relationship between diet and cancer is the ongoing EPIC study (European Prospective Investigation into Cancer and Nutrition), involving more than half a million European subjects. EPIC has confirmed that high testosterone levels in women actually increase their risk of premenopausal and possibly also of postmenopausal breast cancer. Looking at breast-cancer survivors, the study found that women with testosterone levels in the top third had more than a seven times greater chance of recurrence compared with women with testosterone levels in the bottom third.

How do you reduce insulin and testosterone levels? Put into practice all the pointers in this chapter! Doing aerobic exercise regularly; eating a diet with reduced saturated fats; avoiding simple carbohydrates (high GI carbs); and eating generous amounts of fruits, vegetables, beans, lentils and whole grains — all of these things have been shown to lower both insulin and testosterone levels. Moderating your calorie intake also helps to lower insulin levels.

Alcohol and breast cancer

A glass of wine with dinner has become a part of the antipodean culture, and is usually promoted as being a delicious way of safeguarding cardiovascular health. Few women stop to question whether or not their nightly tipple could be detrimental to their health . . . and whether it could in any way affect their risk of becoming a breast-cancer statistic.

For a long time, the link between alcohol consumption and breast cancer was unclear. Now it is generally accepted that there is indeed a connection between the amount of alcohol a woman consumes and her risk of developing breast cancer. The large American Cancer Society Cancer Prevention Study (CPSII) followed a group of American women for over 14 years, and found that amongst postmenopausal women who drank a single alcoholic beverage a day, the risk of dying of breast cancer increased by 30% compared with the risk for non-drinkers.

Interestingly, they did not find any association between alcohol consumption and increased breast-cancer mortality amongst premenopausal women.

Before getting too excited (and pouring another glass of wine!) it's fair to tell you that while this particular study had good news for premenopausal women, their findings were in direct contrast with those of a number of other studies showing increased mortality for premenopausal women with alcohol consumption. As in the case of so many nutrition/breast cancer issues, more research is needed.

The next obvious question is just how much alcohol is it safe to drink before your breast-cancer risk begins to rise? We still don't know for sure, but it seems that even fairly small amounts of alcohol cause risk to rise. One study found that for each 10 g of alcohol consumed a day, the lifetime risk of a woman developing breast cancer increases by almost 10% (and keep in mind that in one typical alcoholic drink there are approximately 15 g of alcohol).

A 2004 study in the *Journal of the American Medical Association* reviewed recent research on the question of alcohol and breast-cancer risk. After reviewing studies using different populations from around the world, from 1977 onwards, the authors found that there is consistent evidence that breast-cancer risk is higher amongst women consuming moderate to high levels of alcohol (three or more drinks daily) than amongst abstainers. They also found that as few as 1–2 drinks daily increases risk. In overviewing these numerous studies, they concluded that it makes no difference whether you are premenopausal or postmenopausal, or what type of alcoholic drink you consume. Risk is the same in the case of wine, beer or spirits, so there's no use fooling yourself that because you drink red wine, complete with its abundant antioxidants, the risk will go away.

The general consensus amongst those in the know is that alcohol consumption and breast-cancer risk are linked, but it's still not fully understood what it is about alcohol that increases

Green-light foods for breast-cancer prevention

Make these foods frequent staples in your diet.

Fresh fruits and vegetables and antioxidant-rich foods, especially:

* berries
* black grapes
* cranberry juice and black grape juice
* leafy green vegetables
* cruciferous vegetables (broccoli, cauliflower, bok choy and Brussels sprouts)
* garlic
* onions
* mushrooms (maitake and shiitake)
* seaweeds — kombu, nori, wakame
* turmeric
* green tea

Phyto-oestrogen-rich foods, especially:

* nuts
* lentils
* flax
* whole grains
* seeds
* beans
* soya

Omega-3 fatty acids:

* oily fish (salmon, sardines and herrings, and, in moderation, tuna)
* flax oil
* avocados
* nuts and seeds

Omega-9 fatty acids:

* cold-pressed extra virgin olive oil

our risk. There are two main theories to explain the relationship. The first relates to the fact that alcohol increases the levels of oestrogen in the blood, especially in postmenopausal women who generally have low oestrogen levels. In women who drink regularly, breast cells are exposed to increased levels of oestrogen, which may trigger oestrogen-sensitive breast cells to become cancerous. The second theory relates to alcohol's effects on the B-vitamin folate. Low levels of folate are associated with increased risk of a range of cancers, and drinking alcohol increases our excretion of this vital nutrient. Some studies suggest that women

Red-light foods for breast-cancer prevention

Minimise your intake of the following foods:

* processed or refined foods
* foods with artificial colourings, additives, preservatives
* alcohol
* caffeine
* meat
* preserved meats (containing nitrates)
* chicken (unless organic)
* dairy products
* saturated fats (meat, dairy, palm oil)
* trans-fats (margarine, peanut butter, snack foods, French fries, potato chips, commercial baked goods)
* polyunsaturated fats containing predominantly omega-6 fatty acids (corn, soya bean, safflower, cotton seed oils)
* sugar and foods containing added sugar
* stale or rancid foods
* charred or highly browned meats
* high Glycaemic Index (GI) carbohydrates

who have low levels of folate in their diet and also drink alcohol are at increased risk of breast cancer compared with women who consume a high-folate diet (lots of fresh fruit and vegetables) and drink alcohol.

So:

* If you don't drink alcohol already, don't start.

* If you are a woman who has, or has had breast cancer, don't drink alcohol.

* If you are a woman who wants to do absolutely everything possible to reduce the risk of breast cancer, don't drink alcohol.

* For other women, occasional alcohol consumption (a glass once or twice a week) is unlikely to increase your breast cancer risk significantly, if at all.

Nutritional supplements and the prevention of cancer

Just as following the perfect 'breast-friendly' diet will not guarantee you absolute protection against breast cancer, swallowing a daily handful of nutritional supplements or herbs cannot be considered a guaranteed insurance policy either. That said, there are several nutritional supplements and herbs which affect our biochemistry in ways which are potentially very beneficial to our breast health.

A word of wise warning: never fool yourself into believing that swallowing nutritional supplements or herbs atones for a lifestyle which breaks all the rules of healthy living. There is not a pill in existence which can make up for a consistently poor diet, cigarette smoking, or a sedentary lifestyle . . . and be wary of anyone who ever tries to convince you otherwise with the intention of selling you a 'miracle elixir'.

I3C and DIM

If you have read the section on the benefits of eating cruciferous vegetables for breast health, you will already have come across reference to the phytonutrient I3C (indole-3-carbinol) which occurs naturally in cruciferous vegetables, especially broccoli. Once ingested, this compound is broken down into multiple compounds, one of which is DIM (di-indolylmethane). Both I3C and DIM are available as nutritional supplements, and much confusion over the relative merits of each exists in the minds of consumers. In truth it is I3C which has been widely tested, and for which human studies are available. In the case of DIM, on the other hand, there is little in the way of scientific studies verifying its effects in the human body.

Both I3C and DIM have been shown to exert an effect on human breast-cancer cells. In the case of I3C supplements, these effects have all been found to be favourable in terms of breast-cancer prevention. DIM, on the other hand, seems to be less predictable, exerting different effects (not always favourable) depending on the dose in which it is administered.

I3C is the parent molecule from which DIM is made in the body. When we digest I3C, about 6% of its metabolites are DIM, and the remaining 94% of metabolites are accounted for by a range of other chemicals, each with their own unique anti-cancer qualities.

I3C studies have uncovered a myriad of exciting ways in which this compound can inhibit the development of cancers, including breast cancer. These include: protection of cellular DNA from oxidation and damage; detoxification of carcinogens; increasing the activity of tumour suppressor genes; and modulation of oestrogen receptors in such a way as to reduce the likelihood that they will stimulate cell proliferation and cancer. There is also some evidence that I3C reduces the likelihood that breast-cancer cells will move from the breast to invade surrounding tissue.

I3C and DIM change the way in which your body breaks

down oestrogens, encouraging the production of more of the 'safe' $_2$OH metabolites (instead of the potentially troublesome $_{16}$OH metabolites). The ratio of the relative amounts of these two oestrogen metabolites in your body appears to influence the risk of developing breast cancer. This effect appears to be more pronounced with I$_3$C supplementation, compared with using DIM. The effects of DIM on oestrogen metabolism are not so clear-cut, with studies suggesting it can work as both an oestrogen modulator and as an oestrogen stimulator, depending on dosage. I$_3$C, on the other hand, always works to downregulate oestrogen receptors.

When evaluating effects of I$_3$C and DIM on oestrogen-negative breast-cancer cells, another important difference comes to light. I$_3$C retards the growth of such cells, while DIM has no proven effect on oestrogen-negative breast-cancer cells.

Vitamin E

Vitamin E is not just one vitamin, rather it is a complex. In food, vitamin E occurs as a complex of different tocopherols and tocotrienols, which are rarely available all together in a supplement. This complex has powerful antioxidant properties, which can protect cells (including those of the breast) from free-radical damage. Unfortunately, many of the studies looking at the efficacy of vitamin E as a breast-cancer protector have used the isolated alpha-tocopherol form of the vitamin, and results have been disappointing. Several of these studies have assessed the effects of standard alpha-tocopherol supplements, even at high doses, and have found no protective effect against breast cancer. Given the evidence of a breast-protective effect with a diet naturally high in foods that are rich in vitamin E, these findings suggest that it is the synergistic effect of the complex of tocopherols and tocotrienols which is of benefit to breast health.

In contrast, there is exciting news concerning a high dietary intake of vitamin E. The Harvard Nurses' Health Study showed that premenopausal women with a family history of breast cancer and a high dietary intake of vitamin E showed a risk reduction of 43%. This compared with a reduction of only 16% in breast-cancer incidence amongst the women with no family history of breast cancer, suggesting that dietary vitamin E protects against genetically predisposed cancer more powerfully than against environmentally induced cancer.

However, those studies which have looked at dietary intake of a form of vitamin E called alpha-tocopheryl succinate have produced encouraging results, with high dietary intake offering breast protection. Risk reduction amongst women with the highest dietary intake varies from 30% for postmenopausal women with a history of breast cancer to 90% for similar women of a premenopausal age. In the lab, vitamin E succinate has been shown to be a potent inhibitor of human breast-cancer cell growth in culture.

Of all the vitamin E forms, it is tocotrienols which have shown the most significant protective effect against breast cancer. Studies in cultures have shown that tocotrienols inhibit the growth of breast-cancer cells that are oestrogen-receptor-positive by up to 50%. In cell cultures, tamoxifen reduces oestrogen-receptor-positive breast-cancer cell proliferation by 50%. Amazingly, when tocotrienols were added along with the tamoxifen, the dose of tamoxifen needed to produce a 50% reduction in cell proliferation was lowered by a massive 75%. Tamoxifen can also reduce cell proliferation in oestrogen-receptor-negative cancer cells by 50% (in a test tube), and when tocotrienols are added to the mixture, the amount of tamoxifen required to produce this inhibitory effect drops by 95%. Surprisingly, the addition of alpha-tocopherol (the usual vitamin-E supplement) actually increased the amount of tamoxifen needed to have a therapeutic effect, suggesting that alpha-tocopherol supplements may actually be detrimental rather than useful in breast-cancer patients who are taking tamoxifen. Tocotrienol supplements are derived from either palm oil or rice bran oil, and it is the rice bran derivative which has demonstrated the breast-protective effects.

(When taking tocotrienols it is important to take them with a meal containing fat, or at the same time as evening primrose or fish oil supplements.)

Fish oil

See the section on dietary fats and breast cancer.

Coenzyme Q10 (ubiquinone)

CoQ10 is one of the most powerful antioxidants occurring naturally in the body. As well as protecting cells from free-radical damage, CoQ10 is involved in the production of energy in every cell in the body. This powerful antioxidant has a scientifically proven list of benefits in the prevention and treatment of heart disease. What is less widely known is the distinct possibility that CoQ10 has cancer-fighting properties. To date, the number of studies investigating cancer and CoQ10 in humans has been small, and according to the National Cancer Institute, some of these studies have design flaws. Nevertheless, there is enough evidence to get excited! While more research remains to be done on the CoQ10/cancer connection, what is clear is that cancer patients taking this nutrient experience increased energy and well-being, and decreased weight loss . . . and experience no toxicity problems or side effects from CoQ10 supplements.

When a cell becomes cancerous, it becomes resistant to the normal programmed process of cell death, called apoptosis. This allows cells to proliferate wildly, forming cancerous tumours. When CoQ10 is added to cancerous cells in a culture, the normal process of apoptosis is restored, inhibiting the unchecked growth of breast-cancer cells and at the same time strengthening and stabilising the normal breast cells. In human subjects, some small studies have demonstrated regression of breast-cancer tumours and an improved survival time in patients whose cancers had spread too far to be completely removed by surgery.

Research on rats has suggested that CoQ10 may be a powerful addition to tamoxifen treatment. Four groups of rats with breast cancer were treated with either tamoxifen alone; CoQ10 alone; tamoxifen plus CoQ10, or received no treatment at all. The most significant tumour-suppressing effect was seen in the group receiving both tamoxifen and CoQ10 together. (Rats with breast cancer are usually found to have very high levels of cancer-causing free-radicals, and low levels of naturally occurring antioxidants (free-radical fighters). When CoQ10 is added to tamoxifen therapy, free-radical levels decline and antioxidant levels increase. More in-depth human studies are required to definitively state that CoQ10 has a cancer-fighting ability but there is enough evidence from test-tube and rat research to strongly suggest this.

Selenium

Can supplementing with selenium reduce the risk of breast cancer, or help to fight the disease if you already have breast cancer? Interesting questions . . . with murky answers! In theory, the connection is very plausible. In practice, there are a number of animal and laboratory studies which suggest a relationship, but when it comes to human studies, in general, the link between selenium and breast cancer has not been substantiated. Some studies suggest a correlation between low selenium levels and increased incidence of breast cancer . . . and other studies demonstrate no such correlation.

A large geographical study showed an inverse relationship between selenium and breast-cancer incidence. That is, women in areas with the highest selenium intake had the lowest incidence of breast cancer. US studies looking at the selenium content of soil and the incidence of breast cancer have shown that those areas with the lowest soil-selenium content are also the areas with the highest incidence of breast cancer.

In contrast, the Harvard Nurses' Health Study failed to show a correlation between selenium levels and breast-cancer incidence. However, critics of this trial suggest the way in which selenium levels were measured (through toenail clippings) has subsequently been found to be a poor way of measuring selenium status.

The National Prevention of Cancer Trial was a large, respected and well-designed trial which investigated the effect of giving a selenium supplement (200 mcg of selenised yeast daily) to a large population and then measuring the incidence of a range of different cancers. They discovered a 25% reduction in total cancer incidence, and a 51% reduction in total cancer mortality.

A recent Polish study found an exciting connection between selenium supplementation and a reduced incidence of DNA damage (a precursor to cancer) in women carrying the BRCA1 gene. Women with the gene were supplemented with 275 mcg of sodium selenite a day for two months. Their blood lymphocytes were checked for DNA damage at the start and end of the study. As a control, women who were relatives of these women, but who did not have the BRCA1 gene, were also tested. At the start of the study, the BRCA1 women showed an average number of chromosome breaks per cell of 0.63, whereas the control women showed an average of 0.39 breaks per cell. After two months of selenium supplementation, the chromosome breaks in the BRCA1 group had declined to normal levels of around 0.40 per cell.

While the data relating to selenium and human breast cancers is still not definitive, animal and laboratory studies have demonstrated a strongly favourable cancer-protective effect with the use of selenium supplements.

In human studies showing favourable results in the treatment or prevention of breast cancer, it is the sodium selenite form of selenium which has shown the greatest effect, usually in doses of 200 mcg per day. As New Zealand soils are lacking in selenium, supplementation with this vital mineral is strongly recommended for optimum health.

Turmeric (curcumin)

There's not a single respectable kitchen in India that would dream of being without this pungent, bright yellow traditional spice. Used generously in a number of Indian dishes and curries, turmeric is now coming under the scientific spotlight and revealing itself as a treasure-trove of healing properties. Turmeric functions as a powerful antioxidant and some studies suggest that it has both preventative and therapeutic properties when it comes to a range of different cancers.

Mice studies at the M.D. Anderson Cancer Center in Houston suggest that (in mice at least!) turmeric may help prevent the spread of breast cancer to the lungs. Curcumin was found to inhibit the production of an inflammatory protein that promotes cancer-cell growth by dampening the signals of the hormone neurotensin, which spurs production of the protein. In the mice studies, administering turmeric along with the common cancer drug taxol reduced the incidence of lung metastases from 75% when taxol was given alone, down to 22%. People who eat diets naturally rich in turmeric have a lower incidence of breast, prostate, lung and colon cancer.

Curcumin has demonstrated a powerfully protective effect on breast cells. By filling certain receptors on breast cells, curcumin blocks the ability of potentially carcinogenic chemicals such as dioxins from stimulating these cells. It's not just the negative effects of chemicals which are reduced by this wonder spice. In studies in which rats were irradiated with the specific intention of inducing breast cancer, those rats receiving curcumin had only one-quarter the risk of developing breast cancer, compared with the risk measured in the non-supplemented rats.

Curcumin protects cells from cancer through a number of different mechanisms. Not only does it block chemical receptors, but it also improves the body's immunity, thus stimulating the body's ability to search for and destroy cancer cells. Tumours always need a new and extensive network of blood vessels to thrive. Turmeric reduces the formation of these new blood vessels, thus depriving tumours of nourishment.

Some studies suggest that curcumin has the most potent ability to inhibit the growth of breast-cancer cells when it is combined with isoflavonoids (phyto-oestrogens such as occur naturally in soya products).

The addition of a single teaspoon of turmeric powder to your daily diet gives you adequate quantities for cancer-fighting effects. Sprinkle in soups, salad dressings or pasta dishes.

Calcium d-glucarate

This nutrient occurs naturally in a range of fruits and vegetables including apples, grapes, grapefruit, bean sprouts, lettuce and cruciferous vegetables such as broccoli and cauliflower. Calcium d-glucarate is also available as a nutritional supplement, and has been shown to be extremely safe and without side effects, while possibly helping protect the breasts from cancer.

To date there is limited data available from human studies looking at calcium d-glucarate and breast cancer. Animal studies are producing exciting results, however. Rats specifically bred to develop breast cancer showed a 70% reduction in the incidence of breast tumours when fed calcium d-glucarate in their diet, and those that did develop tumours still exhibited a 73% reduction in the number of tumours, compared with the rats that did not receive the supplement. The treated rats also showed a reduction in the levels of oestradiol (the form of oestrogen implicated in many breast cancers) in their blood.

Calcium d-glucarate is involved in the process called glucuronidation, which the body uses to break down toxic and carcinogenic substances, and then rid itself of these. Glucuronidation is a complex chemical process through which the body combines carcinogens and toxins with water-soluble substances, allowing them to be excreted more easily through the gut and bladder. There is an enzyme called b-glucuronidase which the body uses to reverse this process of glucuronidation. Calcium d-glucarate actually inhibits this enzyme, thus maximising the detoxifying effect of glucuronidation, and allowing the body to more effectively rid itself of carcinogens. This supplement also helps to prevent the reabsorption of oestrogen from the gut back into the bloodstream, through its ability to decrease levels of b-glucuronidase.

This is an extremely safe supplement which has produced no evidence of side effects or toxic effects, even when it is administered at very high dosages of 10 g a day to women at high risk of breast cancer.

B-vitamins / folic acid

Folate is a B-vitamin found in a range of foods, including beans and peas, leafy green vegetables and fruit, citrus fruit, wheat, beef, liver and milk. It is also available in supplemental form (folic acid) on its own, or as a part of a multivitamin complex. Most women think of folic acid in relation to its use during the first trimester of pregnancy to prevent spina bifida.

A number of studies suggest that a high dietary intake of folate reduces breast-cancer risk (but as is usually the case with nutritional medicine, still other studies have been unable to find any such association). A large study reported in the *Cancer Research Journal* involving nearly 3000 women in America and China found that the 20% of women consuming the most dietary folate had a significantly lower risk of developing breast cancer compared with the 20% with the lowest folate intake. This risk was even further reduced in women who were also consuming generous amounts of the other nutrients needed for proper utilisation of folate, such as methionine, B6 and B12.

One branch of the Harvard Nurses' Health Study, in which 80,000 nurses were followed for 16 years, looked at the relationship of folate intake and breast-cancer incidence. A similar correlation between folate intake and breast-cancer risk was observed. In women who were drinking one or more alcoholic drinks a day, the risk of breast cancer was highest among those with a low folate intake. Women with the highest folate intake and who were drinking one or more alcoholic drinks per day were found to be 89% less likely to develop breast cancer compared with women who had a low folate intake but were drinking the same amount of alcohol. Interestingly, in women consuming alcohol, the use of a daily multivitamin supplement (containing folic acid) was associated with a lower risk of breast cancer. Premenopausal women with higher intakes of vitamin B12 also appeared to be at lower risk of breast cancer, but no such correlation was found in postmenopausal women. High B6 levels also correlated with lower breast-cancer risk.

Can stress cause breast cancer?

That stress can in some way cause breast cancer is a widespread popular notion, but one which has little in the way of definitive scientific evidence to back it up. Despite much study into the connection between stress and cancer, an irrefutable link has yet to be established. Many breast-cancer patients I have worked with have experienced significant stress, trauma or shock in the two to five years prior to their breast-cancer diagnosis. Despite this empirical observation, numerous well-designed studies have failed to show a definitive link between stress and the development of breast cancer; or a link between stress and risk of breast-cancer recurrence.

A British study following 170 women with breast cancer for several years found that stressful life experiences in the year before a breast-cancer diagnosis had no effect on breast-cancer recurrence, nor did depression. Amazingly, the women who had the most significant stresses in the five years after their diagnosis, had almost half the incidence of tumour recurrence of their less-stressed peers.

In general, published studies reveal very mixed findings. A long-term study looking at women who had endured the ultimate stress of losing a child found no increased incidence in breast cancer over a 16-year period An eight-year follow-up of one branch of the Harvard Nurses' Health Study, involving 70,000 women, found that perceived stress was not related to breast-cancer incidence.

In direct contrast, other studies have found (amazingly) that high levels of stress appear to reduce a woman's risk of breast cancer. While I am personally very sceptical of this particular claim, study authors suggest that high stress levels may reduce the oestrogen levels in premenopausal women, and thus lower their breast-cancer risk. It has also been suggested that these 'highly stressed' women may be more engaged with health-promoting behaviour (in order to cope with their stress levels) such as exercising, getting regular sleep, and so on.

While the scientists continue to debate the impact of stress on breast-cancer risk, it makes sense to make lifestyle choices to minimise adverse stress as much as possible. Life is always unpredictable and often, despite our best attempts at balanced living, an unexpected shock or trauma will shatter our tranquility and tip us over into stress mode. Having acknowledged that, we can still minimise our stresses through good nutrition, regular exercise, plentiful sleep, work/life balance, regular active de-stressing activities (for example, meditation, yoga, or tai chi), social support systems and friendships.

Traditional Chinese medicine and the connection between stress and breast health

Traditional Chinese medicine has long acknowledged a connection between the mental and emotional state and breast health. From the perspective of traditional Chinese medicine, lumps and tumours are always the end result of years of stagnation or blockage in the flow of energy (qi) through the energy meridians in the body. In the case of breast tumours, it is a stagnation of energy in the liver meridian in particular which is an underlying issue. Emotions can contribute strongly to stagnation of qi. Liver qi is affected by repression of emotion, anger, frustration and resentment. (See Chapter 4 for more information.)

The mammogram debate

While many medical investigations require some type of informed consent, women attending for screening mammograms are seldom provided with objective information on the risks and benefits.

Trevor Smith
Auckland breast surgeon

We constantly hear the message that in order to prevent breast cancer, women between the ages of 40 and 69 (or 50 and 59, depending on whom you listen to) should have regular mammograms. Of course, mammograms cannot actually prevent breast cancer, but are used to detect cancer (hopefully early) once it is present. In New Zealand, women over the age of 40 are encouraged to have regular mammograms, and between the ages of 45 and 69 mammographic screening is provided free of charge, every two years. While private breast clinics encourage women over the age of 40 to have regular screening, the Cancer Society doesn't recommend regular mammograms for women under the age of 50. This conflicting advice highlights one of the most debatable aspects of mammographic screening, namely that of its benefit in terms of reduced mortality for women under the age of 50.

Women in this part of the world are generally unaware that beyond New Zealand's shores, the past decade has seen researchers and advocacy groups embroiled in a passionate and confusing debate over the merits of routine mammographic screening, most especially for women in the under-50 age group.

Mammographic screening involves giving every healthy woman in the right age bracket a regular mammogram, regardless of whether she is exhibiting any potential symptoms of breast cancer. In theory, mammograms are able to detect breast lumps when they are too small to be detected by manual, self- or clinician examination. Common sense would suggest that through early detection, mammographic screening programmes would reduce the number of women dying from breast cancer. Contrary to this expectation, a significant number of large and reputable studies have failed to find any significant reduction in breast-cancer mortality with screening programmes.

Despite the consistently positive media message we are constantly fed, mammography is an imperfect science, and not without risk. Most women are completely unaware that there is controversy over the benefits of mammographic screening, or that there could possibly be any form of negative consequence to such a programme. US experts, including researchers at the National Institutes of Health, believe that women should be made aware of the debate around the key questions 'Does regular mammographic screening translate into improved breast-cancer mortality'? and 'Do women younger than 50 and older than 65 benefit from regular mammograms?'

Long a subject of debate, the controversy was refuelled in 2001 by a Danish study published in the prestigious journal *Lancet*, in which seven large studies of mammography conducted over the past few decades were reanalysed. The findings showed that the earlier studies, which demonstrated a benefit from mammography, were flawed. Study authors Dr Gotzsche and Mr Olsen claim that five of the seven studies failed to meet agreed-upon standards for well-conducted and reliable research. In their *Lancet* paper they said that women who had mammograms were just as likely to die from breast cancer as those not screened. Also, the screened women had more mastectomies, more radiation therapy and more surgery. The extra treatment, without a demonstration of overall benefit, made the researchers question the widespread use of mammography.

Following the release of their paper, a riot ensued. In response to vehement attack by many of their peers, Gotzsche and Olsen reanalysed their data using an even more stringent statistical analysis model. The reanalysis confirmed their initial findings, and *Lancet* editor Richard Horton concluded that 'at present there is no reliable evidence from large randomised trials to support screening mammography programmes'.

Before the debate had settled, the National Cancer Institute and the American Cancer Society reiterated their positions that women over the age of 40 should have regular mammograms, as the test saves lives (a stance reflected in New Zealand as well). A Government Task Force stressed that there was a clear mortality benefit with mammography, claiming that with mammography the breast-cancer death rate was reduced by about 16%.

Two different papers on the subject of mammography published in the *Annals of Internal Medicine* further confused the issue. One paper, by the United States Preventive Services Task Force, concluded that the pooled data from randomised trials continued to support mammography every one to two years for women aged 40 to 74.

In an editorial accompanying the report, Dr Steven Goodman, a biostatistician at the Johns Hopkins Kimmel Cancer Center, wrote 'if we are still unsure after looking at something like half a million women, that points to how small the risks are and how much smaller the benefit is in absolute numbers'. Dr Harold Sox, editor of the *Annals*, commented in his editorial that 'the big picture message is that the effect of screening in any age group is limited at best'. He commented that there appeared to be a small benefit in women starting at 50, but for women in their forties, it is not clear whether there is any benefit at all.

A second paper summarised findings of a large Canadian study involving 90,000 women. It reported that women in their forties reap no benefit from mammography and also have real risks of harm from unnecessary treatment. The study, which had been running for 16 years, showed that even after such a lengthy period mammography had not saved any lives and had led to excess treatment. In the group receiving regular mammograms there were 120 breast-cancer deaths, while the control group (who didn't have mammograms) experienced 111 deaths.

In January 2002 the American expert group responsible for

writing information for the National Cancer Institute's online database concluded that evidence was insufficient to show that mammograms prevented breast-cancer deaths. Concurring with the findings of the Danish researchers, the group agreed that seven large studies of mammography had serious flaws, casting doubts on the studies' validity.

Further doubts were cast by a Swedish study that compared 21,088 women who had mammograms with 21,195 who served as controls. After nearly nine years, 63 women in the mammogram group had died of breast cancer compared with 66 in the control group — an insignificant difference. Mammograms did not lead to fewer mastectomies — in fact, quite the reverse. During the course of the study, 424 women in the mammography group had mastectomies compared with just 339 in the control group. This may be explained by the fact that doctors aggressively treated some tiny tumours found in mammograms, which might otherwise never have developed into cancer or might never have been noticed in a woman's lifetime.

More recently, the July 2005 issue of the *Journal of the National Cancer Institute* found that mammographic screening was not effective in decreasing the death rate from breast cancer. Regardless of the risk level of a woman, and her age, there was no association found between breast-cancer mortality and screening history. In other words, women of all ages and risks who had regular mammographic screening were just as likely to die of cancer as their matched peers who were not taking part in mammographic screening.

While these pronouncements from respected journals and researchers are damning of mammographic screening, other equally prestigious studies show reduced mortality (albeit small) in some age groups of women. Are you confused? Yes, even the experts who argue endlessly about the pros and cons of screening are confused! The October 2005 *New England Journal of Medicine* published an extremely sophisticated statistical analysis to invest-igate the reduction in breast cancer in the USA from 1975 to 2000.

The investigators concluded that an improvement in therapies and mammographic screening were equally responsible for the decrease in deaths. In direct contrast with this plethora of negative findings, a Danish study published in the *British Medical Journal* in 2005 showed that women participating in their national screening programme demonstrated a 37% decrease in mortality.

Breast Screen Aotearoa's website says that for women over the age of 50, mammograms make a significant impact on breast-cancer mortality. They comment that overseas studies show that when a woman is 50 and older, and is given a regular two-yearly mammogram, her chances of dying from breast cancer are reduced by at least a third. The same efficacy cannot be claimed, however, when screening women under the age of 50.

Other studies have discovered benefits for some age groups and lack of benefit for others. In 2002, Swedish researchers carried out a review of four large mammographic screening trials carried out in Sweden up to 1996. They found that there was a small benefit for women aged 55–69 at the start of the screening trial. For women aged 55–59, the reduction in mortality as a result of screening was 24% (29 deaths per 100,000 woman years versus 38 deaths per 100,000 woman years in the control group which received no mammograms). This rose to 32% for women aged 60–64 and 65–69. No statistically significant reduction in breast-cancer mortality was seen for women outside the ages of 55–69.

October 2006 saw the publication of another significant review of studies into the pros and cons of routine mammographic screening. The review, published in *The Cochrane Library*, pooled together findings from six randomised controlled trials (the gold standard for scientific trials), involving half a million women. The study found that women who have regular mammographic screening are 15% less likely to die of breast cancer than women who do not have mammograms. The reviewers estimated that for every 2000 women who are invited to get mammograms for 10 years, one woman's life will be prolonged as a result of detecting and treating a potentially lethal cancer.

The review also stresses the very real downside to screening. In order to reap this rather moderate decrease in mortality, women also face a 30% increased likelihood of receiving a breast-cancer diagnosis and treatment, for a form of cancer (ductal carcinoma *in situ*) which in the absence of screening would most likely never have posed a threat to their life.

What is obvious to anyone who has seriously investigated the pros and cons of mammographic screening is that there remains, after 35 years of widespread use, no clear, absolute and definitive evidence of decreased mortality resulting from routine screening.

If benefit is difficult to definitively prove, is there a 'downside' to taking part in mammographic screening programmes . . . beside there being no clear evidence of benefit? Many experts argue that there are clearly defined drawbacks to mammographic screening.

Mammographic screening can lead to an overdiagnosis and overtreatment of breast cancer. Breast Screen Aotearoa estimates that up to 10% of cancers detected through mammographic screening in New Zealand are overdiagnosed and overtreated.

Ductal carcinoma *in situ* (DCIS) is a very common, often non-invasive form of breast cancer, most cases of which are detected through mammograms. In fact, DCIS accounts for approximately 30–40% of all breast cancers detected by mammograms. Once discovered, it is almost always treated with surgery (lumpectomy or mastectomy), despite the fact that it is not known whether surgical treatment of this form of cancer extends the life of the patient. Some researchers question the validity of this aggressive treatment for a form of cancer which is often not life-threatening. The advent of mammographic screening has led to a massive increase in the detection and treatment of this form of cancer, which sometimes can go on to become invasive breast cancer, but in the majority of women does not seem to do so. Autopsies performed on women who died from all causes show that up to

16% of them had undiagnosed DCIS at the time of their death, suggesting that many women live with this condition without knowing about it, and without it threatening their life.

Assessing the drawbacks of mammography is partly an age-related issue. The age of the patient greatly influences the probable accuracy of a mammogram. Postmenopausal women are more accurately screened than younger, premenopausal women. Prior to menopause, the breast is very dense and cancerous growths are easily obscured on a mammographic X-ray. Postmenopausally, the breast becomes less dense and more fatty, making cancers more visible on a mammogram. Consequently, premenopausal women

New guidelines for mammographic screening

On 3 April 2007 the American College of Physicians released new clinical practice guidelines for mammographic screening for women aged between 40 and 49 years. These guidelines were formulated after evidence from 118 different trials had been evaluated. The guidelines stress that the benefit of screening mammography for women in this age group needs to be discussed **individually** with a patient's doctor, taking into account the patient's **individual** level of risk and the possible benefits and harms of undergoing screening.

New recommendations to physicians for best practice emphasise the need to:

✳ perform individual assessment of breast cancer risk for each patient in the 40- to 49-year age group in order to help guide the woman's decision whether or not to undergo routine mammographic screening

✳ inform all women in this age group of the potential benefits and harms of screening mammography.

have much higher rates of false-positive results (results saying they have cancer when they actually don't) and false-negative results (results saying they don't have cancer when they actually do). A false-positive obviously brings with it huge amounts of fear and anxiety, as well as further invasive investigations such as a biopsy. Sometimes biopsy can damage breast tissue and cause scarring, which in turn makes future mammograms more difficult to interpret.

While false-positives are traumatic, what is of most concern with premenopausal mammograms is the very real potential for missing the detection of present breast cancer (false-negative). In women between the ages of 40 and 49, as many as 25% of breast cancers fail to show on mammograms. This false-negative rate drops dramatically to around 10% for women aged 50–59. Women using HRT are also at increased risk of false-negative results. The potential for false-negatives is one of the most powerful arguments for women also performing their own regular manual breast examination, and having an annual breast check with their doctor.

As scientific debate continues, confused women are left to make their own decisions regarding mammograms. Contrary to what we are generally led to believe, women need to understand that while mammograms have until now been the gold standard in breast-cancer detection, they are not invincible and will not guarantee protection against breast-cancer mortality. (That said, the addition of ultrasound along with your mammography can greatly increase the accuracy of screening.) We also need to understand that mammograms sometimes lead to unnecessary biopsies and even mastectomies, for abnormalities and small cancers that would never become life-threatening.

If we take a step back this controversy looks almost Swiftian when we consider that even under the most optimistic assumptions, mammography still cannot prevent the vast majority of breast-cancer deaths

... There will come a time when all the study patients
have been followed up, all the analyses have been
done, all the expert groups have met, and all the
editorials have been written, and we still won't be sure
how much benefit and how much harm are caused
by mammography. We must find good ways to help
women deal with this uncertainty, for that time is
imminent.

Steven Goodman MD
Biostatistician
Johns Hopkins Sidney Kimmel Cancer Center

Take-home messages

By now you are probably thoroughly confused: should you have
regular mammograms or not? In truth, the benefit and risk ratio
will vary from woman to woman, and should be discussed on
an individual basis with your health provider. The following
important points may help you to make an informed choice
regarding mammographic screening.

* The fact that the benefits of mass mammographic screening
  are controversial, and for some age groups may be totally
  ineffectual, does not mean that mammograms cannot be a
  useful diagnostic tool if breast cancer is suspected.

* The benefits of mammographic screening before
  menopause are controversial. The risk of false-negatives
  (missed diagnosis of present cancer) is high. The addition
  of ultrasound reduces the rate of false-negatives.

* Postmenopausally mammogram results are more reliable,
  but even for women older than 50 both false-positive and
  false-negative results occur.

* Postmenopausal women taking HRT have an increased
  risk of false-negative results.

✳ If you are a premenopausal women, try to schedule mammograms for the week following your period when breast tissue is at its least dense.

✳ Never rely solely on mammograms. Always perform manual breast self-examination every month (see Chapter 1 for details) and see your doctor for a clinical breast examination every year.

✳ Be aware that even if you have a correct negative mammogram, it is still possible to develop breast cancer in the interval between your clear mammogram and your next mammogram. These 'interval' cancers may possibly be detected through monthly self-examination.

✳ It is worth paying extra to have a breast ultrasound at the same time as your mammogram, especially if you are a premenopausal woman or using HRT. Ultrasounds can sometimes detect breast cancers which have been missed by a mammogram.

✳ Mammograms are X-rays and expose the breast tissue to ionising radiation, itself classified as a 'known carcinogen'. Some experts suggest that repeated mammograms marginally increase the likelihood of developing breast cancer. (See *Exposure to radiation* above.)

Thermography (digital infrared imaging)

Breast thermography is now available privately in New Zealand. While the technology is new to our shores, medical infrared imaging has been widely used in Europe, and was first approved by the American FDA as an adjunctive breast-cancer screening procedure 20 years ago. Breast thermography has been widely researched since the late 1950s, and has already been the subject of over 800 peer-reviewed studies, involving well over 300,000 women, some of whom were followed for up to 12 years.

Thermography creates a visual picture of the heat being emitted by the breasts. The detection of breast cancers using thermography is based on the principle that the chemical and blood-vessel activity in precancerous tissue, or in the area around an already existing cancer, is nearly always higher than in healthy breast tissue.

Cancerous tumours increase the circulation of blood and nutrients to their cells by creating a new network of blood vessels; a process which usually results in an increased temperature in the area of the tumour. It is this area of increased heat which theoretically is detected by the thermogram. Thus, advocates argue, breast cancers can be detected in their very earliest precancerous stages, long before they would be detectable by physical examination or mammography.

In truth, there are several other non-cancerous causes for increased temperature in breast tissue. If a 'hot spot' is detected by thermography, it is impossible to know whether it is due to cancerous changes or other causes. Mammography and ultrasound, and possibly biopsy, are needed to confirm diagnosis of any such detections. Thermography is also unable to pinpoint the precise anatomical position of a lesion with accuracy; a mammogram or other diagnostic technique is still required for this.

Thermography is a controversial diagnostic tool for breast cancer. Medical authorities generally argue that its efficacy in detecting breast cancer is unproven, and that it offers no benefits over traditional mammography. Practitioners of thermography argue with just as much conviction in its favour.

What is generally agreed upon is that it is not recommended that thermography be used in place of mammography. However, there is some evidence that it may be a useful adjunctive diagnostic tool, alongside mammograms. Some studies suggest that thermography increases the likelihood of early detection when used adjunctively with mammography.

Preventing breast cancer — a summary

Lifestyle choices

✳ Do not smoke, and avoid inhaling second-hand smoke.

✳ Keep weight within a healthy range.

✳ Keep kilojoule intake in a healthy range.

✳ Exercise aerobically for at least 4 hours a week.

✳ Minimise exposure to ionising radiation such as X-rays and CT scans.

✳ Sleep in a very dark room at night.

✳ Try to get at least 7 hours of sleep a night.

✳ Minimise use of antibiotics as much as possible.

✳ Avoid (or minimise use of) hormone replacement therapy and the oral contraceptive pill.

✳ Choose environmentally friendly cleaning products which are less likely to contain toxic chemicals.

✳ Use plastic gloves and face masks if you are forced to use toxic chemicals, especially if they are sprayed.

✳ Always move well away from the car when you are refuelling to avoid inhaling petrol fumes.

✳ Use safety-conscious personal care products that contain no parabens.

✳ Avoid hairspray, nail polish and perfume containing phthalates.

✳ Avoid underarm antiperspirants containing aluminium; instead use aluminium-free deodorants (still controversial).

* Breastfeed your babies.

* Avoid cooking or storing foods in plastics; using plastic kettles; wrapping food in clingfilm.

* Go without a bra whenever possible to allow unimpeded blood and lymphatic circulation in breasts.

* Aim to have at least 15 minutes of sun exposure every day, at the lowest ultraviolet times of the day (before 10 a.m. and after 4 p.m.).

Nutritional choices

* Eat organic foods as much as possible to minimise intake of potentially oestrogenic or carcinogenic spray residues.

* Eat 9 or more servings of organic fruits and vegetables every day.

* Always wash fruits and vegetables well before eating.

* Eat brassica vegetables every day (broccoli, cabbage, cauliflower, Brussels sprouts).

* Drink 3–6 cups of green tea daily.

* Eat leafy green vegetables daily to boost intake of folate.

* Minimise or avoid drinking alcohol.

* Eat a high-fibre diet containing plentiful amounts of fruits, vegetables, whole grains, nuts and seeds.

* Add 10 g of flax seeds to your daily diet.

* Include in your diet a moderate amount of soya foods, as in an Asian diet, and a wide variety of other phyto-oestrogen-rich foods. (See *Tofu or not tofu . . . that is the question* above for more detailed information about soya, and its contraindications.)

* Decrease intake of saturated fats, trans-fats and omega-6-rich polyunsaturated fats, and increase intake of omega-3 and omega-9 fatty acids from fish, flax oil, flax seed, avocado, nuts and seeds, and olive oil.

* Reduce intake of red meat and increase fish-based or vegetarian meals.

* Avoid processed meats that contain carcinogenic nitrates.

* Never eat charred or burned foods. Minimise consumption of barbecued meat.

* Support friendly gut bacteria with unsweetened low-fat *acidophilus* yoghurt or probiotic drinks.

* Choose low-GI carbohydrates and minimise intake of sugars and processed foods that contain added sugar, which cause insulin spikes.

* Cook with generous amounts of turmeric and garlic.

* Consult a naturopath or nutritionist for advice on nutritional supplementation and breast cancer.

Part Two

Getting Well

A–Z of women's health

Amenorrhoea

Healthy women of a reproductive age (approximately 13–50 years) should have a period every month, unless they are pregnant, breastfeeding, nearing the menopause or have just started menstruating (at which times menstruation can be erratic). If the periods stop and their absence cannot be explained by pregnancy, breastfeeding, menopause or the use of artificial hormones, the condition is called *amenorrhoea*. Sometimes a seemingly healthy woman will stop menstruating, but more often a lack of periods is part of an overall picture of ill health which may include being underweight, suffering from extreme stress, nervous exhaustion, iron-deficiency anaemia or polycystic ovarian syndrome. This type of amenorrhoea occurring after years of healthy menstruation is called *secondary amenorrhoea*. *Primary amenorrhoea* is the name given to a condition in which a teenage girl has never had periods.

Causes of secondary amenorrhoea

If you miss the occasional period during times of great stress or when travelling, the chances are you don't have much to worry about. Your monthly loss of blood is the end result of an intricate interaction between the brain (pituitary gland in particular), female hormones, and the ovaries and uterus. This delicate interaction is easily thrown into disarray by long-term or severe stress. In most cases, once the stress dies down, menstruation spontaneously begins again. If, however, you have missed a period three or four times in a row, it's time to do some serious detective work.

Start by looking at the obvious causes. Are you an exercise addict? If you go to the gym at every possible opportunity, or consider marathon running a form of relaxation, your amen-orrhoea may be the result of exercise-induced underweight. Contrary to the Western notion that the ideal female form is an emaciated one, a healthy woman needs at least 18% body fat for normal hormonal balance. If your body fat drops below this level, you may be the envy of body-conscious female friends but your periods will disappear. Ballet dancers, aerobics teachers, triathletes and other super-fit sportswomen often live without periods for years at a time. While it saves them the inconvenience and mess of menstruation interfering with their active lifestyles, they ultimately pay a big price with potentially serious health consequences.

Long-term amenorrhoea signals very low oestrogen production, often comparable with that of a postmenopausal woman. Along with low oestrogen comes increased cardiovascular risk, infer–tility and rapid bone demineralisation leading to early-onset osteoporosis.

Crash dieting is another sadly common cause of amenorrhoea. Trying to lose too much weight too quickly can leave your hormones knocked out of kilter, and unable to stimulate ovulation and menstruation.

Amenorrhoea is a common symptom of malnutrition and iron-deficiency anaemia, resulting from frequent dieting, a poorly balanced vegetarian diet, or plain bad dietary habits. Iron-deficiency anaemia is a common problem among New Zealand and Australian women. Traditionally, the richest dietary sources of iron were red meat and whole grains. With the decline in red meat consumption and the proliferation of refined grain products such as white bread, iron deficiency is now a significant issue for women in their reproductive years. A diet that is extremely low in protein will also lead to amenorrhoea, although this is not a common scenario for Western women unless they are living on unbalanced weight-loss regimes.

If you exercise sensibly, have a healthy body weight, good nutrition and a relatively stress-free life, a sudden absence of periods may signal an underlying undiagnosed health condition. Diabetes, overactive or underactive thyroid, hepatitis, Addison's disease and Cushing's disease (both adrenal gland disorders) or polycystic ovarian syndrome can all cause periods to stop. In very rare instances amenorrhoea may result from an ovarian or pituitary tumour.

Various forms of contraception can stop menstruation. Depo-Provera injections will inhibit menstruation, sometimes for months or even years after the injection has been used. Similarly, progesterone-releasing IUDs such as the Mirena will often cause periods to disappear. Women coming off the oral contraceptive pill can find that it takes several months before normal menstruation returns.

A monthly period is evidence of normal functioning and inter-relation between the hypothalamus and pituitary gland (in the brain), the thyroid and adrenal glands, and of course the ovaries and uterus. Problems in any one of these organs or glands can cause a lack of periods.

Undiagnosed hypothyroidism is surprisingly common and it is not unusual for a woman to exist for years in a state of chronic 'unwellness' because of a sluggish thyroid gland. Ask your doctor for a thyroid function test if you are troubled by:

* dry hair and skin, and hair loss

* excessive sensitivity to the cold

* poor immune function, and susceptibility to colds and infections

✳ exhaustion and apathy

✳ foggy thinking, inability to concentrate, depression and
anxiety

✳ tendency to gain weight easily.

It is always advisable to have a medical check to rule out any
potentially serious underlying conditions before embarking on a
programme of self-help for amenorrhoea.

A traditional Chinese perspective of amenorrhoea

Traditional Chinese medicine places huge emphasis on menstruation, believing that a woman's menses are a powerful reflection
of her health in general.

According to traditional Chinese medicine, in the weeks
following a monthly bleed the body manufactures blood which
fills the uterus, and 'spills over' as the next menstrual period. If
the quantity and quality of blood is poor, there will be insufficient
to fill the uterus . . . and consequently no 'spilling over'!

Amenorrhoea usually results from a deficiency of blood or
the other vital life force called qi (pronounced chi); or from a
stagnation of blood which impedes its flow. The spleen, kidney
and heart meridians are central to the production of blood.
If any of these meridians are deficient, 'blood deficiency' can
occur. Kidney and spleen energy is weakened by the following.

✳ Overwork, lack of relaxation, exhaustion, overindulgence
in sex. (Yes, traditional Chinese medicine believes you can
definitely have too much of this good thing!)

✳ Chronic fear or anxiety.

✳ Overuse of the mind (for example, worry or excessive
study).

Medical treatment

This varies dramatically depending upon the cause of your problem, and may involve pharmacological treatment of an underlying condition such as diabetes or thyroid disorders. Where there is a clear psychological component, antidepressants or tranquillisers may be prescribed. Hormonal imbalances may be treated with synthetic hormones. Surgery is possible in the case of a tumour on the ovaries or pituitary gland.

* Poor dietary habits: a lack of nourishment, excess of cold foods or sweet foods; eating at irregular times, and skipping meals.

Blood stagnates usually because of a weakness of qi — as qi is the force that moves the blood. Qi is weakened through 'wrong living' as described above. Blood can also become 'stuck' or stagnant due to the congealing effects of the cold. The Chinese firmly advise against women exposing themselves to cold air or cold water before or during their periods. At this time the uterus is especially vulnerable to 'taking cold'. Going for a swim in cool waters around the time of menstruation is definitely not advisable.

Traditional Chinese medicine can be very effective in the treatment of both primary and secondary amenorrhoea. Acupuncture and herbs are used to nourish the blood by strengthening and balancing the qi in the kidney, spleen, heart and liver meridians. In the case of stagnation, qi flow is strengthened and cold blockages are removed through application of heat to acupuncture points with the warming herb moxa.

Self-help

If you've had all the tests and there is still no explanation for your lack of periods, it may be time for some honest self-analysis. The body/mind connection is nowhere more significant than in the realm of female hormonal imbalance. If you're living under a permanent load of almost intolerable stress, drastic measures may be called for. Establishing new boundaries and saying 'no' to requests for help from others while you lighten your own load is a prerequisite for finding your balance again. Maybe you need to take serious stock of your work/life balance and make some changes even if they mean fewer dollars in the bank. Put regular time aside for 'active de-stressing' activities such as yoga, tai chi, meditation or simply 'time out' alone walking by the sea.

Regular exercise is an important part of your well-being, but both too little and too much exercise can contribute to hormonal imbalance. If you are over-exercising and excessively lean, it may be time to reduce the aerobic content and increase stretching and relaxation exercises, such as yoga or Pilates. If you're not exercising, begin a gentle programme to stimulate your endocrine system and normalise hormones. Simply going for a half-hour brisk walk three or four times a week will produce beneficial results.

Diet and nutritional supplements

Read the healthy diet outline in Chapter 2. Pay particular attention to your protein and fat intake. An excessively low-fat diet can lead to underproduction of oestrogen. While it's a good idea to moderate intake of animal fats, 'healthy' fats such as those found in nuts and seeds, avocados, oily fish, flax and olive oil are a daily necessity.

Deficiencies of vitamin B6 and zinc are common among women with inexplicable amenorrhoea. These deficiencies are especially likely to occur in women on unbalanced weight-loss regimes; those consuming a 'junk-food' diet high in refined carbohydrates;

or those on a vegetarian diet. A balanced multivitamin supplying 20–50 mg of B6 and 15–20 mg of elemental zinc each day is a useful addition to a 'period-friendly' diet. Most multivitamins also contain vitamin B12 and folic acid, a lack of which has been implicated in unexplained amenorrhoea.

Herbal help

Primary amenorrhoea in adolescent girls can often be helped with a course of herbal uterine tonics such as blue cohosh, rue, false unicorn root, chasteberry, raspberry and squaw vine. These same uterine tonics will help restore normal menstruation in women whose periods are delayed for some unknown reason. They are especially useful to restore a normal menstrual cycle in women who have recently come off the oral contraceptive pill.

Aromatherapy

Aromatherapy oils or herbs which have the ability to promote menstrual bleeding are called *emmenagogues*. Aromatherapy oils with emmenagogue qualities include: sage, basil, German and Roman chamomile, clary sage, lavender, rose, rosemary, peppermint and tarragon.

These oils can be inhaled from an essential oil burner, added to bathwater, or made into a massage oil. Use 100 ml of a cold-pressed oil as a carrier, and add no more than 60 drops (combined total) of essential oils to the base oil. Massage the lower back and abdomen. Obviously this is contraindicated in pregnancy.

Homoeopathy

✳ *Pulsatilla.* The type of amenorrhoea treated by this remedy is usually accompanied by extreme emotional sensitivity and weepiness. There may be migraines and palpitations and a general sense of weakness. Often the periods have been suppressed by exposure to damp, such as may occur in an excessively wet or humid climate or if living in a damp house.

✳ *Dulcamara.* The periods have been suppressed through exposure to damp or cold. There is extreme sensitivity to weather changes, which often result in colds or an attack of sinusitis. Breasts may feel swollen and painful upon pressure.

✳ *Silica.* This remedy can be used if amenorrhoea is accompanied by a tendency to feel the cold and in particular to have poor peripheral circulation. Other symptoms include a general sensation of weakness and often constipation. There are usually skin complaints such as spots with pus or frequent boils.

In addition, there are several homoeopathic remedies that are clearly indicated if the exact cause of the cessation of menstruation is known. For example, menses which stopped after exposure to damp indicate the use of pulsatilla. If exposure to extreme cold or an emotional fright (fear) was the cause, then aconite is the remedy. Periods which stop following an emotional shock of some sort indicate nat mur (*Natrum muriaticum*), while ignatia is more specifically for menses stopped by grief.

Anaemia

Iron-deficiency anaemia

Anaemia can result from a deficiency of iron, folic acid or vitamin B12. The most commonly occurring form of anaemia in women of reproductive age is iron-deficiency anaemia. Between a quarter and a half of all menstruating women have low reserves of this important mineral, partly because of the regular monthly blood and iron loss resulting from menstrual bleeding. Pregnancy and breastfeeding also drain iron reserves and contribute to the much higher incidence of iron-deficiency anaemia in women. During the later months of pregnancy, a growing foetus demands 7–8 mg of iron a day — a large amount when you consider that the average dietary intake is only 15–25 mg a day. Poor dietary practices and frequent weight-loss diets also take their toll on a woman's iron reserves. Adolescent girls are also at increased risk of this form of anaemia due to the combined effects of rapid growth (increasing iron requirements), menstruation and a poor diet. The elderly are another at-risk group for iron-deficiency anaemia, as their reduced hydrochloric acid production in the stomach makes it more difficult for their bodies to absorb iron from dietary sources.

Unless there is acute and severe sudden bleeding such as haemorrhage, iron-deficiency anaemia does not occur overnight. More usually it is the end result of months or even years of dietary iron deficiency, or chronic long-term blood loss such as hidden internal bleeding or heavy, flooding menstrual periods. It is possible (and quite common) to have low iron reserves and yet not display symptoms of anaemia.

Diagnosis

Iron-deficiency anaemia is diagnosed by blood tests including ferritin, measurement of haemoglobin levels, hematocrit and red blood cell count. Serum ferritin is the best test to determine the body iron stores. A ferritin reading of less than 12 indicates iron deficiency. Under a microscope, anaemic blood cells look smaller and paler than normal ones.

Red blood cell count

It is your red blood cells that carry the red pigment (haemoglobin), which is responsible for transporting oxygen from your lungs to your tissues. If you have a low red blood cell count, this function cannot be performed adequately and you are considered anaemic. A normal red blood cell count for an adult woman is about 4 to 5.5 million red blood cells in each microlitre of blood.

Haemoglobin level

This test determines the relative amount of oxygen-carrying pigment in your blood. Even if you have a normal red blood cell count, if your haemoglobin levels are low you will exhibit symptoms of anaemia.

In order for this haemoglobin to bind with the oxygen it transports to your tissues, plentiful supplies of iron are needed. This is why iron deficiency eventually leads to anaemia. Normal haemoglobin levels for women are 12–16 g per decilitre of blood. A haemoglobin level of less than 12 is indicative of anaemia.

Ferritin test

This test allows the cause of your anaemia to be further differentiated. It provides the means of determining whether your anaemia results from lack of iron or from chronic disease, inflammation or infection. This test is a reliable gauge of iron stores.

Symptoms

If you visit your doctor complaining of lethargy and exhaustion, the first diagnostic investigation is often a test for iron-deficiency anaemia. A lack of iron in the body results in a lower than normal number of red blood cells, low haemoglobin levels and lack of oxygenation to all your tissues. No wonder you feel exhausted!

As well as tiredness, there may also be headaches and dizziness, breathlessness, constipation, a poor appetite and poor immune function with frequent infections. You may look pale and have a pale, sore tongue; your skin may itch for no apparent reason and your nails may be brittle and break easily. Mental and emotional symptoms frequently accompany anaemia. These include apathy, irritability and depression, and possibly memory problems. In severe iron-deficiency anaemia there may be a symptom called pica which is a bizarre compulsion to eat strange substances such as ice or clay!

Causes of iron-deficiency anaemia

The most obvious cause of iron-deficiency anaemia is a lack of dietary iron, often as a result of an unbalanced vegetarian diet or stringent weight-loss regimes. Sometimes your dietary intake of iron may be minimally adequate, but other dietary practices may interfere with your ability to absorb and utilise this iron. For example, drinking tea with meals or immediately after a meal can inhibit the absorption of iron by as much as 60%. Eating large amounts of raw grains such as natural muesli can be a problem for iron levels, as raw grains contain a lot of phytic acid which binds iron and passes it in the stools. Calcium supplements can also inhibit absorption of dietary iron, and low stomach acid (which is common in postmenopausal women) will also interfere with iron absorption.

Bleeding is an obvious cause of anaemia. Both massive blood loss from acute trauma, and chronic blood loss over many months — such as a bleeding stomach ulcer; colitis causing intestinal bleeding; or even bleeding haemorrhoids — can all contribute to the development of anaemia. If your menstrual periods are particularly heavy or long, perhaps because of undetected uterine fibroids, then you also run the risk of anaemia. Even a 'normal' period results in the loss of about 18 mg of iron.

The use of pharmaceutical medicines such as tetracycline antibiotics (often prescribed for months on end for teenage acne problems), and prolonged aspirin use can induce iron-deficiency anaemia.

A lack of vitamin C-rich foods, such as fresh fruits and vegetables, can also lead to low iron reserves as this vitamin is essential for the proper absorption of iron.

Treatment
Your doctor will probably prescribe iron supplements containing either ferrous gluconate or ferrous sulphate, and sometimes vitamin C. While ferrous sulphate is an inexpensive and easily absorbed source of iron, it can also irritate the gut, causing constipation and blackened stools. Ferrous gluconate is also cheap and absorbable, and tends not to cause problems with constipation. The usual dosage of either of these forms of iron is around 325 mg two to three times daily. These high doses are

specifically to treat anaemia and shouldn't be used as a general preventative or ongoing supplement.

Other highly absorbable forms of iron include chelated iron such as iron aspartate, ferrous fumerate and ferrous succinate. Whichever forms of iron you end up using, you can further increase absorption by taking vitamin C along with your iron supplement.

It is not advisable to self-administer iron supplements without first having a blood test to ascertain your requirements. Taking an iron supplement simply because you feel a little run-down can lead to iron overload, especially if you are postmenopausal and not losing iron with your monthly period. Excessive iron becomes an oxidant, stimulating free-radical production, as well as promoting inflammation of the fatty plaques in the arteries, thus ultimately increasing risk of heart disease. However, for growing children, pregnant or breastfeeding women, or women with heavy periods, iron supplements in the region of 10–30 mg of iron are often indicated.

Iron and your diet

Lots of foods contain iron, but not all forms of dietary iron are equally useful. There are two types of dietary iron — heme and non-heme iron.

The heme iron is found in food containing animal protein, such as red meat, liver, and other organ meats, and to a lesser extent chicken and fish. This type of iron is readily absorbed and utilised by your body.

Vegetarian iron sources such as whole grains (especially millet, wheat and oats), brown rice, peas and beans, nuts and seeds and fruit and vegetables contain the less readily absorbed non-heme iron. But there are ways you can enhance your absorption of this type of iron, either by eating it along with a little of the heme sources, or else by adding vitamin-C-rich foods. By adding as little as 60 mg of vitamin C to your non-heme meals, you can increase iron absorption by up to 300%. A glass of fresh orange juice, a sliced tomato or a handful of bean sprouts added to your meals containing vegetarian iron will boost absorption.

Foods especially useful for increasing iron reserves include liver, leafy green vegetables, beans, blackstrap molasses, meat and organ meats, dried apricots, almonds, shellfish and spirulina.

You can also increase your iron availability by decreasing your intake of iron-inhibiting foods at the time you are eating your iron-rich foods. Iron-inhibiting foods include tea, coffee, wheat bran, processed foods such as ice-cream, soft drinks, cakes, biscuits and sweets that contain phosphate food additives. (See the chart on p. 72 for information on iron-rich foods.) If you are taking calcium supplements, take them at the opposite end of the day to iron supplements.

Other types of anaemia

Mention the word *anaemia* and everyone thinks of iron deficiency. In truth it is possible (and quite common) to exhibit all the signs of anaemia, including the lab indicators of reduced numbers of red blood cells, while having perfectly adequate iron levels. Vitamin B6, B12 and B9 (folate) deficiencies can all induce anaemia, as can a deficiency of zinc and vitamin E.

If your haemoglobin levels fail to rise despite a lengthy course of iron supplements, the missing link could well be folate. This B-vitamin, found in grains and leafy green vegetables, can boost haemoglobin levels when taken with iron. However, if you are also lacking in vitamin B12 — a common problem in strict vegans and the elderly — supplementing with folic acid will be of little benefit as B12 is essential for the body to change dietary folate into a usable form. Folate deficiency is especially common in women using the oral contraceptive pill, pregnant women or women who regularly consume large amounts of alcohol.

If your anaemia fails to improve despite all these measures, see a nutritionally oriented health professional for more detailed guidance and a solution to your health problem.

Cervical dysplasia

Waiting for the results of a Pap smear can be nerve-racking. If you are then told that you have an abnormal reading, or cervical dysplasia, it can be easy to go into panic mode. Don't! Cervical dysplasia means that some abnormal cells have been found on the surface of your cervix . . . it does not mean that you have cancer! Dysplasia is considered to be a precancerous condition, which in time, if left untreated, could develop into cervical cancer. Between 30 and 50% of women with cervical dysplasia will go on to develop cervical cancer if the condition is left untreated. This progression is usually (but not always) slow, and takes between three and seven years. Cancer of the cervix is one of the most common cancers affecting women, so having regular Pap smears can literally save your life, as dysplasia is treatable almost 100% of the time.

Cervical dysplasia, or CIN as it is referred to, is graded according to its severity, from grade 1 (mild and moderate changes) to grade 3 (most severe, and including carcinoma *in situ*).

What causes cervical dysplasia? A multitude of different factors may be involved. One of these is sexual activity. Becoming sexually active at an early age and having a history of multiple sexual partners increases the risk of cervical dysplasia significantly (because of the increased likelihood of exposure to human *Papilloma* virus, HPV). Cervical dysplasia could almost be thought of as a sexually transmitted disease (STD), in the sense that a number of infectious agents which are sexually transmitted can stimulate the development of abnormal cervical cells.

The two main infective agents involved in the development of dysplasia are both viruses — herpes simplex type II; and HPV, the virus also responsible for genital warts. HPV infection is pandemic amongst sexually active women with multiple partners. While there are about 200 different strains of the virus (40 of which affect the genital area), only a few of these strains have been linked to abnormal cervical cell development. Of these, it is the HPV16 strain which is found in 50–70% of all cervical dysplasia cases. Very often there are no symptoms to suggest that you have been in contact with HPV. Sometimes, even if you do contract HPV, the virus disappears on its own in time, without causing any cervical cellular changes . . . but sometimes it does trigger cervical cellular changes which occasionally go on to become cervical cancer. Using a condom during sex will reduce the likelihood of contracting HPV, but not eliminate the risk altogether as the virus can still exist on skin areas not covered by the condom.

Long-term use of the oral contraceptive pill is associated with an increased risk of cervical dysplasia. Female smokers with dysplasia are more likely to go on to develop carcinoma *in situ* than are non-smokers. If you are diagnosed with dysplasia, it's in your best interest to stop using the pill or smoking cigarettes.

Nutritional deficiency of vitamins A, B6, C, folate, and beta-carotene can also increase your susceptibility to dysplasia.

And what of treatment? (See Chapter 1)

If you have cervical dysplasia classified as CIN 1, your doctor will probably simply recommend a repeat smear in six months' time. Dysplasia rated CIN 2 and above is usually further investigated, and some form of treatment performed to remove the abnormal cells. This is usually laser surgery or cryosurgery (where the cells are frozen off). Removing cells which are significantly abnormal is a good idea. However, it also makes sense to take a look at the wider picture and ask yourself if there are any changes you can make to safeguard and improve the health of your cervix. Stopping smoking, coming off the pill (if it is safe for you to do so) and improving your diet are three such sensible changes.

Nutrition and dysplasia

When it comes to reducing your risk of dysplasia, or treating it through nutrition, the nutrients supreme are humble folic acid (part of the B-complex of vitamins) and vitamin C. Folic-acid deficiency is the most common nutrient deficiency in the world, and is particularly prevalent in pregnant women or those using the oral contraceptive pill. Studies have shown that folic-acid supplements taken in high doses of 10 mg a day for at least three months can either improve or normalise Pap smears in women with dysplasia. After three months of this high dose, reduce the dose to 2.5 mg of folate per day, until your smear comes back normal. Even if this treatment fails to cure the dysplasia, the folic acid may reduce the risk of the dysplasia developing into cervical cancer. It is important to always supplement with a balanced B-complex containing B12 at the same time as using high-dose supplements of folic acid.

Whenever there is any kind of cell abnormality, or cancer, vitamin C is always one of the first nutritional supplements to think of. Clinical studies have repeatedly shown women with dysplasia to have lower intakes of vitamin C than women without dysplasia, and some researchers go so far as to suggest that a low dietary intake of vitamin C is an independent risk factor for cervical dysplasia and cancer. Keep your vitamin-C intake high by eating at least nine servings of fresh fruits and vegetables daily, as well as taking a vitamin-C supplement regularly. If you are diagnosed with dysplasia, supplement with up to 5000 mg of vitamin C daily. (See Chapter 2.)

Beta-carotene is the plant-based form of vitamin A. There is a very strong inverse relationship between beta-carotene intake and dysplasia risk. The more beta-carotene you consume, the lower your risk of dysplasia. Women with low beta-carotene levels are three times more likely to develop severe dysplasia than women with adequate levels. For treating dysplasia, supplement with between 25,000 and 50,000 iu per day. This is a safe non-toxic form of vitamin A, and is even safe to use during pregnancy.

Some studies have found that women with dysplasia have lower levels of antioxidants in their body compared with healthy controls. It is not clear, though, whether the low levels of antioxidants actually cause dysplasia, or whether the dysplasia itself leads to a drop in antioxidants. However, from what we know about antioxidants and cancer, it is advisable to increase dietary antioxidants (see Chapter 6), and in addition to use an antioxidant formula containing antioxidant nutrients, such as turmeric, green tea extract, pine bark or grape seed.

Other useful supplements in the treatment of dysplasia include vitamin B6 (25 mg three times daily); vitamin E (preferably a mixed tocopherol formula supplying 200 iu per day) and selenium (200 mcg per day).

Preventing the development of cervical cancer obviously involves a great deal more than simply swallowing a few nutritional supplements every day. A high-fat diet is associated with increased cervical cancer risk, so take a look at your fat intake and take steps to reduce the unhealthy forms of fat you eat, while increasing beneficial fats in your diet. (See the discussion of fats in Chapters 2 and 6.)

Aim for nine servings (or a minimum of five) of fresh fruits and vegetables daily, to increase dietary supplies of folate, beta-carotene and vitamin C.

Cystitis

Do you rush to the toilet every 10 minutes, and still feel as though your bladder is full? Does your urine burn like fire-water? If your answer to these questions is 'yes', the chances are that you are suffering from a urinary tract infection, commonly called cystitis. For mostly structural reasons, women are many times more likely than their male partner to suffer from cystitis. Most cases of simple cystitis are caused by bacteria which find their way from the outside world into the urethra, from where they travel the short distance to the bladder. Females have a very short urethra in comparison with males, resulting in an increased propensity to bladder infections. The opening to the urethra is also situated close to the anus in the female, again making infection more likely, as most of the more-common infecting organisms responsible for cystitis live in the gut and bowels.

Symptoms

The most usual symptoms of cystitis include:

* frequent urge to urinate, night and day

* blood in the urine (in severe cases)

* sensation that the bladder is never empty, even after passing water

* burning sensation when voiding

* pain just above the pubic bone or in the lower back

* general malaise.

Causes

In a healthy person, the urine is completely sterile. A diagnosis of cystitis is usually made by collecting a mid-stream urine sample, and testing for the presence of bacteria. In 85% of cases of cystitis, *Escherichia coli (E. coli)* bacteria (normal inhabitants of the colon) are found in the urine. In the remaining 15% of infections, staphylococcal and streptococcal bacteria are found.

Diagnosing urinary tract infections (UTIs) based on the results of mid-stream urinary testing is not always accurate. Only around 60% of women with symptoms of a UTI actually have significant amounts of bacteria in their urine. Generally, a woman presenting with all the symptoms of a UTI, but with a negative urinary analysis, will still be treated as if she has a urinary tract infection. However, in these cases, additional cultures to check for possible STDs are often carried out.

In recurring cases of urinary tract infection, further testing is carried out to rule out underlying problems such as anatomical abnormalities, urinary reflux or kidney stones. Often there is no obvious underlying cause for recurrent infections. People in this group of chronic cystitis sufferers often become frustrated with traditional medicine which has little to offer them besides repeated courses of antibiotics.

There are a number of commonly acknowledged causes of cystitis, such as those discussed here. However, if these are the 'causes' of cystitis, it seems sensible to ask why all women don't suffer frequently from urinary tract infections. How come there are very many women in the world who have never experienced a bladder infection?

The answer is that our susceptibility to any form of infection is largely related to our overall health and the strength of our immune system. Cystitis is an infection, and as with all infections, women with poor nutritional status, poor cellular health and lowered immunity will be more susceptible to its threat. Not everyone develops a case of cystitis each time a few stray *E. coli* bacteria find their way into their bladder. As is the case with many of the other genito-urinary infections, it is common for us to play host to potentially troublesome bacteria for weeks, months or even a lifetime, without them proliferating into an active infection. It is only when our systemic health is lowered (for example during a period of great stress, such as during a divorce or after the death of a loved one), that the bacteria undergo a sudden population explosion.

If you suffer from more than the occasional bout of cystitis, making some holistic changes to increase your total well-being, rather than simply focusing on your bladder in isolation, may prove to be a turning point in the frustrating battle against never-ending bladder infections. Ultimately, a whole-person approach may be a more effective way of reducing the frequency of cystitis attacks than spending your life frantically trying to avoid possible sources of infection.

So what are the causes of cystitis?

Since *E. coli* bacteria normally live in the bowel, incorrect toilet procedure can transfer the bacteria to the vagina or urethra. After a bowel movement, always wipe away from, rather than towards, the vagina. This is important, too, if you suffer from frequent attacks of vaginal thrush, as the *Candida* fungal spores often exist in the bowel. *E. coli* can also be transferred from the bowel if your partner touches your anus with any part of their body, and then goes on to touch your clitoris or vagina, during lovemaking.

With even the best of hygiene, the act of sexual intercourse can be followed 36 hours later by an attack of cystitis. The thrusting motion of the penis, combined with the tiny distance from the outside world to the female bladder, makes it possible for bacteria to be literally pushed up towards the bladder. This is particularly likely in the traditional 'missionary' position of intercourse.

Weak pelvic floor muscles allow the bladder to prolapse and bulge forward into the wall of the vagina. If the back part of the bladder droops below the neck of the bladder, it becomes virtually impossible to empty the bladder completely during urination (something akin to weeing uphill!), leaving a permanent reservoir of urine in the bladder. This stagnant urine provides a haven for bacteria to multiply and irritate the bladder.

What goes in at one end of the body must come out at the other end. An overdose of hot curries, coffee and alcohol can cause irritation to the delicate tissues lining your bladder and urethra.

Women who 'hold on' when they get the urge to pass water are more prone to bladder infections. It's important to drink plenty of water and urinate frequently (when you feel the natural urge). This reduces the opportunity for pathogenic bacteria to multiply in the urine.

Waste materials are excreted from the body through several different channels:

* the bowel — in the form of faeces
* the lungs — in the form of carbon dioxide
* the skin — in the form of perspiration
* the kidneys and bladder — in the form of urine.

If any one (or several) of these 'garbage collectors' is lazy, it places an excessive load on the others. If you only manage a half-hearted bowel movement every two or three days, you are placing an undue load on your kidneys and bladder, as accumulated toxins are passed out through these organs instead. So in this sense there is a direct link between constipation and cystitis!

When we are children and teenagers, each of our abdominal organs is tidily tucked in its designated rightful position. Unfortunately, having children, growing older, carrying a spare tyre of fat, having a poor posture and spinal problems all conspire to wreck this perfection. Eventually the transverse colon which lies across the abdomen from right to left may begin to sag in the middle. The sagging weight of the transverse colon in turn squashes and compresses all the organs beneath it, including the bladder. Blood flow is impeded and the long-term result is congestion and a downgrading of tissue health.

A bladder starved of oxygen and nutrients is a bladder ripe for infection. This same kind of poor tissue health can occur as a direct result of chronic spinal problems. Each pelvic organ receives nerve impulses from the spine. A back problem, anywhere from level with the bottom of the shoulder blades down to the coccyx (tail bone), can affect the health of the bladder. If you suffer from chronic urinary tract infections it is always worth a visit to a registered osteopath or chiropractor to check for spinal misalignment that may be contributing to your bladder problems.

Medical treatment

Sometimes cystitis will spontaneously cure itself in the first 24 hours, so if you suspect that you have an infection wait a day before visiting your doctor. During that time, try the self-help measures discussed below.

The medical treatment of simple acute cystitis is a course of antibiotics, from 1 to 10 days in duration. Relapse within a couple of weeks is common, and may be due to the initial offending bacteria not being completely wiped out by the antibiotics.

From what you now know, you can understand that there are many underlying factors (besides the presence of bacteria) which contribute to the recurrence of UTIs. Ironically, one of the problems of repeat antibiotic use is that the treatment itself may contribute to further UTIs. Broad-spectrum antibiotics are indiscriminate killers, wiping out the friendly gut and vaginal bacteria which work to keep a healthy balance of 'friendly' and 'unfriendly' bacteria living uneventfully side by side. Once the delicate gastrointestinal and vaginal microflora are upset, less-desirable strains of bacteria (such as *E. coli*) are left to proliferate virtually unchecked. In turn, future re-infection and problems with cystitis become more likely.

If you do take antibiotics for UTIs, it is important to replace the 'friendly' bacteria in the vagina and gut. Taking an oral probiotic formula for 4–6 weeks after a course of antibiotics will restore a healthy gut environment. To replace friendly bacteria in the vagina, simply insert an *acidophilus* capsule high into the vagina nightly for two weeks.

Self-help treatment

Long-term preventative changes are important if you suffer from frequent bladder infections. To reduce the risk of future bladder infections, do the following:

* Wipe from front to back after a bowel movement.

* Change pads and tampons frequently during a period.

* Encourage your partner to wash thoroughly before sexual contact, and try to avoid the transfer of bacteria from the anus to the vagina during sex play.

* Avoid tight-fitting jeans, and nylon pants and tights. Cotton pants and crotchless tights or stockings and suspenders allow more air flow and ventilation.

* Make a habit of drinking more water, rather than tea or coffee. Aim for seven or eight glasses of water a day. This

keeps your urine diluted, and less favourable to bacteria. It also keeps the urine flowing frequently, thus washing out any problematic bacteria.

* Empty your bladder frequently. Women who ignore their urge to urinate and hold on for long periods of time are more likely to develop cystitis. When you need to go, go straight away!

* Pass water immediately after sex. This helps flush away any bacteria that may have been pushed up the urethra during intercourse.

* See a registered osteopath or chiropractor if you think you may have spinal problems which might be contributing to recurring cystitis.

* Eat wisely, exercise regularly and relax frequently — in short, apply the recommendations for healthy living found in this book!

* If you are using the oral contraceptive pill and are suffering from chronic cystitis, consider another form of contraception. Women who use the oral contraceptive pill are at greater risk of cystitis then non-users. Poor-fitting cervical caps or diaphragms can also lead to bladder irritation.

Self-help for acute cystitis

So you have promised yourself you will make all the long-term changes, but right now you're in agony and want some relief — quickly! What can you do? Start drinking and drinking and drinking. Stay away from tea, coffee and alcohol, instead choosing water, parsley tea (which will really get you running to the toilet), and cranberry juice.

In New Zealand it is difficult to find unsweetened cranberry juice, but dried cranberry capsules are available and will serve the same purpose as cranberry juice. These can be taken in high doses of up to three capsules, three times daily during a bladder infection. The cranberries change the pH of your urine, making it more acidic and therefore less hospitable to bacteria. Cranberries also contain a high concentration of a strong antibacterial called hippuric acid. This acid makes the lining of the bladder very slippery and prevents unfriendly bacteria from gaining a foothold on the walls of the bladder.

Recent studies have discovered that blueberries also contain hippuric acid, and are helpful in the prevention or treatment of UTIs. The therapeutic dosage of cranberry juice needed to reliably prevent UTIs is 450 ml per day. Both cranberry juice and vitamin C acidify the urine, but when taken together, this acidifying effect is much greater.

If you can't get hold of cranberry juice or cranberry tea, try drinking buttermilk (*acidophilus*), or a glass of water with two teaspoons of apple cider vinegar — they all perform the same acidifying function.

During a bladder infection, cut out completely all sugar, refined carbohydrates, alcohol, coffee, tea, soft drinks and full-strength fruit juice.

If your urine stings you when you void, try sitting in a bowl of warm water to urinate, or spray your vulva with warm water as you pass water.

Nutritional supplements

Increase your intake of vitamin C up to your bowel tolerance, with repeated doses two-hourly. Use the ascorbic acid form of vitamin C to help acidify the urine. Because you are fighting an infection, your vitamin-C tolerance will probably be very high. You may find that you can take as much as 5000 to 10,000 mg (5–10 g) in a day without it causing diarrhoea. Vitamin C concentrates in high levels in the urine, and exerts a direct bactericidal effect as well as supporting the function of your immune system systematically. Vitamin C activates neutrophils, the white blood cells most involved in the front-line defence against infection.

It also increases production of lymphocytes, important for co-ordinating immune function at a cellular level.

Supplement with vitamin A (such as halibut liver oil capsules) up to 50,000 iu a day during the acute phases of infection (don't take this dose for more than three or four days). *If you are pregnant, or even if there is a remote possibility that you could be pregnant, avoid the use of vitamin-A supplements as they can cause foetal abnormalities.* Instead use beta-carotene supplements (the plant form of vitamin A) in doses of up to 200,000 iu a day during the acute phase of infection. Vitamin A and beta-carotene help protect the mucous membranes from irritation during infection, as well as improving antibody response and white blood cell functions.

The mineral zinc is essential for supporting the increased immune activity which occurs during infection. Zinc improves cell-mediated immunity by helping to regulate the function of the white blood cells. During acute infection, approximately 50 mg of elemental zinc can be taken each day (along with 50 mg of B6 to aid absorption).

Herbs

Many herbs can be used as urinary antiseptics. These include buchu, golden seal, juniper berries, and garlic. Demulcents are herbs which sooth inflamed mucous membranes (such as the inside of the bladder and urethra). These include such herbs as marshmallow root, couchgrass and cornsilk.

An old naturopathic cure for burning urine involves mixing together equal parts of fennel, burdock and slippery elm. Steep a teaspoon of this mixture in a cup of boiling water for 20 minutes. Drink when cold, one cup before each meal and before bed.

Two herbal teas for cystitis are particularly effective. They are flax seed tea, and a tea made up of equal parts of uva ursi and buchu. Make the teas using 1 teaspoon of dried herbs to a cup of boiling water. Allow to steep for 15–20 minutes, and drink one cup three or four times a day.

Homoeopathy

* *Cantharis.* For cystitis characterised by frequent, painful and burning urination, accompanied by violent spasms of shooting pain. This is the best remedy for the majority of cystitis cases.

* *Causticum.* For chronic cystitis accompanied by loss of bladder control.

* *Sarsaparilla.* For cystitis with pain that is worse on completing urination.

* *Mercurius.* For classic cystitis with a frequent urge to urinate, burning urine, and dark urine when passing in small

Traditional Chinese medicine and urinary tract infections

Traditional Chinese medicine can be very effective in treating both acute and chronic UTIs. In the case of an acute infection, favourable results are only likely if treatment is given quickly at the onset of symptoms. When UTIs are chronic, a longer course of acupuncture is required to gently restore balance to the meridians which influence the bladder. Simply treating with acupuncture during an acute infection without treating on an ongoing basis is a short-sighted and symptomatic approach.

The most common energetic cause of bladder infections from a traditional Chinese medicine perspective is the accumulation of damp and heat in the bladder. Often there is a weakness of the qi or energy flowing in the kidney and spleen meridians. A weakness of spleen energy leads to the formation of damp in the body, which in turn leads to a stagnation or blockage of qi and the development of heat symptoms (such as cystitis). The energy of the spleen is weakened through the overconsumption of sugary, sweet foods, or chilled, cold, or raw foods. Drinking endless glasses of chilled water is a common summer pastime amounts. The pain is worse when not passing water, or at the start or finish of urination. All the symptoms are worse at night.

* *Nux vomica.* For burning or pressing pain during urination. Cystitis accompanied by extreme irritability and bad temper.

* *Apis.* For cystitis that creates a strong urge to urinate, but the ability to pass only a small amount of urine. Characterised by burning urine. Abdomen is very sensitive to pressure.

* *Arsenicum album.* For acute cystitis with burning pain and frequent urge to urinate. Symptoms are relieved by heat or warmth, for example the application of a hot-water bottle.

---

in this part of the world, and the end result is weakened spleen energy. Overeating and drinking with meals also damages spleen qi. Students are great candidates for spleen energy weakness as overuse of the mind, particularly through chronic anxiety or worry, also depletes spleen energy.

When the cooling yin energy of the kidneys is weakened, heat in the bladder (what we in the West diagnose as cystitis) becomes more likely. Kidney yin naturally weakens as we age, but can be diminished prematurely through a typical Western lifestyle. Long-term overwork, overactivity, stress, exhaustion, overconsumption of alcohol, too much sex, all deplete this vital kidney energy.

A traditional Chinese acupuncturist will usually recommend dietary and lifestyle changes to augment the beneficial effects of the acupuncture. Chronic cystitis sufferers may need weekly or twice-weekly acupuncture treatment for a period of several weeks. An acute attack of cystitis may be helped by two to four acupuncture sessions, on consecutive days.

✳ *Pulsatilla*. Indicated more for mild but chronic cystitis. The
patient is usually thirstless, and cannot stand any kind of heat.

Hydrotherapy

Traditional hydrotherapy for cystitis involves the use of hot sitz
baths or hot compresses over the bladder. Simply dip a small
hand towel in a basin of water as hot as you can bear. Wring
out and quickly apply to the area just above your pubic bone.
Repeat the process as the cloth cools, applying the compress eight
or nine times, on two or three occasions throughout the day. For
a sitz bath, fill a small tub with water as hot as you can tolerate.
Add five or six drops of bergamot oil to the water. Sit so that the
water covers your pelvis and lower abdomen, for half an hour.
Keep replenishing with fresh hot water to maintain an even
temperature. Do not use hot sitz baths if you have a weak heart
or high blood pressure, or if you are pregnant.

Aromatherapy

Bergamot oil is most effective for treating cystitis. The lower
abdomen (just above the pubic bone) can be massaged gently
with an oil containing essential oils of bergamot, lavender and
German chamomile.

Packs

A hot-water bottle over the lower abdomen and another over the
lower back will help any aching pains.

Dysmenorrhoea

Dysmenorrhoea (period pain) can severely disrupt a woman's
life, resulting in lost hours at work, and strain at work and in
relationships. Dysmenorrhoea is a widespread problem, and while
there are no figures available for its incidence in New Zealand,
we most likely are comparable with the USA, where half of all
menstruating women suffer regularly from period pain.

Symptoms

Period pain can range from a nagging ache in the lower abdomen or lower back, through to severe, incapacitating cramping similar to birthing pains. When the pain is severe, it may be accompanied by other symptoms such as fainting, trembling, pallor, vomiting or nausea.

Causes

There are two main classifications of dysmenorrhoea — primary and secondary. *Primary dysmenorrhoea* usually begins within the first few years of menstruation. Gynaecological examination fails to find any kind of disease of the uterus. The cramps usually begin a few hours before or after bleeding starts. This is by far the most common type of period pain. The pain is the result of the uterus contracting (in much the same way as it does during childbirth) under the influence of a type of local inflammatory hormone called a prostaglandin.

Secondary dysmenorrhoea is the result of some organic abnormality of the uterus, such as endometriosis, pelvic inflammatory disease, fibroids, polyps, cancer, or the presence of an intrauterine contraceptive device (an IUCD). This type of menstrual pain tends to start as a dull aching in the abdomen, sometimes for as long as 10 days before the actual onset of the period. The pain may go away when your period starts, or it may persist right to the end of the period.

So what actually causes the pain?

A major breakthrough in the understanding of period pain came with the discovery of prostaglandins in the 1930s. These local hormones regulate the tone of smooth muscles such as the uterus, blood vessels and intestines. The smooth muscles contract, depending on the type and amount of the prostaglandins we produce.

The lining of the uterus produces prostaglandins E and F, with the highest concentration occurring when the menstrual bleeding starts. When the uterus produces too many prostaglandins, or when type F is produced in excess of type E, it causes the uterus to become overactive. It contracts excessively and causes cramping and the all-too-familiar pain.

The uterus is designed to carry and then expel a baby, and as such it is a very powerful muscle. During menstrual cramps it contracts so powerfully that it compresses the blood vessels in the uterus, literally cutting off its own blood supply. When a muscle is deprived of oxygen in this way (as also occurs during an angina attack), the pain is excruciating.

Once they have wreaked havoc with your sanity, these same uterine prostaglandins can escape into the bloodstream and go on to affect other smooth muscles in your body. For example, the intestines may be overstimulated and contract too quickly, causing diarrhoea. The blood vessels may dilate and allow blood to pool in your legs and feet, which in turn deprives the brain of blood and oxygen, and may cause you to faint.

It's hard to imagine that so much suffering can be attributed to the effects of one tiny chemical imbalance, but this seems to be the case. Women who suffer from dysmenorrhoea have five times as much prostaglandin in their menstrual blood as their non-suffering peers.

Medical treatment

If your doctor diagnoses primary period pain, he or she may well recommend the contraceptive pill. By preventing ovulation, the pill prevents the thickening of the lining of the uterus (endometrium) and thus reduces the production of prostaglandins in the uterus.

The Mirena is a progesterone-releasing IUCD. By releasing synthetic progesterone into the uterus, the Mirena prevents the thickening of the endometrium, and so reduces prostaglandin release. Many women find their periods become much lighter with use of the Mirena, and in some cases, stop altogether.

If you don't want to take the pill (or can't because you fall in the high-risk category), you will probably be prescribed some type of painkilling drug, such as aspirin, ibuprofen, naproxen or mefenamic acid. These drugs all belong to a group of drugs called 'non-steroidal anti-inflammatories'. Such drugs appear to help period pain by slowing down or stopping the production of prostaglandins in the uterus, and consequently reducing the hard contractions.

Mefenamic acid is marketed in New Zealand and Australia under the trade name of Ponstan, and is available as a non-prescription item from your chemist. It inhibits prostaglandins in the same way as aspirin, and many women find it extremely effective in controlling menstrual pain. However, some users report symptoms of nausea, diarrhoea and indigestion, and its use is contraindicated for asthmatics.

Nutrition

Clinical nutrition has much to offer in the alleviation or prevention of period pain.

Magnesium

A dietary magnesium deficiency is common among New Zealand women, partly as a result of our low soil-magnesium content. Women who consume a high-meat diet, eat few green vegetables, regularly drink alcohol, or use calcium supplements which are not balanced with magnesium are especially at risk. Common signs of deficiency include muscle cramps; feelings of anxiety and depression; twitching muscles and eyelids; insomnia; rapid heart beat; and poor memory.

Magnesium is the first nutritional supplement to think of whenever there is muscle cramping pain, such as occurs in dysmenorrhoea. Magnesium is usually taken in conjunction with vitamin B6 and calcium, in the range of 300–400 mg of elemental magnesium per day during the period. It is advisable to use magnesium supplements for a week before the expected onset of bleeding if pain is a regular occurrence. Taken prior to menstruation (along with B6), magnesium will usually reduce common PMS symptoms such as irritability, tension and depression, and breast tenderness.

Calcium and vitamin E

Calcium is nature's painkiller. It greatly increases our pain tolerance. Like magnesium, calcium is often lacking in our diets, and is often poorly absorbed. Calcium and magnesium are best taken in combination in a balanced formula supplying twice as much calcium as magnesium.

Aspirin and mefenamic acid are both pharmacological prostaglandin inhibitors. Nature's version of the same is simple vitamin E. As well as inhibiting these pain-causing chemicals, vitamin E increases blood circulation and increases the amount of blood carrying oxygen to the uterus.

It is suspected that the cut-off of oxygen to the muscles of the uterus during a contraction is partly responsible for the cramping pain. As little as 100 iu of vitamin E taken daily throughout your cycle can reduce your period pain. On your painful days you can increase your dose up to 500 or 1000 iu, as long as there are no contraindications (see Chapter 2). The most effective vitamin-E supplements contain 'mixed tocopherols' rather than alpha-tocopherol alone.

Essential fatty acids and period pain

So far we have only talked about the prostaglandins which cause the uterus muscles to contract. In truth, not all prostaglandins are trouble-makers. PGE1 prostaglandins are also made by the uterus, but these chemicals inhibit cramping.

The body produces enzymes which act on different essential fatty acids to produce prostaglandins. The series 2 prostaglandins, which cause inflammation and cramping, are made from a fatty acid called arachidonic acid, found in animal fats such as meat, butter and other dairy products. Arachidonic acid can also be made from another fatty acid called linoleic acid, found in polyunsaturated oils such as corn, soya and safflower oil.

The 'anti-cramping' PGE1 and PGE3 series prostaglandins are made using different essential fatty acids, in particular alpha-linoleic acid, EPA, DHA (known as omega-3 fatty acids). Dietary sources of omega-3 fatty acids include cold-water fish such as salmon, sardines, herrings, pilchards and tuna; most nuts and seeds; and flax oil. These oils block the production of the inflammatory series 2 prostaglandins, instead favouring production of series 1 and 3 'anti-inflammatory' prostaglandins. Evening primrose oil and borage oil contain large amounts of linoleic acid and gamma-linoleic acid which produce a similar increase in prostaglandin 1 and 3 series, with a decrease in the inflammatory 2 prostaglandins.

You can manipulate your body's production of prostaglandins by decreasing your intake of the raw materials used to form the 'cramping' prostaglandins, and increasing your intake of the raw materials needed to make the 'relaxing' PGE1 prostaglandins. Cut down on animal fats, red meat and dairy products and increase intake of flax and fish oils, nuts and seeds.

Evening primrose oil supplements taken in doses of 3000 mg per day, throughout the month, are also recommended.

Herbal help

'Women's' herbs such as raspberry leaf, squaw vine, cramp bark and blue cohosh have provided relief from menstrual pains for hundreds of years. Even something as simple as drinking a strong infusion of raspberry leaf tea every day can help reduce menstrual pain. This herb is a gentle but effective uterine tonic, and is traditionally used during pregnancy, as a birth preparer. Ginger tea combined with chamomile tea is also useful to ease period pain and calm the nerves. Allow approximately 1 inch of grated fresh ginger root for each cup of tea.

Hydrotherapy

Hot sitz baths have traditionally been used to ease the misery of menstruation. Fill a small tub with hot water (38 °C), and submerge your bottom and lower abdomen for about half an hour. Keep topping up with hot water to maintain a regular temperature. You can try adding herbal infusions or a few drops of essential oil to the bath water to enhance its effect.

A strong brew of chamomile tea or lemon balm tea added to the bath water will both help relax you and lessen the cramps. Remember also that these herbs will benefit you if taken internally as a tea.

Aromatherapy

Antispasmodic and painkilling essential oils are appropriate for the treatment of period pain. Useful oils include: aniseed, Roman chamomile, clary sage, juniper berry, sweet marjoram, peppermint and rosemary. For pain which feels dull, dragging and widespread, think of Roman chamomile and cyprus. Spasmodic or cramping pain is treated with peppermint, lavender or clary sage. Add a few drops of the chosen oil to a vegetable oil and massage gently into the abdomen. Cover with a hot pack or hot-water bottle wrapped in a towel.

Homoeopathy

In order to use homoeopathy to treat your period pain effectively, you must determine the exact timing and nature of your pain, so that the correct remedy can be selected. First, does your pain occur mostly before you begin bleeding? If it does, you will probably find your remedy in the following group.

* *Belladonna.* Symptoms for which belladonna is indicated are that the face is usually flushed red. There is great sensitivity to any kind of movement or touch, which makes the period pain worse. The pain feels like a very heavy dragging sensation in the lower abdomen and pelvis.

* *Calcarea.* Indicated when the pain is often accompanied by a sensation of weakness and general 'unwellness' and

nausea. The pains are colicky and often accompanied by noticeable sweating.

* *Chamomilla.* Indicated for great emotional sensitivity, with a sense of great anger and intolerance of noise or other people. Pain is severe and colicky before the onset of bleeding. This may be accompanied by vomiting, diarrhoea and fainting.

Another group of remedies is indicated if your pain occurs once your menstrual period actually begins.

* *China.* This remedy is indicated where the periods are heavy and clotty, and often early. Along with the low-abdominal, cramping, colicky pains, there is a feeling of great exhaustion, sometimes to the point of collapse.

* *Graphites.* Again the pain is sharp and cramping, but often is in the left ovary area. The pain is accompanied by nausea, generalised body aches and chest pain.

* *Nux vomica.* This type of pain is more in the lower back, and accompanied by constipation but with an urge to urinate frequently. There is often nausea and a very irritable and angry disposition.

* *Phosphorus.* There are a lot of emotional symptoms with dysmenorrhoea for which this remedy is indicated. The severe contraction-like pains felt in the back are accompanied by anxiety and fearfulness. Headaches and an inability to get warm also accompany the pain.

Exercise and period pain

Regular exercise, throughout the month and while you are menstruating, can make a dramatic different to the intensity of period pain. Exercise improves blood circulation, increases the oxygenation of cells (including those in your pelvis and uterus), and generally assists in decongesting the pelvic area. A brisk walk or jog three or four times a week is an important part of your self-help programme. Lower back and abdominal stretching, or yoga, are also useful.

Massage

Acupressure and massage are very useful tools to help you cope with period pain. Firm massage to the lower back and sacrum area will help to decongest the uterus. Using a little oil (perhaps with some added essential oils — see above), ask your partner to press and rub either side of the spine, and over the sacrum (the triangular-shaped bone at the bottom of the spine), for

---

Traditional Chinese medicine and dysmenorrhoea

Traditional Chinese medicine understands period pain as resulting from an imbalance of qi or blood. The pain is usually the result of a blockage of qi or blood, or the retention of heat, wind or dampness (these are Chinese concepts used to describe different patterns of symptoms). Qi and blood stasis causes symptoms such as bloating, severe stabbing menstrual pain and dark, clotty blood. Alternatively, period pain can result from 'deficient' conditions in which qi or blood is deficient. Likely symptoms with deficiency include scanty bleeding, pale blood and pale complexion, fatigue, and pain which responds to pressure and warmth.

While acupuncture can offer symptomatic relief when you are actually in the midst of menstrual pain, by far the most effective approach to the problem involves regular 'preventative' acupuncture, designed to balance qi and blood and restore pain-free menstruation. Depending on the severity of your symptoms, three or four months of regular treatment may be required.

10 minutes or so. The relief is wonderful. The following acupressure points are also useful:

* *Spleen 6.* On the inside of the lower leg. The point is four finger widths above the tip of your ankle bone (that is, the part of the ankle bone that juts out). The point is found just behind your shin bone.

* *CV4.* This point is found on the lower abdomen. Find the halfway point between the naval and the crest of your pubic bone. Now move down about 1.5 cm from this point. This is the level of CV4, and the point lies exactly on the midline of the abdomen.

* *Spleen 8.* On the inside of the lower leg. The point is one-and-a-half hand widths below the knee crease. The point is found just behind your shin bone.

Using the tip of your thumb, apply firm downward pressure to the point. Maintain the pressure for 20 seconds before gradually releasing. Repeat the process six or seven times. If pain persists, acupressure can be used repeatedly until symptoms abate.

Acupuncture and osteopathy

Self-help may be all that's needed for mild cases of dysmenorrhoea, but for more severe cases, osteopathy and traditional Chinese medicine may both help significantly.

The uterus receives nerve impulses from the spinal nerves which emerge from the lower vertebrae of your spine. If you have a lower back problem (which you may not even be aware of) these spinal nerves are impinged, blood circulation and lymph drainage in the pelvis are reduced, and over a period of years the health of your uterus may diminish. A check-up with a registered osteopath or chiropractor may pay huge dividends in terms of pain reduction.

Endometriosis

Endometriosis affects 10–15% of all menstruating women. Hundreds of thousands of women in the 25- to 45-year age group suffer the pain and infertility caused by this illness. Forty per cent of all sufferers are unable to conceive.

Endometriosis can wreak its permanent damage in a sinisterly silent way. Months and years of gradual damage may have occurred before symptoms are considered unusual or severe enough to be investigated. Once symptoms do occur, it may be years (if ever) before the woman acknowledges she has a health problem and seeks help. Many women accept even crippling period pain (and a whole host of other 'women's' problems) as simply 'our lot', and fail to seek medical attention.

What is endometriosis?

The lining of the uterus is called the endometrium. In a healthy woman, this lining gradually thickens between periods in preparation for receiving a fertilised egg. If this egg doesn't arrive in the uterus, the blood-rich lining is sloughed off and flows from the body as a period.

Endometriosis occurs when stray fragments of the endometrium find their way into the pelvic cavity and attach to various organs and tissues. It is still not understood how exactly this occurs, but the most popular theory to date is that during a period, fragments of the endometrium flow backwards up through the fallopian tubes and out into the pelvic cavity. Interestingly, many women experience this retrograde menstruation without going on to develop endometriosis, so merely the presence of the endometrial tissue in the abdomen is not enough to cause endometriosis. In women who do develop endometriosis, the stray tissues embed and grow on the ovaries, fallopian tubes, bladder, bowel, cervix and the ligaments that hold the uterus in place. Endometrial growths can also form in C-section scars and laparoscopy scars. In rare cases, endometrial tissue has been known to travel as far afield as the spine, lungs and brain! There is also some evidence that abnormal cells may be present in the abdominal cavity from birth, making endometriosis a congenital condition, although this is not a widely recognised theory. Researchers are also searching for an 'endometriosis' gene.

There is compelling evidence that endometriosis may be an auto-immune disease. In women with endometriosis there are immune abnormalities. For example, macrophages whose job it would normally be to destroy the stray endometrial tissue, instead contribute to their colonisation. T-cells and natural killer cells are also abnormally low. Women with endometriosis also experience a higher than usual occurrence of auto-immune diseases such as rheumatoid arthritis and lupus.

Environmental pollution, specifically xeno-oestrogens, also seems to play a part in the development of endometriosis. We are all exposed to these oestrogen-mimicking chemicals, through daily living. Even those of us who are not directly using synthetic hormones such as the pill or HRT are nevertheless exposed to powerful oestrogenic-like substances. In many countries (but not New Zealand) synthetic oestrogens are used in the raising of livestock, and these hormonal residues are passed on to us through the food chain. Many pesticides, herbicides and fungicides mimic the effects of oestrogen when they find their way into the cells of the human body. When you paint your nails or remove your nail polish you breathe in a good dose of xeno-oestrogens, as you do whenever you use a solvent or put on clothes freshly cleaned at the drycleaners. Car exhaust fumes, and a wide range of chemicals used in personal care products such as make-up and shampoo expose us to xeno-oestrogens. Do you wrap your food in cling film, heat dinner up in a plastic container, or reuse plastic drinking bottles? You've guessed it — more xeno-oestrogens. Endometrial implants are stimulated by the presence of oestrogen. When we are exposed to regular doses of xeno-oestrogens it can lead to a relative excess of oestrogen in our body compared with the amount of progesterone we are producing. (See *Avoiding xeno-oestrogens* below for tips on how to reduce exposure to these chemicals.)

Genetics may also increase endometriosis risk. If you have a first-degree relative with the problem, your own risk of developing endometriosis is increased 10 times.

Irrespective of how these rogue endometrial cells find their way into the pelvic cavity, once there they behave as if they were still growing inside the uterus. As such they are still under the control of female sex hormones, and mimic the 'plumping and sloughing' cycle that occurs monthly in the uterus. The blood that is released into the pelvic cavity has no exit and simply settles and hardens on tissues in the pelvic cavity. The formation of scabs and cysts causes inflammation, and scar tissue eventually forms. At this point, a woman's fertility is greatly reduced. These misplaced endometrial tissues also have the ability to grow and spread to neighbouring pelvic organs.

Symptoms

How do you know if you have endometriosis? As many as one-third of endometriosis sufferers have no symptoms, and only become aware of its presence when they are unable to conceive.

For the remaining two-thirds of sufferers, the number one symptom to look for is pain. Be suspicious of periods that become painful after many years of little or no pain. The pain may be dull aching, cramping, or bearing down pressure felt in the lower abdomen or back. The pain tends to worsen with time and often begins progressively earlier in the cycle. Severe sufferers may have as little as one pain-free week out of each month. The pain of endometriosis doesn't just occur before or during a period. There may be pain during ovulation; during sexual intercourse (a sharp, shooting pain); during urination; or during bowel movements while menstruating. Other symptoms include infertility, abnormally heavy or irregular periods, and unexplained exhaustion and lethargy. Abnormal bowel motions during menstruation are also common with endometriosis and may range from constipation to diarrhoea and pain with bowel motions. Endometriosis wreaks an emotional toll too, and depression, anxiety, irritability and anger are common.

Who is most likely to suffer?

Ironically, endometriosis often affects women who have otherwise normal, healthy menstrual cycles. Women with a history of non-ovulation, or irregular and missed periods, are least likely to suffer from the additional problem of endometriosis. It is the women who ovulate regularly and postpone having children until they are well into their thirties who are the most likely to develop endometriosis. Given the changed demographics of our society, with the widespread delaying of childbirth until later in life, it's not surprising that we are seeing an upsurge in the incidence of endometriosis.

Medical treatment

If your doctor suspects that you may have endometriosis, the only truly definitive diagnosis is through a minor surgical procedure known as a *laparoscopy*. MRIs and ultrasounds can sometimes detect large and widespread growths, but will usually miss small clumps of tissue.

During a laparoscopy, a slender telescope-like instrument is passed into the abdominal cavity (either through a small puncture wound beneath the navel, or by being passed through the upper vagina). This telescope allows the size and number of abnormal implants to be estimated. There is no other definitive way to diagnose and assess the extent of endometriosis.

There are several different treatment options if your diagnosis is endometriosis. Sadly, none of them are perfect, and many have side effects. Treating endometriosis through conventional or holistic therapies can be a challenging process.

Depending upon your circumstances and age, having a baby may be an answer to your problems. Of course this is not always practical or desirable (or even possible if you have already become infertile), but many women find their endometriosis is greatly improved by pregnancy. Nine months of no ovulating tends to shrink the stray endometrial tissues. Pregnancy is not a panacea, though, and some women report no change, or even a worsening of their problems.

Pain relief may be achieved with the use of painkillers or anti-inflammatories. Neither of these medications 'fix' the problem, but simply offer some symptomatic relief when the monthly pain arrives.

A range of hormonal preparations is also used in the treatment of endometriosis. The most simple of these is the oral contraceptive pill which alleviates (but doesn't cure) symptoms by suppressing ovulation and inhibiting the growth of the endometrium (and of course the stray endometriosis growths too), in much the same way as pregnancy.

Synthetic progesterone such as Provera or Primolut similarly suppresses the endometriosis implants and allows them to shrink. The contraceptive injection Depo-Provera and the progesterone-releasing IUCD called the Mirena are also used in the symptomatic control of endometriosis. Side effects with progesterone therapy are common and can include acne, bloating, spotting, breast tenderness, depression, dizziness, moodiness, nausea and weight gain. Not all women are affected, however, and for some, side effects are minimal. One commonly used therapy, Danazol (see below), can cause masculinisation as a side effect, as well as weight gain, voice deepening and facial hair growth.

Another type of hormonal treatment which may be offered is the use of GnRh agonists. This group of drugs has been used for over 20 years, and the drugs are a synthetic version of a naturally occurring hormone known as a gonadotropin-releasing hormone, which helps to control the menstrual cycle. GnRh agonists come in the form of injections or nasal sprays. They work by suppressing the production of oestrogen in the body, thus depriving the endometrial implants of the stimulatory effect of oestrogen, causing them to shrink. GnRh agonists stop your menstrual periods, but these usually return within three months of cessation of the medication. There are side effects with this medication, which effectively nudges your body into a menopausal state. Not surprisingly, side effects mimic those of menopause and include such things as hot flushes, night sweats, vaginal dryness, mood swings, depression, acne, muscle pains and dizziness. By far the most worrying side effect is thinning of the bones, in particular the bones of the spine. Typically bones have thinned by 4–6% by the end of a six-month course of GnRh agonists. Most of this bone loss is replaced after the treatment has been completed, but potentially this drug-induced bone loss may be detrimental for women with a family history of osteoporosis or with several risk factors. Sometimes low-dose oestrogen or progestogen is prescribed in tandem with this medication, to offset some of the side effects, without interfering with the effectiveness of the treatment. GnRh agonists are usually prescribed for three to six months, with a six-month course offering a longer period of endometriosis remission after coming off the medication. In time, the endometrial growths regrow, and a second course of therapy may be required.

Before the advent of GnRh agonists, Danazol was the most commonly used drug in the treatment of endometriosis. It is a synthetic male hormone or androgen. Not surprisingly, side effects associated with its use are 'male' in nature. These include the growth of facial hair and deepening of the voice, weight gain, acne; the drug also has a tendency to adversely affect cholesterol levels. Danazol causes male hormone levels to increase and oestrogen levels to decrease, thus stopping menstruation and causing endometrial implants to shrink. Most women stop menstruating and ovulating by the second month of treatment, which is about the time it takes for the symptoms of endometriosis to begin to abate. Periods usually resume within a couple of months of stopping treatment.

A typical course of Danazol therapy lasts anywhere from three to nine months. Although hormonal treatment provides relief from symptoms during the course of therapy, when the hormones are stopped it is not uncommon for endometriosis symptoms to gradually develop again over the ensuing months or years. Thirty to forty per cent of women using Danazol experience a recurrence of endometriosis within three years following cessation of medication.

Surgery is another treatment option for endometriosis. Conservative surgery aims to improve or relieve symptoms by surgically removing as many endometrial growths as possible. Scar tissue and adhesions are also removed. The latest laser techniques combined with 'key-hole' surgery allow endometrial growths to be vaporised without causing any harm to surrounding healthy tissues. Conservative surgery is often undertaken if infertility is a problem, and between a third and a half of all women who undergo this surgery will conceive in the following three to six months.

A few women with long-term and extensive endometriosis may choose radical surgery as an end to their suffering. This involves removing the uterus and the ovaries. Obviously, this is a very traumatic type of surgery, and a last-resort form of treatment, and there is no guarantee that even this drastic step will cure endometriosis.

Natural progesterone cream

Saliva testing frequently shows that endometriosis sufferers have low progesterone levels. Natural progesterone cream increases progesterone levels, decreasing the relative excess of oestrogen which is a factor in many cases of endometriosis. (See Chapter 5 for more information on natural progesterone.)

Natural alternatives

Many endometriosis sufferers find relief from a range of gentle holistic therapies. These may include dietary change, nutritional supplements, herbal medicine, acupuncture, homoeopathy and osteopathy.

Diet and nutrition

Dietary change is a vital component in managing endometriosis. An 'endometriosis-friendly' diet is one which encourages a reduction in the levels of oestrogen circulating in the bloodstream. It is also a diet rich in foods which encourage the production of anti-inflammatory substances, series 1 prostaglandins. (See section on dysmenorrhoea for more information.)

* A vegetarian diet is the ideal. If you cannot stick to a strictly vegetarian diet, then reduce your intake of red meat and chicken to no more than once a week each. Try to eat organic meat whenever possible.

* Eliminate or strictly limit your intake of dairy products (cows' milk, cheese, yoghurt, ice-cream). If you do use dairy products, use the lowest-fat versions such as trim milk, cottage cheese, and so on. Dairy products (and red meat) contain saturated fat which increases circulating oestrogen levels as well as increasing the production of series 2 inflammatory prostaglandins.

* Change to a 'fat-friendly' diet. Avoid saturated (animal) fats such as meat, dairy products and palm oil (read labels for this one, commonly used in processed foods). Instead use 'friendly' fats such as flax, avocado, and olive oil, nuts and seeds, and cold-water fish (for example, salmon, sardines, herrings and pilchards). These fatty acids all encourage the production of the series 1 and 3 anti-inflammatory prostaglandins.

* Avoid processed, hydrogenated fats which are full of trans-fats, and consequently pro-inflammatory. That means no traditional margarine, French fries, commercially baked cakes and biscuits and commercial peanut butter.

* Avoid refined carbohydrates such as white bread, cakes, biscuits, refined and processed foods. These foods are not

only devoid of many nutrients, but they also play havoc
with your insulin levels, causing blood-sugar fluctuations
and hormonal imbalance. Choose carbohydrates with a
low GI rating, which break down into sugars slowly and
gradually, such as fruits and vegetables, nuts and seeds,
whole grains and basmati rice. (See Chapter 2.)

* Increase intake of fresh organic vegetables and fruits.
Organic produce has not been sprayed with pesticides and
herbicides derived from petrochemicals, and is therefore
virtually free of xeno-oestrogens. The fibre supplied by a
high intake of fruits and vegetables binds with oestrogen
in the gut, and helps to excrete it from the body, thus
lowering circulating oestrogen levels. Eat cruciferous
vegetables daily as they help to promote the production of
'friendly' oestrogen metabolites in your body, and decrease
production of the oestrogen metabolites associated with
endometriosis and breast cancer. These vegetables include
broccoli, cauliflower, kale, Brussels sprouts and cabbage.

* Limit caffeine and avoid alcohol. Caffeine increases the
excretion of B-vitamins which hampers the liver's ability
to break down and detoxify oestrogen. Alcohol places a
detoxifying stress on the liver, and optimum liver function
is essential for the management of endometriosis.

* Increase dietary phyto-oestrogens (see list in Chapter 6)
such as miso, tempeh, tofu, soya milk, flax oil and flax
seeds, beans, lentils, legumes, nuts and seeds. Phyto-
oestrogens block the enzyme aromatase, which is required
by rogue cells growing outside the uterus to make
oestrogen. Phyto-oestrogens also work as a natural anti-
inflammatory in the case of endometriosis.

Avoiding xeno-oestrogens (See Chapter 6)
* Change to organic fruits, vegetables, grains, dairy products
and meat.

* Change to natural, safe herbicide and pesticide products in your own garden.

* Avoid exposure to solvents, dry-cleaning vapours, nail polish, hairspray and perfumes.

* Use 'safety conscious' personal-care products that are free of additives with an oestrogenic effect, such as parabens.

* Avoid the use of plastic whenever possible. Store food in ceramic or glass containers. Never use plastic to heat food in the microwave, and never cover food with cling wrap when microwaving.

* Do not re-use plastic drink bottles.

Nutritional supplements

There are a number of nutritional supplements commonly pre-scribed to help control the symptoms of endometriosis, either through enhancing oestrogen breakdown and elimination, or through limiting inflammation and cramping.

Supplementing with a high-potency B-complex will support the liver in breaking down and detoxifying oestrogen. Look for a formula which provides at least 50 mg of thiamin, riboflavin, niacin and pantothenic acid, 30–50 mg B6, 400 mcg folic acid and 200 mcg of biotin. Vitamin B6 is a godsend for any woman suffering from pre-menstrual syndrome or endometriosis. Doses of 50–150 mg of B6 daily can greatly reduce the severity of hormonal symptoms such as headaches, exhaustion, irritability, breast tenderness and abdominal bloating. Remember that vitamin B6 is only one part of a whole complex of different B-vitamins that work together. Use a B-complex supplement and, if you wish to increase B6, take a separate B6 tablet along with the complex.

Vitamin E naturally balances oestrogen levels, and is useful for the hormonal imbalances common among endometriosis sufferers and menopausal women. This vitamin also helps to keep the pelvic scar tissue soft and pliable, and consequently reduces pain from abdominal adhesions, as well as functioning as a natural antispasmodic. Women with heavy periods often find that vitamin E reduces their blood loss. Use a combined tocopherol formula in doses of 400–800 iu a day. (See section on vitamin E in Chapter 2 for further information and contraindications.)

Evening primrose oil is rich in gamma-linolenic acid which promotes the production of anti-inflammatory prostaglandins. Regular daily doses of 2000–3000 mg of evening primrose oil help reduce symptoms of pain, along with depression, fatigue, breast tenderness and bloating.

Antioxidant supplements are important to reduce the damage resulting from inflammation, and to lessen cramping. Use a combined antioxidant formula containing vitamin C and E, beta-carotene, selenium, and zinc. Pine bark extract, grape seed extract and turmeric are powerful herbal antioxidants, and are included in some of the more sophisticated antioxidant formulas, providing great benefit.

Additional vitamin C taken in high enough doses acts as a natural antihistamine and anti-inflammatory. A formula containing bioflavonoids and a complex of different forms of vitamin C is useful. Doses of 500–1000 mg can be taken three to four times daily.

I3C, taken in doses of 200–300 mg a day, encourages the production of less-active oestrogen metabolites, thus reducing the effect of oestrogen dominance common in endometriosis (see Chapter 6).

Homoeopathy

As is the case when treating any condition with homoeopathy, there are no 'set' remedies specifically for endometriosis. Remedies are selected based upon the exact and specific symptoms of the individual. With a complex condition such as endometriosis, it is preferable to consult a registered homoeopath rather than trying to self-prescribe.

Herbal help

Endometriosis can be helped a great deal through the use of herbal medicine. Due to the chronic and difficult nature of this problem, it is advisable to consult a medical herbalist for individualised herbal treatment.

Fibrocystic breast disease/chronic cystic mastitis/ mammary dysplasia

Once upon a time, if you presented to your doctor with lumpy, painful breasts, you were likely to be told you had fibrocystic breast disease (FBD). This somewhat old-fashioned term is less frequently used now. Dr Susan Love, author of *Dr Susan Love's Breast Book*, refers to fibrocystic breast disease as being a 'wastepaper basket diagnosis'. In other words, it's the label you're given to describe uncomfortable or lumpy breasts, whatever the underlying cause of the condition.

Lumpy breasts affect around half of all menstruating women at some time in their lives, most commonly between the ages of 30 and 50, although younger women and women using HRT can also suffer from FBD. These benign lumps usually cause shock and anguish when first discovered. They can range in size from one tiny nodule the size of a pea, through to masses of painful lumps the size of a grape or even a golf ball.

Symptoms

Symptoms usually follow one of two patterns. Lumpiness and breast tenderness may be spread throughout the breasts, and usually worse in the week or so before the onset of your period. After your period you will notice a decrease in pain and lumpiness. Or there may be one or several clearly defined cyst-like lumps (often affecting only one breast), varying in size from a pea to a golf ball. These lumps are also often more painful pre-menstrually.

Causes

Breast pain and lumpiness usually have a hormonal basis. Cyclical breast tenderness and lumpiness are common features of pre-menstrual syndrome, and are partly the result of a relative excess of oestrogen. Many women with this condition also have elevated levels of the hormone prolactin, the chief function of which is to regulate the development of the breasts and milk secretion during and after pregnancy.

While FBD or cystic mastitis is a benign condition, the presence of fibroadenomas (smooth, firm, benign tumours which feel slippery and move around the breast easily) may increase the risk of breast cancer where there is a family history of the disease. Otherwise, there is no clearly proven link between FBD and increased breast-cancer risk.

Many women who eliminate caffeine from their diet (coffee, tea, chocolate, caffeinated soft drinks and energy drinks) notice a definite improvement in their breast symptoms. A diet high in saturated fats also appears to aggravate FBD symptoms for many women. Reducing saturates and increasing omega-3 fats and GLA in the form of evening primrose oil quickly improves cyclical breast discomfort and lumpiness.

Medical treatment

The first step in treatment is to establish that lumps or cysts are actually benign and not cancerous. A mammogram may be suggested, but in premenopausal women especially, results are not always accurate. For this reason, it is advisable to have an ultrasound along with the mammogram. (See Chapter 6.)

Sometimes a fine-needle biopsy may be performed. This procedure involves inserting a needle into the cyst with the aim of withdrawing a little fluid for testing. A breast biopsy may be performed, in which a small amount of the cystic tissue is removed for analysis. If there are one or two largish lumps, surgical aspiration may be performed, during which the trapped fluid and dead cells are withdrawn from the lump, through a fine needle.

Pain killers and anti-inflammatories offer symptomatic relief from cyclical breast pain, but do little to address the problem itself. Sometimes the oral contraceptive pill is suggested, and for some women this significantly reduces breast pain. Danazol is a hormonal drug which has been shown to relieve breast pain in 70–80% of women. Unfortunately, it creates a number of very unpleasant side effects including irregular periods, loss of libido, leg cramps, weight gain, and, in some women, a deepening of the voice and hairiness. Bromocriptine is a drug used to inhibit the release of the hormone prolactin. It has been shown to be effective in around 65% of cases of cyclical breast tenderness. Side effects may include nausea, dizziness, headaches and irritability.

Diet and nutrition

Dietary change can significantly decrease or even eliminate problems with cystic or painful breasts, through changing the underlying hormonal imbalances. An efficient eliminative system is vital for regulating oestrogen levels, and dietary changes are partly aimed at optimising the function of the liver and bowel. A healthy liver more efficiently breaks down circulating oestrogen for elimination, thus helping to normalise the ratio of oestrogen to progesterone. Having regular daily bowel motions is also important for ensuring excretion of oestrogen metabolites from the body. In clinic, I have noticed a strong correlation between constipation or sluggish bowels and FBD.

For optimum liver and bowel function, the ideal diet is rich in fibre from fruits and vegetables, whole grains, beans, lentils, brown rice, nuts and seeds. Refined carbohydrates and processed or 'chemicalised' foods should be kept to an absolute minimum. Minimise your intake of saturated fats in the form of meat, dairy products and palm oil; and increase the amount of omega-3 and GLA in your diet by consuming more oily fish, flax oil, avocado, nuts and seeds and evening primrose oil.

Vegetarian women and women eating a diet low in saturated fat tend to have lower oestrogen levels than meat eaters, and fewer oestrogen dominance symptoms such as FBD, PMS and period pain.

Eat brassica vegetables every day. Choose from broccoli, cabbage, cauliflower, and Brussels sprouts. High in I3C (see Chapter 6), these vegetables help to change oestrogen metabolites into a less potent form, helping to protect breast health.

Until recently there was no proven link between caffeine consumption and breast lumpiness and pain. In 2001, a study published in *Fertility and Sterility* (76: 723–729) confirmed that drinking more than two cups of caffeinated coffee a day boosts oestrogen levels (estradiol). In fact, women consuming four or five cups of coffee a day had 70% higher oestrogen levels in the first half of their cycle, compared with women drinking one coffee a day. For many women FBD improves significantly when caffeine (coffee, tea, chocolate, energy drinks) is eliminated completely.

There is a connection between thyroid function and breast health, and an undiagnosed underactive thyroid may contribute to the development of FBD. Iodine deficiency can contribute to hypothyroidism (as it is used in the manufacture of the thyroid hormone thyroxine), and, interestingly, rats with induced iodine deficiency exhibit all the typical symptoms of FBD. Iodine deficiency is most likely to be an issue if you are a vegetarian, not eating seafoods, and perhaps not using any kind of iodised salt. Adding a little iodised salt to your food, or sprinkling kelp over your dinner, will boost iodine levels. Don't go mad with the kelp though, as you can definitely overdo the iodine boosting and end up causing serious thyroid problems. A half teaspoon of granulated kelp each day should be enough to meet your iodine requirements if you are not eating seafood or iodised salt.

Nutritional supplements

The majority of FBD sufferers experience significant relief from using vitamin E supplements. Vitamin E helps to rebalance the abnormal oestrogen/progesterone ratio common in women with FBD, thus reducing the cyst-promoting effects of excessive oestrogen.

Vitamin E reduces the number, size and pain of breast lumps in approximately 80% of women. In many cases, the FBD completely disappears after several months of regular vitamin-E use. Effective dosage seems to vary from woman to woman, with some responding to as little as 300 iu a day of d-alpha-tocopherol, while others require up to 1000 iu a day.

New Zealand has one of the lowest soil-selenium levels in the world. While it is still not definitively clear, there is a significant amount of research indicating that a deficiency of selenium contributes to the development of FBD, and possibly also to breast cancer. (See Chapters 2 and 6.) B-vitamins are essential for the liver to effectively break down oestrogen. A high-potency, balanced B-complex containing 50 mg of B6 is a useful addition to any clinical nutrition regime for FBD. An additional 50 mg of B6 may sometimes be needed in conjunction with the multivitamin.

Evening primrose oil capsules are slow acting, but often extremely effective in relieving FBD after two to three months of continual use. Doses of 1500–2000 mg three times daily may be required. After three months of this high dose, many women find that they can reduce their intake to 2000–3000 mg a day and maintain the therapeutic effect.

Homoeopathy

* *Plumbum*. Indicated when the whole of the breast feels hard and tender and there is often severe constipation.

* *Carbo animalis*. Indicated when the FBD affects the right breast and results in a clearly defined nodule which produces spasmodic pain.

* *Bryonia*. Hard, heavy breasts with slight heat but severe pain. The symptoms get worse at the time of menstruation.

✳ *Belladonna.* Hot breasts with hard, sore lumps which feel very much worse for any kind of touch, pressure or movement. The pain is shooting and darting in nature.

Herbs

Vitex agnus castus, commonly known as chaste tree, has long been the herbalist's choice for gently relieving FBD problems. *Vitex* decreases prolactin levels which leads to an increase in progesterone levels, in turn helping to minimise the problems of excess oestrogen often associated with FBD. *Vitex* regulates hormones and inhibits the release of FSH and LH (see Chapter 1). This leads to less oestrogen stimulating breast tissue. This extremely safe and gentle herb is often slow acting, and continuous use for three months may be necessary before there is an obvious improvement in symptoms. Do not use *Vitex* if you are on the oral contraceptive pill or pregnant.

The humble dandelion is a herbal favourite for liver cleansing and detoxifying. It has also been a traditional herbal ally in the treatment of both breast cysts and uterine fibroids. Dandelion is best taken as a dried herb or a tincture, rather than using one of the commercial dandelion coffees (which are processed and lacking in active ingredients). Use 10 to 30 drops of dandelion tincture daily, or two capsules of dried herb three times daily.

Phytolacca or pokeroot is a lymphatic cleanser which can be used as a topical application to decrease breast lumpiness and pain. Massage pokeroot ointment into the breasts on the days they are lumpy or sore. Do not use this ointment if you are breastfeeding, as it is highly toxic if ingested by a baby.

Packs

Castor oil packs can work wonders in the treatment of FBD. Use a flannel or towelling facecloth folded over several times and dipped into castor oil until wet but not dripping. Put the cloth over the breast lumps and cover with a piece of plastic or cling film. Next cover with a hot-water bottle, as hot as is comfortable.

Over this place a thick towel. Then just sit back and relax for about an hour. When you have finished with your pack, you can wash the oil from your skin with a solution of water containing two teaspoons of baking soda. Try to use the packs every night, or at the very least three nights a week, until your lumps have gone.

Acupuncture

The liver meridian runs up to the breasts, and from a traditional Chinese medicine perspective this is the meridian most often involved in breast health issues. Lumpy or painful breasts are often the result of a stagnation or blockage of the flow of qi in the liver meridian. Emotional stress and turmoil have a negative effect on liver qi, as does suppression of emotion or frustration. Many women notice that their breast pain and lumpiness worsens with stress, and the resulting disruption to the free flow of qi in the liver meridian.

Acupuncture and Chinese herbs can be used to effectively restore the free flow of liver energy, and can dramatically improve FBD. This treatment is most effective during the early stages of the disease while the breast lumps are still small and few in number.

Natural progesterone cream

Natural progesterone cream is useful to reduce the problems of oestrogen dominance which are common with FBD. Salivary progesterone levels should be monitored before and during use (see Chapter 5).

Fibroids

Fibroids are non-cancerous tumours or lumps that develop in the muscular walls of the uterus. Fibroids can occur in isolation, or in clusters, and can range from the size of a pea to the size of a melon! Fibroids are most common in women in their middle menstruating years, with adolescents and postmenopausal women having a lower incidence. Many women have small uterine fibroids without being aware of them, and it is estimated that as many as 20% of women over the age of 35 have fibroids.

Debate exists over the exact cause of fibroids, although their development and growth seem to be related to the hormone oestrogen. During times of high oestrogen production (such as pregnancy, and when using the contraceptive pill), fibroids develop much more quickly. By the same token, at times when oestrogen levels are low, such as menopause and beyond, fibroids often shrink and disappear on their own. If you're taking a hormonal preparation such as the oral contraceptive pill or HRT, coming off your medication may help to shrink your fibroids. Fibroids, like endometriosis and fibrocystic breast disease, are considered to be an oestrogenic condition, and consequently limiting our exposure to exogenous (outside the body) sources of oestrogen is wise. (See Chapter 6 for discussion of xeno-oestrogens.)

A relative dominance of oestrogen in the body can also occur when women have menstrual cycles in which they do not ovulate, such as is common in perimenopausal women. A lack of ovulation results in a lack of progesterone, and consequently, a relative excess of oestrogen in the body. This oestrogen excess not only stimulates fibroids, but also contributes to the development of fibrocystic breasts, and many of the symptoms of PMS. Natural progesterone cream (when indicated by low salivary progesterone levels) helps to rebalance the progesterone/oestrogen ratio, and may help to shrink fibroids.

There are four main types of fibroid, classified by the area and direction in which they grow.

* *Intramural fibroids* grow within the muscle wall of the uterus.

* *Subserous fibroids* grow outwards from the wall of the uterus, sometimes on a stalk.

* *Submucous fibroids* grow inwards into the uterus. These fibroids can also develop on a stalk, and can sometimes

grow so long as to protrude through the cervix into the vaginal canal.

* *Cervical fibroids* grow in the wall of the cervix. These fibroids are rare.

Symptoms

It is not at all uncommon for women to walk around with a uterus full of fibroids completely unaware of their condition. Fibroids may be quite large (for example, your uterus may be enlarged to the size of a 12-week pregnancy), and still cause no symptoms.

Not all women are this lucky, however. If you have any of the following symptoms, fibroids may be the cause of your problems.

* Excessively heavy or flooding periods, often with large clots. Heavy blood loss may cause iron-deficiency anaemia and symptoms of exhaustion, breathlessness, headaches, dizziness, poor memory and concentration, depression and poor immunity.

* Painful periods. The pain can range from severe cramping (comparable with labour pains), to a dull, constant ache in your lower abdomen and lower back.

* Any change in your usual bowel or urinary habits. For example, you may begin to pass water frequently, develop frequent urinary infections, or have problems with incontinence. Large fibroids pressing on the bowel may cause constipation or haemorrhoids.

* Infertility. Undiagnosed fibroids can sometimes be the cause of infertility.

Diagnosis

If you suspect that you may have fibroids, visit your GP or family planning centre. Usually a vaginal examination, with palpation of the uterus, is sufficient to diagnose fibroids. Your doctor may also suggest an ultrasound scan of your uterus.

Medical treatment

Fibroids are not life-threatening, and sometimes don't even cause any symptoms. In the past, hysterectomy was a first-line, popular choice for the treatment of fibroids, but less so today. If you have asymptomatic fibroids, you can safely leave them where they are. You may well go through the rest of your life with the fibroids causing no problems, and if you are near to menopause anyway, the naturally occurring decline in oestrogen will cause spontaneous shrinking of the fibroids at menopause.

For troublesome fibroids, some form of treatment will probably be necessary. If you are using synthetic oestrogen such as the oral contraceptive pill or HRT, discontinuing your medication is advisable. This alone may be enough to significantly shrink your fibroids.

For large fibroids causing debilitating bleeding or discomfort, surgery is sometimes needed. Endometrial ablation involves the removal of the fibroids through laser surgery and is effective in treating the heavy bleeding associated with fibroids in approximately 90% of women treated. As this treatment destroys the complete lining of the uterus it causes infertility, so it is not a treatment option for women hoping for a future pregnancy.

If fibroids are small it may be possible to remove them (myomectomy) while leaving the uterus intact. This surgery is performed under general anaesthetic, and following surgery there is still a 50% chance of conceiving and carrying a baby to full term. As with any surgery, there are risks involved, and for around 5% of women, the surgery fails to correct heavy bleeding.

If all else fails, the absolute last-resort treatment for fibroids is a hysterectomy in which the uterus is surgically removed. This is major surgery, and should only be considered a last resort. *Do not* be talked into having a hysterectomy before exploring other less-invasive treatment options such as myomectomy or endometrial ablation. If your gynaecologist tells you a hysterectomy is your only option, remember you are free to seek a second opinion before making a decision.

Natural treatments

Naturopathic treatment of fibroids involves a two-pronged approach. First, the aim is to increase the local blood circulation and lymphatic drainage in the whole pelvic region, including the uterus. Osteopathic or chiropractic manipulation is often needed to restore normal function to the lower back and the abdominal organs governed by nerves from this part of the spine. Castor oil packs and hydrotherapy will also improve local blood and lymphatic circulation.

Fibroids are an oestrogen-excess condition, so the second fundamental principle for naturopathic treatment is to regulate hormones and increase detoxification of oestrogen in the body. This usually involves improving the function of the liver and bowels.

Dietary modification is aimed at changing oestrogen metabolites to their least oestrogenic form, thus reducing the oestrogenic stimulation to the uterus (see Chapter 6 for a description of different forms of oestrogen), and increasing the detoxification of oestrogen by the liver and the removal of oestrogen from the body via the bowel. The dietary recommendations described in the section on endometriosis are also applicable to the treatment of fibroids.

Castor oil packs

Castor oil packs are a traditional naturopathic treatment for a wide range of internal and external ailments. As an external pack, they are useful in the treatment of breast and uterine lumps and ovarian cysts.

To make your own pack, fold a small hand towel several times and soak it in castor oil until it is wet but not dripping. Place it over your uterus (lower abdominal area) and cover it with a piece of plastic (such as a torn-up plastic bag). Wrap the whole of your lower abdominal area in a large sheet of plastic. Then place a hot-water bottle (as hot as is comfortable) on top and cover the whole area with a towel. Lie down in a comfortable position and rest for about an hour before removing all your layers and the pack. Repeat this process three to four times a week and persevere for a couple of months if needed. When you have finished with your pack, you can wash the oil from your skin with a solution of water containing two teaspoons of baking soda.

Hydrotherapy

The most effective hydrotherapy for uterine fibroids involves regular alternate hot and cold sitz baths. Sit in a small tub of hot water, making sure that your bottom and lower abdomen are submerged, for no more than 10 minutes. Then repeat the process in another tub containing cold water. Stay in the cold tub for 30 seconds to one minute before returning to the hot tub. While sitting in the hot tub, have your feet submerged in the cold tub, and vice versa. Repeat the process three or four times. For best results use sitz baths two or three times a day. Do not use hot sitz baths if you have a weak heart or high blood pressure.

Herbal help

Herbal help for uterine fibroids involves the use of herbs to rebalance female hormones (*Vitex*, black cohosh, black haw); support liver detoxification functions (dandelion, burdock and yellow dock); and reduce troublesome symptoms such as heavy menstrual bleeding (shepherd's purse, red raspberry).

Homoeopathy

* *Belladonna*. Indicated when the menstrual period is characterised by heavy flooding or bright red blood and clots. Any kind of movement or touch makes you feel worse.

* *Tarentula*. Indicated for heavy periods, accompanied by severe pain and restlessness resulting from multiple fibroids.

* *Aurum mur*. Indicated for heavy periods with a yellowish vaginal discharge throughout the rest of the cycle. The uterus is physically enlarged from the presence of the fibroids.

Acupuncture

Traditional Chinese medicine can effectively treat smaller fibroids, and reduce symptoms such as heavy menstrual bleeding. However, treatment of very large fibroids with acupuncture is not always effective.

Natural progesterone cream

Natural progesterone cream is useful to reduce the problem of oestrogen dominance commonly found in women with fibroids. Salivary progesterone levels should be monitored before and during use (see Chapter 5).

Genital herpes

There isn't much good news about this painful and virulent sexually transmitted virus. There is no successful medical treatment, and no guaranteed effective natural treatment. Once you are infected, you carry this virus for life. It is a case of prevention being better than cure.

Causes

Genital herpes is caused by infection by the herpes simplex virus (HSV). There are two types of virus, known as type I and type II. Both can cause cold sores around the mouth and lips, or sores around the genitals; however, the vast majority of genital herpes is caused by the HSV-II strain.

The herpes simplex virus is extremely virulent, and can be transmitted by infected sexual partners even when they are not experiencing an acute attack of genital herpes. This asymptomatic transmission occurs most often during phases in which there is 'viral shedding' — that is, the virus is active and infectious but not producing symptoms in the host. The virus can be active before a sore erupts, and for months after the sores have healed and disappeared. Condoms do not offer 100% protection, although they are an essential protective measure that greatly reduces infection rates for all sexually transmitted diseases, including genital herpes. Genital herpes can also result from receiving oral sex from a partner with an active oral cold sore.

Symptoms

Symptoms usually occur for the first time within three days to two weeks of contracting the virus. The first attack is usually the most virulent, with subsequent attacks generally becoming decreasingly painful. In some instances, there is only ever an initial attack, with the virus becoming dormant thereafter. Women who have ever had oral cold sores prior to contracting genital herpes tend to have less painful attacks.

An acute herpes attack starts as a tingling or burning feeling or an itchy rash in the genital area. The whole of the vulva may swell and become inflamed. Tiny fluid-filled blisters erupt in the genital, anal or buttock areas. These blisters burst to form greyish sores with red edges, lasting about 10 days before healing. Sometimes the blister stage may be missed completely and ulcers may appear like cracks or cuts in the skin. There may be an accompanying vaginal discharge.

Genital herpes sores are painful, with a sharp burning sensation which is particularly severe when you urinate. The first attack of herpes can leave you feeling as if you've been run over by a bus. The sores are often accompanied by a flu-like illness with fever and swollen glands. Once you recover from the initial attack, you will probably never experience such a severe attack again, although the chances of you suffering another attack are still high — there is a more than 50% likelihood of another attack within the next six months. Subsequent attacks seem to be most likely at times of increased emotional or physical stress. Women often find they are more prone to attacks during menstruation, and excessive or vigorous sexual intercourse can also trigger attacks.

Women who have had genital herpes, and who also are infected with HPV virus (see cervical dysplasia) are two to three times more likely to develop cervical cancer. However, being infected by the HSV-II virus without also carrying the HPV virus does not increase cervical cancer risk at all.

Women who have an active outbreak of genital herpes at the time of giving birth can readily transmit the virus to their baby. For this reason, Caesarean birth is necessary if an active infection is evident at the time of birth.

Medical treatment

There is no magic elixir to prevent herpes, although the drug acyclovir (Zovirax) taken at the onset of an outbreak will reduce the severity of symptoms, and reduce the frequency of subsequent outbreaks.

The sores should be kept clean through bathing with a saline solution (lukewarm water with a little table salt dissolved in it). After saline baths, dry the area thoroughly with a gentle warmth from a hair drier. Warm sitz baths with baking soda added to the water will provide symptomatic relief from pain or burning. It may also help to lessen the pain of urination if you sit in a bowl of warm water to urinate, or spray the vulva with water as you urinate.

Complementary therapies

After your first attack of herpes, subsequent outbreaks are most likely to occur at times when you are under increased stress, feeling run-down or exhausted or are lacking sleep. These are the times when you may be already fighting an infection such as a cold or flu, or when your immune system is hampered through stress and late nights, overwork and poor diet. The secret to living painlessly with herpes is to optimise your systemic health, in particular the strength of your immune system. Once you have the herpes virus you have it for life, but you can have a significant impact on how frequently the virus makes its unpleasant presence felt, by making the right lifestyle choices. Making the right choices for your health may involve a fairly radical lifestyle overhaul, including dietary change, regular exercise, stress management, and the use of nutritional supplementation.

Dietary assistance

L-lysine is an amino acid (building block of protein) which may help to prevent acute attacks of herpes when taken regularly as a supplement. L-lysine is antagonistic towards another amino acid called l-arginine. The herpes virus needs l-arginine to thrive. By increasing your intake of lysine (and in turn inhibiting the absorption of arginine), you can create less-favourable conditions for the herpes virus. Preventative doses of lysine need to be in the range of 2000–3000 mg per day. This should be coupled with a low arginine diet (see below). Dietary sources of l-lysine include: potatoes, soya products, dairy products, chicken, meat, eggs, fresh vegetables and brewer's yeast. High-arginine foods (to be avoided) include all nuts and seeds, raisins, brown rice, oatmeal, and (tragically) chocolate.

Other vital ingredients of a preventative regime include zinc and vitamin C. Oral supplementation with 50 mg a day of zinc has been shown to effectively reduce the frequency, duration and severity of herpes attacks. A vitamin-C formula containing bioflavonoids should be taken daily between attacks, in doses of 2000–4000 mg per day. In an acute attack, vitamin-C intake can be increased to bowel tolerance (see section on vitamin C in Chapter 2). To achieve this, keep taking vitamin C every two hours until you develop slight diarrhoea, then cut back your intake slightly until your stools return to normal. Keep up this dosage until the acute attack has ended, before gradually decreasing your intake back down to your maintenance dose. You may be surprised just how much vitamin C you can take before you reach bowel tolerance — up to 10,000 mg a day is not uncommon!

Other powerful immune-supporting supplements include bovine colostrum; green foods such as spirulina, chlorella and barley grass; mushroom extracts such as codyceps and ganoderma; and olive leaf extract.

During an acute attack, vitamin-A supplements will help speed healing of the ulcers. A safe supplementary dose is 15,000 iu a day, with one halibut liver oil capsule containing around 4900 iu. Vitamin A is best taken after a meal containing a fat source. *If you are pregnant, do not use vitamin-A supplements as this vitamin can cause foetal abnormalities, if taken in excess. Instead use beta-carotene as a safe supplemental source of vitamin A.*

Acupuncture

Acupuncture cannot cure herpes, but it is effective in reducing the length of an acute attack. Regular acupuncture treatment between outbreaks can stimulate immunity and greatly reduce the frequency of genital herpes outbreaks.

Topical applications

One of the most effective topical applications for the treatment of genital herpes blisters is a cream containing extract of lemon balm (*Melissa officinalis*). Some studies, such as one published in the journal *Phytomed* in 1994, have found that using the cream on the initial outbreak of blisters in the first attack prevents any future attacks. Find a friendly medical herbalist who will make you a cream with a 70:1 concentration of lemon balm.

Essential oil of melissa can also be used. As soon as the blisters appear, dab one drop of pure melissa oil onto them, three times on the first day. The blisters will usually disappear within 24 hours. Take care not to apply the oil to surrounding skin.

Invest in a jar of 500 iu vitamin-E capsules, and keep them in your fridge. Pierce a capsule and apply the oil to your herpes blisters to decrease the pain and itching, and decrease healing time. Apply the oil two or three times daily. Alternatively, buy a good-quality vitamin-E ointment that contains at least 30 iu of vitamin E per gram of base. To this add some powdered vitamin C, and then apply to the sores two or three times daily.

Several herbs make useful topical applications. Pure aloe vera gel will reduce stinging and pain and itching, as will diluted calendula tincture. Slippery elm powder can be made into a thick paste with a little water and applied topically to soothe the area.

Herbal antibiotics such as myrhh, echinacea and golden seal can also be applied, either as tinctures (but be warned, this may sting badly), or as powder mixed with water to form a paste.

Herbal medicine

Taken orally, herbs can effectively boost immunity, as well as acting as specific antivirals. Commonly used herbs include: garlic, echinacea, golden seal, myrrh, red clover, olive leaf, and St John's wort (do not use this if you are on antidepressants or blood-thinning medication).

Homoeopathy

✳ *Graphites.* Used when there is an acute attack of painful, red, weeping blisters in the genital area. The weeping fluid is clear or yellow and causes itching, but not burning, sensations.

✳ *Nitric acid.* Indicated when there is marked ulceration of the genitals and/or mouth causing local cracking and tenderness. Especially useful for ulcers on the corners of the mouth.

✳ *Rhus tox.* For blisters which cause a lot of itching and discomfort and local redness. Symptoms are made better with applications of heat and with movement.

✳ *Sulphur.* Used in chronic cases characterised by burning pain and secondary infection. Pain is very much worse with any type of heat.

Incontinence

If you can't go to aerobics because your bladder leaks when you do the jumping exercises; or if your bladder leaks whenever you cough, sneeze or laugh, you are suffering from urinary stress incontinence. Men can also be afflicted with this embarrassing problem, but it is many times more common amongst women. This is partly because of the physical trauma to the pelvic area during pregnancy and childbirth, and partly because of uniquely female hormonal factors, most especially the decline in oestrogen experienced from menopause onwards.

Causes

Stress incontinence is more common in women who have had a baby. During pregnancy, the increased abdominal load is supported by a thick sheath of muscle known as the pelvic floor. The growing weight of a pregnancy places an added load on the pelvic floor, sometimes causing stretching and weakening. With age and successive pregnancies, the pelvic floor loses tone, and if you don't give it a regular workout in the form of pelvic floor muscle exercises, it will lose its strength and tone in the same way as any other muscle in the body will. A weakened pelvic floor leads to a generalised sagging of the abdominal organs and a weakening of the urinary sphincter.

A stretched and weakened pelvic floor may not become immediately apparent, or may only cause slight leaking of urine occasionally. Postmenopausally, lowered oestrogen levels tend to aggravate the weakness, making it increasingly noticeable. Women who have had several pregnancies, long or difficult labours, a forceps delivery, large babies or large vaginal tears are especially at risk. Other risk factors include obesity (especially abdominal fat), and poor abdominal tone from lack of exercise.

Temporary incontinence is common following a traumatic emotional experience, such as a great fright or shock, or an emotional loss such as a divorce or the death of a loved one. In these cases there is obviously a very strong mind–body connection, and with time and emotional healing, the bladder usually rights itself with no further intervention needed.

Symptoms

Inability to hold urine in the bladder, especially during exercise or when coughing or sneezing. Symptoms can range from an occasional trickle to complete involuntary emptying of the bladder.

Medical treatment

In the past, women with postmenopausal stress incontinence were frequently treated with hormone replacement therapy (HRT). Since the demise of its popularity based on its proven health risks, long-term HRT use is now much less common. Oestrogen vaginal cream can sometimes improve symptoms of postmenopausal incontinence.

In severe cases of incontinence, surgery is used to repair the sagging and weakened pelvic floor muscles. This operation does not offer a 100% cure, and failure rates are usually around 10–20%. In some cases, incontinence can be improved through the daily use of a small rubber device called a pessary. This device is inserted into the vagina and stretches from the back of the pubic bone to the top of the vagina, acting as a sort of trampoline to hold prolapsed organs in place.

Alternative treatment

If your incontinence is due to pelvic floor weakness, there are few real alternative treatments to try, besides a faithful adherence to a regular regime of pelvic floor exercises. (See Chapter 1.)

Acupuncture

Acupuncture can be very effective in helping restore normal bladder function in mild cases of stress incontinence. Prolapses of any kind are usually related to a weakness of spleen energy in traditional Chinese medicine. Spleen qi is vulnerable to worry and overuse of the mind (including studying); an excess of cold or chilled foods and drinks; and too much sugar in the diet.

Vegetarians are especially prone to spleen qi deficiency. Besides using acupuncture, you can strengthen your own spleen energy by stilling the mind through meditation or relaxation; eating more lightly cooked vegetables and reducing intake of salad and raw fruit; and staying away from all chilled food and drink, and sugars. Root vegetables, chicken broth, well-cooked rice and warming herbs such as ginger, black pepper and chillies also strengthen the spleen qi.

Infertility

Little girls still grow up with the expectation that one day they will meet their Prince Charming, have children and live happily ever after. In reality, for increasing numbers of modern women, the fairytale ending comes tragically unstuck. Partly this is the result of the modern female expectation that we can have it all: a stimulating career, travel, independence, and — when the time suits us — children. While society no longer frowns on a 40-year-old pregnant woman, biology still does not approve. From the spectacularly young age of 26, female fertility begins to decline; with a precipitous drop between the ages of 35 and 40 and an even more radical decline after the age of 40.

Contrary to common belief, it is not unusual for around 20% of perfectly healthy couples to take at least a year to conceive. By the end of the first year of trying, 80% of couples have conceived. Of the remaining 20%, 9 out of 10 couples will have a physical explanation for their infertility. Approximately 35% involve male issues, with female causes accounting for another 35%. Twenty per cent of infertility cases involve a combination of male and female factors, and the remaining 10% fall into the 'unexplainable' category.

New Zealand and Australia both boast internationally recognised assisted fertility technology. Treatment of infertility is available through both private clinics and state-funded treatment programmes.

What causes infertility?

Male infertility can result from a number of different physical causes, including: varicose veins in the scrotum; physical abnormalities with sperm-carrying ducts; immunological abnormalities; hormonal imbalance; testicular failure and infections (such as undetected *Chlamydia*); heavy metal contamination (lead, cadmium, arsenic and mercury). Sperm abnormalities — including low sperm count, poor motility, or excessive numbers of abnormal sperm — are an increasingly common cause of male infertility. The past 50 years have seen a shocking 50% decline in the average male sperm count. Many experts believe this precipitous decline to be the result of increasing environmental contamination with synthetic oestrogenic substances called endocrine disruptors. Plastics, car exhaust fumes, pesticides (PCBs, dioxin and DDT) and heavy metals in food and water cause impaired semen quality. Dioxins, commonly produced during the manufacturing of plastics, have been shown to be especially damaging. Heavy metals such as lead and cadmium interfere with the reproduction of genetic information in sperm, and aluminium decreases sperm motility.

To understand the myriad of possible causes of female infertility, it helps to first understand exactly how conception takes place. In order for conception to occur, there must be present a healthy female egg (ovum) and male sperm. In healthy women, an egg is released from an ovary approximately every 28 days, with ovulation occurring about 14 days after the start of the menstrual period (in other words, mid-cycle). Once released from the ovary, the egg begins its mammoth 10 cm journey through the fallopian tubes to the uterus — a journey that takes four days to complete. Conception can take place at any stage of the journey, if the egg meets sperm. If the egg is fertilised, it embeds itself within the thick, nutrient-rich lining of the uterus, where it begins its nine-month miraculous transformation into a fully formed human being.

Problems can arise at any stage of this process. A lack of ovulation means there is no egg to fertilise. If ovulation does occur but the fallopian tubes are blocked or damaged (often as a result of pelvic inflammatory disease, STDs or endometriosis), the released egg may not be able to complete its journey to the uterus.

Sometimes hormonal imbalances are the cause of fertility problems. An abnormally short second half of the menstrual cycle (called a luteal phase defect) can mean that the lining of the uterus doesn't have sufficient time to prepare itself to successfully sustain an implanted egg. If the time from ovulation until the start of a period is less than nine days, it is considered to be a luteal phase defect, and a cause of infertility.

Other hormonal imbalances, usually centred at the level of the hypothalamus (the master controlling gland in the brain), can result in failure to ovulate.

If eggs and tubes are healthy, problems can still occur if the vaginal mucus is excessively acidic. High acidity will effectively paralyse sperm and prevent them completing their journey. In about 20% of cases of unexplained infertility, female immunological factors are the problem. Inflammatory cells and their secretory products are involved in the processes of ovulation and preparation of the endometrium for implantation of a fertilised egg. A problem with the immune system can interfere with these normal reproductive processes and can cause infertility.

Polycystic ovarian syndrome (PCOS) is an increasingly common cause of female infertility. PCOS leads to the formation of multiple small cysts on the ovaries which interfere with ovulation and normal hormonal levels. Common signs that PCOS may be a cause of infertility include irregular or absent periods, easy weight gain, excessive hairiness and acne.

Nutritional deficiencies can lead to reduced fertility in both men and women. Common deficiencies effecting fertility include: vitamins A, E, B2, B5, B6, B12, folic acid, vitamin C, iron, zinc, magnesium and essential fatty acids.

Plan of action

If you have been having regular unprotected sex (at the right time of the month!) for a year or more and you are not pregnant, it is probably time to visit your GP for some preliminary detective work. An initial consultation will probably involve sperm analysis, checking the sperm count, motility (how well they swim) and the percentage of abnormally formed sperm; and looking for the presence of 'anti-sperm' antibodies. Sperm tests should always be done prior to embarking on the more difficult and invasive investigation of female fertility.

If sperm results come back fine, then it's time to begin checking the female side of the equation. This will involve an internal pelvic examination, Pap smear and blood tests to check hormone levels and ovulation, thyroid function, and so on. An ultrasound of the pelvic area may be performed to check the shape of the uterus and how it is lying, and to ensure that there are no fibroids or polycystic ovaries. Further down the track, if conception still doesn't occur, a laparoscopy is sometimes performed to check for internal adhesions, or endometriosis. As this involves a general anaesthetic, it is not a first line of investigation.

Blocked fallopian tubes are sometimes a cause of infertility. This is especially likely if there are problems with endometriosis, pelvic inflammatory disease or a previously 'silent' sexually transmitted disease such as *Chlamydia*. The only way to determine whether or not the tubes are blocked is to undergo a hysterosalpingogram. During this procedure, a dye is injected into the uterus and tracked by X-ray. When the tubes are healthy and patent, the dye will be seen travelling up through the tubes and into the pelvic cavity, from where the body simply absorbs it.

One of the easiest, but frequently overlooked, tests to be performed is the post-coital test (PCT). If your doctor suggests a hysterosalpingogram before performing a post-coital test, request this test first. It is a lot less invasive and may negate the requirement for the sometimes very uncomfortable hysterosalpingogram. A

PCT is performed around 12 hours after intercourse, during your most fertile time. The mucus high inside the vagina is collected with a syringe. Analysis of the mucus reveals how many live sperm remain after 12 hours of exposure to your vaginal mucus. Healthy sperm should survive for 24 hours, so if there is a high attrition rate after only 12 hours, it signifies a basic incompatibility between your mucus and your partner's sperm. This may be due to inadequate mucus; abnormally acidic vagina pH; high level of sperm antibodies in the mucus; or an abnormality with the sperm itself.

Sometimes the underlying cause of your fertility issues will be discovered quickly, but in some cases there are no identifiable reasons for the inability to conceive. It is for these frustrating cases of 'inexplicable infertility' that complementary therapies can offer some real hope.

Medical treatment

If the cause of fertility problems is irregular or absent ovulation or a luteal phase defect, the first medical solution is often a course of the fertility drug clomiphene citrate (clomid). Clomid will stimulate your ovaries into action, trigger ovulation and a high-quality luteal phase (second half of the cycle). While this drug is useful to stimulate regular ovulation in women who ovulate sporadically, it will make absolutely no difference to your fertility if you are already ovulating regularly. In approximately 60% of women, clomid will trigger ovulation, and in 30% of these pregnancy will occur within three months.

If clomid fails to do its thing, the next drug to try is usually perganol (human menopausal gonadotropin). This is administered by injection for around 12 days of your cycle. Perganol is usually used for women with low oestrogen levels, but is also used in the case of polycystic ovaries and luteal phase defects. Side effects are extremely common, and these include an increase in risk of premature delivery or miscarriage if pregnancy does occur. Other common pharmaceutical approaches to infertility include the use of the drug bromacriptine when prolactin levels are excessively high; or synthetic progesterone if the functioning of the corpus luteum (the part of the egg follicle which secretes progesterone after ovulation) is impaired.

Blocked fallopian tubes may be treated with surgery, although their repair is not always possible. Sometimes undergoing a hysterosalpingogram will actually clear any blockage in the fallopian tube.

High-tech fertility procedures such as insemination by husband or donor; *in-vitro* fertilisation (IVF) or IVF using a donated egg are the last-resort options for infertility. As they are expensive, stressful and often unsuccessful, these high-tech solutions are a last resort after all other treatment approaches have failed.

Self-help for infertility

In every case of infertility, explainable or otherwise, optimising your general health is an important part of fertility enhancement. Take a good close look at yourself. Are you a picture of vibrant health, with abundant energy, a strong immune system, and a relaxed and calm disposition? Or are you stressed, overworked, exhausted, sleep deprived, and struggling with one viral infection after another? If the latter sounds more like you, fertility issues may be just another reflection of suboptimum health.

Body weight and the amount of exercise you do can both impact negatively on fertility. Women need a minimum of 18% body fat to maintain regular ovulation and a normal menstrual cycle. Frequent weight-loss dieters or obsessive exercisers can easily dip below this critical threshold. If this sounds like you, it is vital that you start nurturing yourself by eating a sensible, balanced diet to allow a gradual increase in percentage body fat, up to the healthy and fertile 18% level. Along with more food, reduce exercise levels to a sensible regime which doesn't leave you feeling drained and exhausted.

While we're on the subject of reality checks, take a good, hard look at the pace of your life. If you are working more than

40 hours a week, make a serious effort to shift your work/life balance in favour of more hours of relaxation and pleasure, and less time at the office! Overwork leads to exhaustion, stress, and hormonal changes which can disrupt fertility.

When it comes to stress and fertility there is still much to be learned. In a purely biological sense, it's easy to surmise that a connection exists, as the tiny hypothalamus gland in the brain regulates both stress responses and female hormones. Many women have experienced this connection, with high stress levels causing a missed period. Stress can also interfere with the normal process of ovulation. Faced with excessive stress, the pituitary gland stimulates an overproduction of the hormone prolactin, which causes irregular ovulation.

It's not just female fertility which takes a hammering from stress. Male sperm count is also detrimentally affected by high stress levels. Male prisoners facing the extreme stress of awaiting execution completely stop producing sperm. Admittedly, few men face this degree of stress, but chronic, ongoing, low-grade stress can lower sperm count, reduce libido and cause problems with getting and sustaining an erection.

If it's taking time to conceive, this can become a significant stress in itself. If you have been trying for less than a year, you can take a deep breath, relax, and realise it can easily take a year to get pregnant when you are perfectly healthy. If you've been trying for more than a year, and you're currently going through the trials and tribulations of testing and medical visits, acknowledge just how stressful this can be.

As much as possible, resist the urge to become obsessively focused on your fertility issues, instead creating time and space to spend quality time with your partner. Nurture a loving and supportive relationship, and remember to include some fun in your life together as an important way of countering fertility-related stress. Reintroduce romance . . . something that can quickly take a back seat when you get caught up in the mechanics of temperature taking, ovulation testing and performing on demand.

Weekends away or a romantic night at a hotel, where the focus is on love and communication rather than baby-making, is excellent therapy for body, mind and spirit.

It takes two to tango and it definitely takes two to make a baby. Encourage the male part of your equation to do everything possible to optimise his sperm health. That means that two of life's little pleasures may be kicked into touch — alcohol and caffeine. Too much of either (or both) can play havoc with sperm health. As few as three cups of coffee a day can increase the incidence of abnormally formed sperm. Contrary to what one would expect, caffeine does not motivate sperm to swim faster! In fact, drinking five or more cups of coffee a day has just the opposite effect, making sperm sluggish and unable to swim well.

Alcohol reduces the production of the male hormone testosterone, and also hastens its conversion to oestrogen in the liver, potentially leading to lowered sperm count and a reduced sex drive. Some research suggests that completely abstaining from alcohol for three months results in a significant increase in sperm count for 50% of men with low sperm counts, as well as improving sperm motility (how well they swim). Going alcohol-free is also recommended for women intending to conceive, so support your partner in choosing a fresh juice over a glass of wine in the evenings!

Smoking and conception are definitely incompatible. Cigarette smoking plays havoc with sperm. In men with normal sperm, smoking is associated with a 23% reduction in sperm density, and a 13% reduction in sperm motility. Female smokers are three to four times more likely than non-smokers to take more than a year to conceive. It is impossible to overstate the importance of well and truly kicking this self-destructive habit if you intend to conceive and deliver a healthy baby.

The ideal fertility diet is devoid of processed, refined foods, and additives, colourings and preservatives. Fresh, preferably organic, vegetables and fruit should be eaten in abundance every day, with the aim of consuming nine servings daily (which can include fresh, home-made vegetable and fruit juices). Adequate protein intake is important, but this does not mean sitting down to a steak every night! As well as red meat, protein can come from fish, chicken, dairy products, eggs, brown rice, lentils, beans, nuts, seeds and soya products. High phyto-oestrogen foods such as soya, linseed, tofu and miso are best avoided by men trying to father a child.

To make a complete protein from vegetarian sources, try combining a whole grain such as brown rice, buckwheat, millet, whole wheat or rye products with nuts, seeds and pulses such as lentils, soya beans, legumes or sprouts. Avoid big fish at the top of the food chain, such as tuna and groper, as these are more likely to be contaminated with heavy metals such as mercury.

Dietary fats can interfere with or enhance sperm health, depending on your choices. In order to be fertile, a sperm must have flexible and fluid cell membranes. If the cellular membranes in sperm become too rigid, enzymes are produced which damage the sperm. Membrane health is enhanced by minimising dietary sources of saturated and hydrogenated fats (and consequently trans-fats), and increasing polyunsaturated fatty acids from nuts and seeds, fish, avocado, flax oil and olive oil.

Dietary choices can also influence fertility by changing the pH of the vaginal secretions, making them 'hostile' to sperm. Sperm need an alkaline medium to survive for long enough, and to stay strong enough, to complete the arduous journey up through the vagina to the cervix. A highly acidic diet with an overabundance of grains, meat, fish, eggs, nuts, seeds, coffee and alcohol may contribute to an altered vaginal pH.

Acupuncture and traditional Chinese medicine
Acupuncture can effectively remedy a wide range of fertility-related problems including sperm issues, lack of or irregular ovulation and menstruation, endometriosis, polycystic ovaries, and luteal phase defects. (See box over page.)

Traditional Chinese medicine and infertility

Traditional Chinese medicine placed great emphasis upon treating female and male infertility. Historically in China, a couple who failed to produce at least one son faced catastrophic social consequences, as without a son there was no one to make sacrifices to the gods. Without the sacrifices, there was the prospect of having one's immortality cut off.

The traditional Chinese medicine focus in the treatment of female infertility is very much on normalising the production and circulation of the 'blood' energy in the body. Many female fertility issues are considered to result from a deficiency, stagnation or blockage of this energy.

Blood deficiency results from a weakness or imbalance in one or several of the meridians involved with blood production, including the spleen, kidney and heart.

The heart and spleen involvement in blood production is detrimentally affected by emotional disturbances. The heart cannot create blood if it is 'longing' or broken (usually as a result of unhappiness in a personal relationship); and the spleen is weakened by continued worry, excessive thinking, or years of intensive studying.

The food with which we nourish our body also affects blood production. The spleen function is hampered by excessive amounts of cold foods and drinks. This includes physically cold food such as chilled, iced and frozen foods and drinks, and also cold-energy foods such as fruits and vegetables (especially when they are raw), dairy products and fried foods. Weak spleen qi always requires the elimination of these foods, and the addition of warming foods such as root vegetables, broths, well-cooked chicken and warming spices like ginger and black pepper. How do you know if your spleen qi is weak? Common signs include weight gain, abdominal bloating, loose stools, a pale, swollen tongue, and prolapses such as varicose veins and haemorrhoids.

Weak kidney qi results from long-term overwork and exhaustion, and fear or anxiety. Qi deficiency is almost endemic in our hyper-manic Western culture where we fill every minute of our lives with activity. Our fashion trends don't help strengthen kidney qi either! The penchant for young girls to wear tops which stop at their waist and expose an acre of bare flesh around the lower abdomen and back makes the kidneys vulnerable to cold, which in turn weakens the 'yang' aspect of kidney energy. Common signs of kidney weakness (besides infertility) include dark circles under the eyes; chronic backache in the lower back; cold or stiff knees; frequent voluminous urination; and fatigue. Besides having regular acupuncture, the most important therapy for kidney rejuvenation is rest, rest and more rest.

Liver disharmony is often involved in female health issues, including infertility. Liver qi is responsible for the free flow of energy and blood in the body. Whenever there is a sense of 'stuckness' in the body, you can be sure that a liver imbalance or stagnation of liver qi is involved. Signs of liver disharmony include a range of menstrual problems such as PMS; irregular or painful periods; heavy, clotty periods; breast distension, and pain and volatile moods. Liver qi is affected by stress, and in particular frustration, anger and suppression of emotion. Liver qi stagnation is one of the most common energy imbalances I see in the clinic. It is partly the legacy of the cultural expectation that women should be 'nice' and the peacekeepers at all times. Repeatedly swallowing our frustration without speaking out is guaranteed to stagnate our liver energy. What can you do to stimulate free flow of liver energy? Take regular aerobic exercise; cut back on coffee, chocolate, alcohol and spicy foods . . . and most importantly of all, speak your mind and express your feelings.

Nutritional deficiency and infertility

Essential fatty acid deficiency is one of the most frequent nutritional deficiencies I see in women patients. In our fat-phobic society, eliminating every possible gram of fat from one's diet has become a common goal. In truth, we all need a certain amount of dietary essential fatty acids to stay healthy — and to retain our fertility. Induced EFA deficiencies have produced infertility in laboratory rats (not that I'm comparing women to lab rats!).

Stock up on the right EFAs for fertility by including flax oil, avocado, nuts and seeds, LSA (ground linseed, sunflower seeds and almonds), and cold-pressed virgin olive oil in your diet regularly. Taking a supplement of 1000 mg of evening primrose oil or fish oil three times a day is another useful adjunct to ensure that requirements of these vital fertility-boosting fatty acids are met.

The fat-soluble vitamins A and E are also particularly important for optimum fertility. Both help to maintain the health and cell integrity of the mucous membranes, including the lining of the vagina and the uterus. Vitamin E in particular has been labelled a fertility vitamin par excellence. Once again, laboratory experiments have shown that a diet sufficient in everything except vitamin E produces sterile rats. You also need more of this fat-soluble vitamin in your diet if you are increasing your dietary polyunsaturated fats in an effort to boost essential fatty acid levels. Besides increasing your intake of vitamin-E-rich foods (such as nuts, seeds, wheatgerm, whole grains, avocado, and leafy green vegetables) extra vitamin E can be added with a mixed tocopherol supplement supplying 200–500 iu of vitamin E per day.

Some of the B-vitamins have also been used successfully to treat infertility — in particular, vitamins B6, B12 and folic acid. Vitamin B6 can restore normal ovulation in women with excessively high prolactin levels. Supplementation with 100–200 mg of B6 a day is appropriate for women who fail to conceive because of a lack of progesterone in the second half of the menstrual cycle.

When progesterone levels are low, the lining of the uterus doesn't become thick enough and nutrient-rich enough for the successful implanting of a fertilised egg. Interestingly, most women with this problem also suffer from marked pre-menstrual syndrome, another 'B6-deficiency' problem. When using B6 supplements in these high doses it is best to work with a nutritionally trained health professional.

In clinical trials, supplements of folic acid in the region of 15 mg a day have also facilitated conception in women with reduced fertility, although it is still unclear exactly what the mechanism of fertility enhancement is.

Mineral deficiencies are more common than vitamin deficiencies, particularly deficiencies of zinc and magnesium. Plentiful magnesium is needed to produce the female hormones oestrogen and progesterone. If you have any of the magnesium-deficiency symptoms listed in Chapter 2, a lack of dietary magnesium may be affecting your fertility. Supplementing with 400 mg of magnesium daily (along with vitamin B6) may be of assistance.

How can nutritional therapy help your partner?

It takes two to make a baby . . . so if the male half of your reproductive equation needs some help with the health of his sperm . . . this section is for you.

By far the most common sperm problem is a low sperm count. The past 50 years have seen a worrying downward spiral in the average male sperm count, with most men now only producing 40% of the sperm produced in the average ejaculate in the 1940s. Many scientists believe this decline is the result of increased exposure to environmental contaminants such as heavy metals (for example, lead, mercury and arsenic); organic solvents; and pesticides with an oestrogenic effect. A low sperm count is considered to be less than 20 million sperm in each millilitre of semen. However, it is still possible for conception to occur with sperm counts below this if the percentage of healthy sperm is high, and their motility (swimming ability) is also good.

The nutrient par excellence for male fertility issues is zinc, as it is involved in almost every aspect of male reproduction, including hormonal balance, sperm production and sperm motility. Taken in supplemental doses as low as 50 mg of elemental zinc a day, this mineral can effectively improve the numbers and liveliness of sperm. This effect is especially noticeable when a low sperm count is accompanied by low testosterone levels.

Along with zinc, vitamin C is an antioxidant nutrient which helps protect sperm from damage resulting from free-radical attack. As many as 40% of infertile men have been found to have high levels of free-radicals in their sperm. While free-radicals are constantly produced in the normal functioning of the body, exposure to environmental pollutants such cigarette smoke will exacerbate their production.

Vitamin C is a vital sperm-protecting antioxidant, and a low dietary intake of this vitamin (through a diet lacking in fresh fruits and vegetables) is damaging to male fertility. Cigarette smoking also contributes to a deficiency of this nutrient, greatly reducing levels of vitamin C in the body. A number of studies have found that daily supplementation with as little as 1000 mg of vitamin C results in an increase in sperm count and a reduction in the number of sperm found 'clumping' together (the technical term is 'agglutination'). When they bind together and are unable to move freely, sperm are less able to swim effectively to reach a waiting egg; 1000 mg ascorbic acid supplements taken daily for as little as three weeks can reduce sperm clumping by up to 70%.

Other vital antioxidant nutrients essential for optimising sperm health are vitamin E (a mixed tocopheral form of the vitamin), selenium and beta-carotene. Given in supplemental doses of between 600 and 800 iu a day, vitamin E exerts a beneficial effect on both sperm count and on sperm motility.

L-arginine is an amino acid (building block of protein) which occurs naturally in many protein foods, as well as being available as a nutritional supplement. Arginine is needed in the replication of cells, including sperm. High supplemental doses of arginine, in the range of 4 g a day, have been shown to increase male sperm count and motility (making the sperm better swimmers). L-arginine is most effective in elevating the sperm count when the starting sperm count is 20 million/ml or more. For sperm boosting, arginine is best taken in doses of 2 g, twice daily, for a three-month period. Arginine therapy is contraindicated in people with diabetes.

Korean and Siberian ginseng have both proved effective in the treatment of male fertility problems. In animals, Chinese (*Panax*) ginseng has demonstrated the ability to increase sperm counts, testosterone levels, libido and performance! The *Panax* form of ginseng is considered to be the most potent, and is the form most commonly used by herbalists in the treatment of male infertility.

Dietary and lifestyle choices can make a difference to male fertility. If your partner has fertility issues, support him in making the necessary changes. Go through his drawers and throw out all the tight and sexy underpants (with his consent of course) and replace them with boxer shorts. Testicles need to hang away from the body so as to lower their temperature and encourage sperm formation.

Support him in making the essential dietary changes by adopting the same diet yourself. This involves complete abstinence from alcohol; moderation in the use of or abstinence from caffeine; supercharging intake of fresh fruits and vegetables; swapping to healthy fats; and avoiding processed, refined and coloured foods. If he is a cigarette smoker, kicking the habit is the most important step of all (that goes for use of recreational drugs such as marijuana as well). Overwork, exhaustion, lack of sleep and excessive stress can all play havoc with sperm count, so living a balanced, healthy lifestyle is important for optimising fertility.

If your partner has (or you have) a lot of amalgam fillings (or old fillings), it is worth visiting a holistic dentist to check if fillings are leaching mercury into the body. Sperm are especially sensitive to the toxic effects of mercury.

Suggested supplements for male and female infertility

Female

✳ High-potency B-complex supplying 50 mg of the major B-vitamins, to be taken twice daily with meals, with an additional 200–400 mcg of folic acid daily.

✳ 400 iu of vitamin E (mixed tocopherols or alpha-tocopherol), to be taken with a meal containing fat. Use a supplement which also supplies selenium.

✳ Vitamin C and bioflavonoids: 1000 mg of vitamin C taken three times daily.

✳ Balanced multi-mineral formula supplying at least 50 mg of zinc and 400 mg of magnesium in chelate or orotate form. To be taken between meals.

Male

✳ Multi-mineral formula (as above), supplying at least 50 mg of zinc.

✳ Vitamin E (mixed tocopherols or alpha-tocopherol): 250 iu to be taken three times daily.

✳ Vitamin C: 1000 mg of ascorbic acid to be taken three times daily.

✳ L-arginine: 2 g (2000 mg) to be taken twice daily, not at the same time as food.

Homoeopathic help for infertility

For the treatment of infertility, seek the services of a registered homoeopath rather than self-prescribing. The homoeopath will treat you in your entirety, not just the part of you which is 'infertile'. Consequently, to begin with you may be given a deep-acting homoeopathic remedy that is not especially indicated for

Tips for top fertility

✳ Chart your menstrual cycle with the assistance of a natural family planning (NFP) instructor. (Find out where your local NFP clinic is by contacting your family planning centre.) This will help you pinpoint the exact time of your ovulation. Remember an egg lives only 12–24 hours after ovulation, so timing of intercourse is crucial.

✳ Some sexual intercourse positions are better than others when it comes to making babies. Preferably use a position that allows deep penile penetration such as the traditional missionary position. Raise your hips slightly with a couple of pillows, and stay on your back for at least half an hour after intercourse to give sperm the greatest opportunity to start their marathon journey without fighting the additional effects of gravity.

✳ It's a common scenario that couples who were unable to conceive, and so adopted a child, within a matter of months conceived their own child. This scenario demonstrates the effect that emotional stress and tension can have on our fertility. It's easy to become stressed out and tense when you're trying to conceive, and every lovemaking situation becomes merely another opportunity to conceive, rather than an enjoyable expression of love. If this is the case for you, remember that intercourse is one part of 'making love', and is about mutual sharing and pleasure. Bring back the candles, the romantic dinners, the lounging in the hot tub (although make sure that it's not too hot, and don't stay in for too long — remember the effect of heat on the testicles!), the love and the togetherness. If finances and lifestyle allow, plan regular weekends away or romantic nights at a hotel.

infertility. Once your general level of health and vitality is raised, then a remedy more specifically aimed at the fertility problems may be prescribed.

Menorrhagia

Few women discuss the intimate details of their menstrual blood loss with other women, so it's hard for them to know exactly what is normal, and what constitutes excessive bleeding or menorrhagia. If you have to wear double pads, pass large clots, bleed for more than five days, and find that you build your life around never being far from the nearest toilet, then you are probably losing too much blood. The amount of blood you lose each month (be it heavy or light) should stay roughly constant. Any dramatic change in the amount of blood you lose during a period should be investigated by your doctor.

Even if there are no serious underlying pathological causes for your excessive blood loss, if left untreated this ongoing loss will eventually affect your health detrimentally. When you bleed you also lose iron stores, and heavy bleeding month after month will eventually lead to iron-deficiency anaemia and exhaustion.

Causes

In approximately 50% of cases of menorrhagia, there is no apparent cause. The other half of cases are caused by a variety of problems, such as:

* fibroids
* pelvic inflammatory disease
* endometriosis
* endometrial cancer — usually accompanied by bleeding between periods, too, and most common in postmenopausal women
* endometrial hyperplasia (excessive thickening of the uterine lining)

* severe iron-deficiency anaemia
* anovulation (failure to ovulate)
* sluggish thyroid (hypothyroidism)
* vitamin-A deficiency.

Heavy menstrual bleeding can also be caused by:
* the use of an intrauterine device (IUD)
* the use of the injectable contraceptive Depo-Provera.

There are also several hormonal or physiological imbalances that can cause excessive bleeding, such as problems with the function of the hypothalamus, pituitary gland or ovaries; or chronic kidney or liver problems. One of the most common glandular problems is an underactivity of the thyroid gland (hypothyroidism). The thyroid is responsible for regulating the menstrual cycle, among other things. Around 30–40% of women with hypothyroidism also suffer from excessive menstrual blood loss. If hypothyroidism underlies your menorrhagia, you will almost certainly have other symptoms of hypothyroidism, such as:

* dry skin and hair
* lack of energy and easy exhaustion on exertion
* tendency to gain weight easily
* poor circulation and sensitivity to cold
* depression and inability to concentrate properly
* acne
* recurrent infections
* low basal body temperature (under 36.5 °C).

If you suspect that hypothyroidism may be a problem for you, start by performing the simple but remarkably accurate home thyroid function test, described below.

Test your own thyroid function

This test is most accurate when you perform it on the second and third day of your period. When you go to bed at night, place a thermometer by the bed ready for use in the morning. In the morning, as soon as you awake, take your temperature under your armpit. Leave the thermometer in place for 10 minutes. If your temperature is below 36.6°C (97.8°F), you could well have a problem with your thyroid. Repeat the test the next day.

Medical treatment

It is important that you have your abnormal bleeding or excessively heavy bleeding checked out by your doctor. Even if you don't wish to use drugs to treat your problem, you must rule out any serious underlying problems before deciding on treatment options.

Your doctor may perform a Pap smear and a D and C (dilatation of the cervix and then curettage or scraping out the lining of the uterus) as part of the diagnostic tests. Once all the potentially serious causes of menorrhagia have been ruled out, you may be treated with hormones (progesterone or a combination of progesterone and oestrogen, such as the oral contraceptive pill) to stop your excessive blood loss. Provera (oral progesterone) is often used continuously for various lengths of time (depending on how severe the blood loss is), to completely stop menstruation. The progesterone-releasing Mirena IUCD reduces heavy bleeding and, in some women, completely stops menstrual blood loss.

As an absolute last resort, if all else fails, your doctor may recommend a hysterectomy. A hysterectomy is major surgery, so it is in your best interest to exhaust all non-surgical treatment options (both medical and holistic) before deciding on surgery.

Nutritional therapy

If you have ruled out all the serious stuff, and you're still spending a fortune on pads every month, then a change in diet and some well-chosen nutritional supplements may well help you.

First, have your iron status checked using a simple blood test. Heavy menstrual bleeding and iron-deficiency anaemia share a 'chicken-and-egg' relationship; that is, it's hard to tell which one came first. Heavy bleeding will lead to loss of iron stores and anaemia. In turn, anaemia will exacerbate the heavy menstrual bleeding. If your blood test results show low iron, follow the recommendations listed in the section on anaemia above.

A dietary protein deficiency can also influence menstrual bleeding. Protein is involved in the manufacture of muscle, and smooth muscles play an important part in regulating and then cutting off the flow of blood from the tiny blood vessels lining the uterus. If your muscles are being given adequate protein through your diet, it may be that they are not getting the other nutrients they need to perform their function of contracting and damming blood flow. Such nutrients include vitamin E, essential fatty acids, and the minerals calcium, magnesium and potassium.

After each period, your body must 'heal' the lining of your uterus, stopping the bleeding until your next period. This healing involves other nutrients, especially vitamins A, C and bioflavonoids, and zinc.

Women with heavy periods are often found to have lower than usual serum levels of vitamin A, and supplementing with 25,000 iu of vitamin A daily can sometimes reduce menstrual blood loss to normal. Interestingly, a sluggish thyroid gland (another of the common causes of menorrhagia) will hinder your absorption of vitamin A. *Never self-administer these high levels of vitamin A if you are pregnant or planning on becoming pregnant in the near future, as vitamin A can cause birth defects.*

Another vital wound-healing nutrient, zinc, has an interesting relationship with vitamin A. A dietary zinc deficiency (extremely common among Australian and New Zealand women) will hinder your ability to absorb and utilise dietary or supplemental vitamin A. When supplementing with vitamin A, include generous amounts of zinc-rich foods in your diet, such as whole grains, shellfish, pumpkin and sunflower seeds, and organ meats.

Do you bruise easily and have bleeding gums? If so, a deficiency of bioflavonoids may be partly to blame for your heavy periods. Bioflavonoids enhance the absorption of vitamin C, and are vital to maintain strong blood vessel walls. If you lack bioflavonoids (and vitamin C), the walls of your tiny blood capillaries become fragile and prone to rupture. Consequently, the healing of the uterine lining is also hampered.

Vitamin K used to be given routinely to newborns at birth to lessen their chances of haemorrhage. This blood-clotting vitamin is not available as a supplement, but can be freely obtained from food sources such as leafy green vegetables, egg yolks, kelp, alfalfa, molasses, liquid chlorophyll and fish liver oils.

Essential fatty acids also play an important part in regulating menstrual flow. Women with menorrhagia often have excessively high concentrations of the fatty acid arachidonic acid, concentrated in the endometrial lining. During a period, an increased amount of this fatty acid is released from the endometrium, stimulating the production of a type of local hormone called the series 2 prostaglandins. These inflammatory prostaglandins are implicated in both excessive menstrual bleeding and period pain. By decreasing animal fats in the diet, and supplementing with flax seed or evening primrose oil, the bioavailability of the arachidonic acid may be reduced.

Supplements for menorrhagia

∗ A multi-mineral supplement containing calcium, magnesium, zinc and iron. A chelated or orotate formula is preferable, to enhance absorption.

∗ Vitamin-A supplement, such as halibut liver oil. Use up to 25,000 iu a day.

∗ Vitamin C and bioflavonoid complex, supplying up to 4 g of vitamin C and 1 g of bioflavonoids per day.

∗ Essential fatty acids, supplied in the form of evening primrose oil; use 3000 mg a day.

✳ Liquid chlorophyll as a supplemental form of vitamin K.

✳ Iron, supplying 100 mg of elemental iron per day, *if blood tests show low iron levels.*

Herbal help

Herbal medicine has much to offer in the treatment of menorrhagia. Astringent herbs help to stem excessive blood loss. A holistic herbalist will always prescribe herbs to address systemic imbalance, and any underlying factors which may be contributing to heavy blood loss, rather than simply treating symptomatically with astringents.

One simple herbal self-help measure for heavy menstrual bleeding is the regular consumption of strong infusions of red raspberry leaf tea. Buy a quality loose-leaf tea and make a brew in a teapot. Leave to steep for 10 minutes, turning the pot occasionally. Drink two to three cups of the tea daily throughout your cycle, not just during the period. Raspberry leaf is high in tannins, which accounts for its powerful astringent action and blood-stemming properties. It is also a rich source of iron and helps to replace iron stores depleted by bleeding.

Other useful blood-stemming astringents include: shepherd's purse, cranesbill, cinnamon, beth root, lady's mantle and periwinkle. Shepherd's purse is one of the most effective herbs for stopping blood loss of any kind. Having a bottle of tincture on hand for emergency flooding is a great idea. Remember that this is a symptomatic 'first aid' approach to the problem, and should only be used as part of a broader holistic treatment to address the root causes of your menorrhagia.

Homoeopathy

If you suffer from a heavy loss of blood, and the duration of your menstrual period is more than five days, one of these remedies may help.

✳ *Aconite.* This is indicated when, along with the heavy,

bright red and clotty blood loss, you experience anxiety and faintness. There is a red complexion and a general sense of agitation.

✳ *Nat mur.* To be used when heavy, prolonged periods also tend to be irregular. The sense of dryness of the vagina and other mucous membranes also results in constipation. Cramping lower abdominal pains are also present.

✳ *Sulphur.* Indicated in the case of prolonged, heavy but irregular periods characterised by loss of thick, dark blood which irritates the skin and burns the vulva. There may also be burning-type pains.

Still other remedies are appropriate if your blood loss is excessive but the length of your period is normal (three to five days):

✳ *Belladonna.* Indicated for bright red, clotty, heavy blood flow that is usually early. Again, there is extreme sensitivity to movement or touch, and the complexion is flushed red. Often there is accompanying headache and irritability.

✳ *China.* Early, heavy periods contain black clots, and are accompanied by extreme tiredness and ringing in the ears.

✳ *Ipecac.* Extremely heavy, continuous flow of bright red blood. Menses are usually early and are accompanied by severe, sharp pains in the middle of the abdomen. There is a sense of weakness and vomiting is common.

✳ *Nux vomica.* Indicated for heavy, irregular periods that tend to stop and start. Colicky pains and constipation accompany the irritability characteristic of this remedy.

Acupuncture

Menorrhagia can often be effectively treated with acupuncture. Traditional Chinese medicine differentiates the underlying energetic imbalances causing your particular type of heavy bleeding. These energetic disturbances may include: heat in the blood; heat and dampness in the blood; a stagnation of blood; or a weakness or 'emptiness' of the kidney or spleen energy (qi).

Heat in the blood produces periods with copious amounts of bright red blood that gushes and floods. The periods are often early, and there may be spotting at other times of the month. Quite often, this type of imbalance is accompanied by a tendency to headaches, pre-menstrual tension, and a general feeling of irritability and 'stress' throughout the month. A stagnation of liver energy often underlies this heat condition. Living with chronic frustration or suppressed anger is very damaging to the liver qi circulation. Other factors contributing to the development of hot blood may include an excessive consumption of heating foods (alcohol, red meat, spicy foods) and living a fast-paced, stressful life.

The heavy periods caused by qi deficiency are quite different. Although there is a heavy blood loss, it tends to be paler, more watery blood that 'leaks' rather than gushes. The periods just seem to trickle on for days and days. Deficient heavy bleeding is also accompanied by overall feelings of exhaustion, weakness, and apathy. Often there are feelings of coldness and backache in the lower back. The underlying problem is a deficiency of kidney and spleen qi, usually the result of years of overactivity, lack of rest and relaxation, and excessively high stress levels. Avoid cold or chilled foods and drinks with this 'empty' bleeding. Lightly steamed or stir-fried vegetables are preferable to salads, and drink warm or hot drinks rather than cold water or fruit juice. Well-cooked broths and soups containing chicken and root vegetables are great for tonifying spleen energy. After that, rest, rest, and rest!

Osteoporosis

The word *osteoporosis* literally means 'porous or honeycombed bones'. With ageing there is a natural decline in bone density and mass, as bones are gradually leached of their mineral and protein components. In some cases, this loss of bone density is dramatic enough to result in osteoporosis — weak, fragile bones that fracture easily and are slow to mend. In advanced osteoporosis, the weight of the body itself is enough to cause spontaneous fractures of the vertebrae or hip bones. The simple act of sneezing may be enough to fracture one or several ribs!

Symptoms

Like heart disease, osteoporosis is one of those insidious diseases that you often don't know you have until it's too late. Sometimes, however, there are early warning signs such as gradual loss of height, and a bowing of the upper back, known as dowager's hump. The clearest warning of osteoporosis is a spontaneous fracture.

Osteoporosis has been given its own 'epidemic' status in recent years. Western women now live in fear of spending their twilight years at the mercy of their crumbling bones. While some women undoubtedly develop this severe form of osteoporosis, the statistics showing a massive increase in the incidence of osteoporosis are partly misleading.

Osteoporosis was once defined by the presence of fragility fractures (relatively spontaneous or extremely low-impact bone fractures). In the early 1990s, osteoporosis was redefined as being a bone mineral density (BMD) 2.5 grades less than 'normal' as measured by a DXA machine. In truth, predicting eventual fractures is a lot more complicated than simply referring to a BMD reading, and BMD readings have never been proven to be a reliable predictor of fracture.

Says Gill Sanson in her book *The Osteoporosis 'Epidemic'*, 'low bone density is just one of many risk factors for fragile bones. A diagnosis of low bone density can only accurately predict future fracture in a person who is already deemed to be at high risk because of other fractures.' Many women have what is considered to be a low BMD but will never have a spontaneous fracture . . . they are, however, included in the statistics defining the osteoporosis 'epidemic'. Reviews of evidence in a number of Western countries concluded that bone-density testing is not an accurate way of predicting who will go on to have fractures.

Causes

Bones are living organisms that are constantly being remade as bone cells are dissolved and reformed on a daily basis. The raw materials needed for the formation of bone include a wide variety of minerals and vitamins such as calcium, magnesium, phosphorus, boron, vitamin C and vitamin D. Of these, calcium is required in the greatest quantity. Not only are bones made from calcium, but they also act as large storehouses for this mineral. At all times, your body needs a small amount of calcium circulating in the bloodstream. Blood calcium is essential for muscle contraction, normal blood clotting, and the function of the nerves and brain.

When blood calcium levels are low, stored bone calcium is released from the bones into the bloodstream. With ageing, and especially after menopause (when oestrogen levels are lowered), bones lose calcium more quickly than it can be replaced. Lowered oestrogen levels decrease the body's ability to absorb calcium from the gut and 'fix' it into our bones. If bone density is already low at the onset of menopause, the increased rate of bone loss can eventually lead to osteoporotic bones.

Osteoporosis is not an exclusively female problem, although men suffer from the condition much less frequently, for a number of reasons. The maximum bone density (called peak bone mass) achieved by women is around 30% less than that achieved by men. One of the most rapid times of bone loss is in the five to seven years after menopause — and men don't do the menopause thing!

Even if you are a woman, and postmenopausal, it doesn't necessarily mean that you will develop this condition. There are a number of common factors which contribute to a greater than usual risk. These include:

* having a small frame and being a Caucasian woman

* a family history of osteoporosis

* heavy alcohol or fizzy drink consumption

* consuming too much caffeine in the form of coffee, tea and cola

* eating a lot of meat (especially red meat)

* a high dietary intake of sugar and refined carbohydrates

* having an extremely low calcium intake

* including too much salt in the diet

* suffering from a lack of vitamin K as a result of a diet low in fruits and vegetables

* chronic or repeated dieting

* a history of inactivity and sedentary living

* hormonal problems such as under- or overactive thyroid, and underactive parathyroid glands

* suffering from coeliac disease or rheumatoid arthritis

* long-term use of steroids, anticonvulsants, Depo-Provera, anti-seizure medication, lithium, methotrexate, fluoride

* premature menopause or removal of ovaries at a young age

* cigarette smoking

* low BMD (bone mineral density).

Osteoporosis does not just happen overnight when you become menopausal. The condition of your bones heading into the menopausal years has huge significance. Often, the gradual progression towards menopause begins in our twenties and thirties with pregnancy and lactation. Bones need large amounts of all nutrients, in particular calcium, magnesium and phosphorus, during pregnancy and breastfeeding. Often these increased nutritional demands are not met, leading to the start of bone demineralisation, even at this early age. This early bone damage is increased dramatically after menopause, when we become much more susceptible to the action of the hormone which controls calcium levels in the blood (the parathyroid hormone). Consequently, more calcium is released from the bones than can be easily replaced by the diet.

At the time of menopause, average bone loss is about 2% per year, with this high rate of loss continuing for five to six years postmenopausally. After this 'high bone loss' period, bone demineralisation slows down, until, by the age of 65, bone loss is comparable to that experienced by men of the same age (around 0.2% per annum).

The media and commercial interests would have us believe that osteoporosis is all about calcium deficiency. Nothing could be further from the truth. Simply slurping down litres of milk a day will do nothing to protect you from osteoporosis . . . if only it were that simple! Western women have the highest intake of dietary (and supplemental) calcium of all women, and yet we suffer from the highest incidence of osteoporosis. Asian and African women have a daily calcium intake only a fraction of ours, and yet their osteoporosis rates are dramatically lower. Inuit women eating a traditional diet consume up to a whopping 2500 mg of calcium a day, along with huge amounts of animal protein. Despite their high calcium intake, they have one of the highest rates of osteoporosis in the world. This is because in many ways osteoporosis is a multi-factor 'lifestyle disease'. Take a look at the list of risk factors above, and you'll see how the typical Western lifestyle and diet is a ready-made prescription for bone problems.

The dairy board has been relentless in its promotion of dairy products as the answer to the 'osteoporosis epidemic'. Yes, it's true that dairy products contain lots of calcium, but as you're starting to see, preventing osteoporosis is not just about pouring more and more calcium into our body, be it from food or supplements. People in New Zealand, Switzerland, the UK and Northern Europe have some of the highest levels of dairy consumption in the world and yet they also have the highest rates of osteoporosis. The Chinese, on the other hand, have an extremely low dairy intake (if any), preferring to get their calcium from vegetables. Their typical diet provides half the dietary calcium intake of the average Kiwi diet, and yet their incidence of hip fracture (a common marker for osteoporosis) is one of the lowest in the world.

The much quoted Harvard Nurses' Health Study (USA) found that women with the highest dietary intake of dairy products also had the highest rate of fracture. Bones need a lot more than just calcium to generate themselves. Other minerals and trace elements are also important, such as magnesium, vitamin D, manganese, boron, zinc, vitamins A, C, E and B-complex, and essential fatty acids.

With the heavy marketing of dairy products in connection with bone health, it's easy to forget that there are other ways of getting your dietary calcium besides consuming milk products. Leafy green vegetables are very high in absorbable calcium, especially broccoli, kale, bok choy and mustard greens. Other calcium-rich foods include: figs, beans, oatmeal, tofu, calcium-enriched soya milk, bony fish (salmon, sardines, herring), almonds, sesame seeds and tahini, and seaweed.

There is a certain amount of genetic lottery involved in determining your risk of osteoporosis. Bone density is partly pre-determined genetically. If you are Caucasian, your bone density is likely to be up to 20% less than if you are African, Maori or Pacific Islander. Body shape also has an impact . . . finally here's something to make all the more curvaceous women of the world jump for joy! If you are tall and/or larger built or more curvaceous, you are at a lower risk of osteoporosis than your dainty, petite friend whom you have always envied!

Medical treatments

Up until three years ago, HRT was considered the gold-standard pharmaceutical preventative agent for osteoporosis. Menopausal or perimenopausal women were routinely prescribed long-term hormone replacement, to stave off the bone-demineralising effects of postmenopausal 'oestrogen deficiency'. Since the negative findings of the Woman's Health Initiative study, long-term HRT use has fallen distinctly out of favour.

In place of HRT, a number of other pharmaceutical drugs have become increasingly popular. Bisphosphanates such as Fosamax, Didronel, Actonel, and Boniva are non-hormonal drugs which slow down the normal rate of bone resorption, by poisoning the bone cells responsible for remodelling (osteoclasts). By killing the cells responsible for bone breakdown, these drugs temporarily increase bone density. Unfortunately, the cells responsible for the creation of new bone (osteoblasts) are stimulated in their task by the presence of osteoclasts. When osteoclasts are killed, slowly but surely, osteoblasts also begin to die. There is increasing concern that long-term use of these drugs may actually contribute to the very thing they are trying to cure; that is, an increase in bone brittleness and fracture.

Bisphosphonates are not without potentially serious side effects. Unlike many other drugs, the worrying thing about this class of drugs is that they have a half-life of 10 years in the body. That means if you take them and experience serious side effects, and then stop the medication, the drug will remain active in your body for this period of time or longer.

Side effects include: gastrointestinal problems; chronic, severe joint and bone pain; muscle cramping and stiffness and difficulty walking; and, most frightening of all, necrosis (bone death) of the jaw.

Coupled with this, the anti-fracture benefits of taking the medication are very small. Spinal fracture reduction has only been proven in women with severe pre-existing osteoporosis, and a previous spinal fracture. A review, published by *Osteoporosis International* in 2005, of 11 clinical trials of at least three years' duration failed to find any non-spinal fracture benefit at all from Fosamax.

Self-help treatments

Prevention is always better than cure, especially in the case of osteoporosis, and preventing osteoporosis means making the right lifestyle choices, preferably from a young age.

Prevention of postmenopausal osteoporosis begins back in the teenage years, with a bone-healthy diet coupled with regular exercise. I am a mother of two girls, one of whom is a teenager, so I know just how difficult this can be. The most powerful way of influencing our daughters is by leading by example and modelling healthy lifestyle practices in our own lives.

Swallowing a calcium tablet every day and believing that all your osteoporosis worries are over is foolish, to say the least. Our bones increase in density until our mid-thirties, so it is vital to take advantage of this bone-building phase by supplying the body with *all* the raw materials it needs for the job . . . not just calcium.

Of course it is important to have an adequate supply of calcium-rich foods in your diet, but it's just as important to avoid those dietary practices which increase calcium release from the bones, or which inhibit the uptake of dietary calcium.

A steak on the barbecue is a part of our national identity, but too many steaks may leave your bones in a sorry state in the years to come. Meat contains 20–50 times more phosphorus than calcium. Since phosphorus and calcium must be balanced in the body, calcium is leached out of the bones to maintain the proper blood balance of these two minerals. Animal proteins are also rich in sulphur-containing amino acids which tend to acidify the blood. The body restores a normal blood pH by releasing bone calcium into the bloodstream. Vegetarians and vegans tend to have less risk of osteoporosis despite often having a low dietary intake of calcium.

If you wash that steak down with a fizzy drink, you are further compounding your troubles. A study from the Harvard School of Public Health confirmed that a liking for soft drinks can cause bone damage. Out of 5398 women, the cola drinkers were found to be about twice as likely as non-cola drinkers to suffer a first bone fracture at the age of 40. This is because, like meat, fizzy drinks contain large amounts of phosphorus. Try drinking mineral water or fresh fruit juice instead. Drinking a glass of fruit juice with a calcium-rich meal will enhance absorption of calcium.

Very few Australian and New Zealand women suffer from a lack of dietary protein (unless they are living on unbalanced weight-loss regimes); in fact, the opposite is more likely to be true. A certain amount of protein is needed for the absorption of calcium. However, too much protein can work against you by depressing the retention of calcium in your bones.

To prevent osteoporosis

* Eat a minimum of five-plus servings of fresh fruits and vegetables daily, to obtain vitamin C, vitamin K and magnesium.

* Minimise your intake of animal protein, especially red meat, and maximise your intake of vegetarian proteins such as tofu, lentils, nuts and seeds, soya beans and grains.

* Have regular exposure to sunshine, during the low-ultraviolet times of the day (before 10 a.m. and after 4 p.m.), to enable your body to manufacture its own calcium-fixing vitamin D.

* Include plenty of calcium-rich foods in your diet, but don't overdo the dairy consumption. Choose plant-based dietary sources such as calcium-enriched soya milk; nuts and seeds (especially almonds, sesame seeds and tahini); corn; peas; broccoli; leafy green vegetables; and bony fish (salmon, sardines, herrings).

* Don't overdo the 'low fat' thing. Fats are essential for calcium absorption, so eat healthy fats every day, such as avocado, olive oil, flax oil, nuts and seeds.

✳ Exercise regularly, especially do weight-bearing exercise such as walking, weight training and resistance training.

✳ Use restraint when it comes to coffee and tea, sugar, soft drinks, and salt.

✳ Don't smoke: cigarettes cause calcium to be lost from the bones.

And what of calcium supplements?

There is a place for calcium supplementation according to many studies. However, it's important to realise that prevention of osteoporosis is much more effective if lifestyle and dietary change are a part of the programme, along with the calcium supplement.

Calcium supplements do make a difference to your chances of developing osteoporosis, if your dietary intake of calcium is low. After years of debate we now know that supplements make a difference to you, even if you are postmenopausal or already have osteoporosis. Postmenopausal calcium supplementation slows the rate of bone loss by 30–50%, and significantly reduces the risk of hip fractures. Starting calcium supplementation in the perimenopausal years has also been shown to make a significant difference to osteoporosis risk. It's not just any old calcium supplement that is needed though . . . read on for details of how to choose your calcium supplement.

First, what not to buy. I recommend that you avoid supplements of bone meal or dolomite (ground-up mountains), and oyster shell (nothing to do with oysters, and is actually mined from fossilised limestone quarries). These forms of calcium may be contaminated with toxic substances such as lead, mercury and arsenic.

The most common forms of supplemental calcium are calcium carbonate, phosphate, gluconate, citrate, orotate and chelate, and a relative newcomer, coral calcium. When weighing up the pros and cons of the different forms of calcium, there are two main considerations. First, how much usable calcium is provided by each tablet? And, second, how absorbable is the calcium?

To work out just how much calcium you are really getting from your supplement, it's important to know how to read the label. What you are interested in is not the amount of calcium in each tablet, but the amount of 'elemental calcium' listed. This refers to the amount of calcium that is actually available for your body to absorb. For example, a 2000 mg tablet of calcium lactate will chemically break down to 860 mg of milk sugar, and only 140 mg of elemental calcium. Calcium carbonate contains the most elemental calcium (40%) followed by calcium citrate (21%), calcium lactate (13%) and calcium gluconate (9%).

In terms of value for money, calcium carbonate would seem to come out on top. However, we need to look at the issue of absorption as well. Which form of calcium is your body most able to absorb? Across the board, calcium tends to be a poorly absorbed mineral, whether it's supplied as a supplement or in a natural food form, with between 10 and 40% absorption, and with postmenopausal women absorbing as little as 7% of their calcium. Calcium absorption becomes even poorer with age and declining stomach acidity. Supplementing with other minerals such as iron or zinc in high doses can also interfere with your absorption of calcium.

In general, calcium citrate is one of the most absorbable forms of calcium, with approximately 25% more absorbed than in the case of calcium carbonate. It is also one of the most effective forms of calcium for building bones, and offers the best overall compromise of price, percentage of elemental calcium and absorption. Other highly absorbable forms of calcium include calcium orotate and chelate.

In its natural form, calcium never occurs in isolation. To get the most from your supplemental calcium, it's important to use a formula which includes other nutrients to enhance absorption. These include magnesium, phosphorus, manganese, boron, silica and vitamin D.

Having found a quality, balanced calcium supplement, take your supplements in split doses two or three times a day, rather than swallowing several tablets at once. Your body can only absorb a finite amount of calcium at any one time. Take your tablets with a glass of orange juice or warm water with the juice of a lemon, to enhance absorption. Calcium citrate is best taken on an empty stomach, while carbonate is better absorbed when taken with food.

Exercise — the other important preventative

The single most beneficial thing you can do to safeguard your bone health is to exercise regularly, throughout life. High-impact activity such as jogging or running is especially effective as a bone-density builder. Pressure placed on bones during exercise stimulates bone building. Without the force of gravity, astronauts in space lose about 200 mg of calcium a day from their bones. Similarly, while we here on Earth lie at rest, our bodies are not fighting the effects of gravity, and calcification of the skeleton stops. In fact, calcium is released from the bones during sedentary times and while we are sleeping at night. There are now many studies that have clearly demonstrated the beneficial effect of regular weight-bearing exercise on bone mass and bone density. Weight-bearing exercise and resistance training can actually increase bone density, not just slow down bone loss.

To change your bone density effectively, you need to perform weight-bearing exercise for one hour, two to three times a week (but of course, take time to work up to this level if you are frail, sick or unfit!). Weight lifting, jogging, hiking, stair climbing, step aerobics, dancing, racquet sports and other activities that require your muscles to work against gravity will all benefit bone density. Such exercise not only slows loss of bone density in pre- and postmenopausal women (even in the years immediately after cessation of periods, when maximum bone loss occurs), but can actually increase the bone density . . . even after menopause. A review of many of the studies looking at the effect of exercise on pre- and postmenopausal women concluded that regular exercise prevented or reversed bone loss from the spine and hips, at the rate of approximately 1% a year. While it's never too late to exercise for bone health, it's also never too early to start a regular exercise programme. Regular exercise is vital for stimulating a high peak bone mass in young women, and teenagers and children who exercise regularly are more likely to have a higher peak bone density than their sedentary peers.

There is some evidence that natural progesterone cream may be of assistance in reducing the rate of bone loss before and after menopause. Salivary progestone levels should be monitored before and during use (see Chapter 5).

Pre-menstrual syndrome (PMS)

Approximately 40% of women suffer from PMS during their child-bearing years. Many of them lead a kind of schizophrenic existence. For three out of every four weeks they are calm, capable, high-functioning superwomen. Then in the fourth week they undergo a complete and sometimes devastating personality transformation. Gone is the confident superwoman and in her place appears a tired, clumsy, impatient, irritable, moody, weeping impersonator. This is the human face of PMS or pre-menstrual syndrome — the technical term for the myriad of physical and emotional symptoms often associated with the hormonal shifts prior to menstruation.

For approximately 10% of PMS sufferers, their condition may be serious, debilitating and even life-threatening. Women are most likely to be committed to psychiatric institutions, be caught committing a crime, have a car accident, abuse their children or try to commit suicide during their pre-menstrual week.

In theory, any menstruating woman can suffer from the hormonal swings of PMS, but PMS is much more common amongst women leading stressed and pressured lives. Western women suffer from PMS more often than women from any other culture, and it is often in her mid-thirties that a woman begins to notice a worsening of PMS symptoms.

Symptoms

Suspect that you have PMS if you experience physical or emotional symptoms that appear cyclically, in the days before your period. Your symptoms will most likely occur each month, some time after day 14 (ovulation) of your cycle. They may last for anywhere from 2 to 14 days, disappearing on or just after the day you start your period. The list of PMS symptoms is long and varied, with women tending to experience 'groupings' of symptoms. These clusters of symptoms have traditionally been grouped under four different types of PMS.

* *Type A*. A stands for *anxiety*. This type of PMS is the most common symptom category, accounting for 80% of PMS symptoms. It is characterised by emotional symptoms of anxiety, irritability and mood swings.

* *Type C*. C stands for *carbohydrate cravings*. If you would put your raincoat on and drive to the dairy in the middle of a wet and blustery winter night to satisfy your cravings for a bar of chocolate, then you probably suffer from Type C. Along with sugar cravings come exhaustion and headaches, and maybe fainting and heart palpitations (all symptoms of low blood sugar or hypoglycaemia).

* *Type D*. D stands for *depression*. Depression is often accompanied by mental confusion, an inability to think clearly, poor memory, lack of concentration and clumsiness.

* *Type H*. H stands for *hyperhydration* — in simple speak, puffing up like a water-logged balloon. If you need to keep a special 'fat' wardrobe for the PMS days, and your rings cut into your fingers at this time of the month; breasts swell and go up a bra size or two, then you have Type H PMS.

It is rare for PMS sufferers to experience symptoms exclusively from one of these categories. Much more commonly, there is an overlap of symptoms from different groups, with one group predominating.

Causes

There are still a lot of things we don't know about PMS. What is for certain is that PMS results from hormonal imbalance, and is not 'all in your head' as some uninformed people may suggest.

Type-A PMS seems to result from an abnormal balance between the progesterone and oestrogen produced in the second half of your cycle, with a deficiency of progesterone relative to the amount of oestrogen.

About 60% of PMS sufferers report Type-C symptoms. These 'craving' symptoms are indicative of abnormal fluctuations in blood-sugar levels. PMS-C sufferers appear to experience an alteration in the way insulin works in their body in the pre-menstrual days. This leads to blood-sugar fluctuations and symptoms of hypoglycaemia. If you are stressed, or nutritionally deficient (especially if you have a deficiency of B-complex vitamins and magnesium), hypoglycaemic symptoms will be aggravated. The quality of your diet has a direct bearing on these problems too. Women with PMS-C consume around two and a half times the amount of refined carbohydrates that non-sufferers eat. Some studies point to a deficiency of the prostaglandin PGE1 in the pancreas of PMS-C sufferers. (See also discussion of evening primrose oil for PMS.)

If you are a puffed-up PMS-H sufferer, it is the hormone aldosterone which is making your life a bloated misery. This hormone indirectly instructs the kidneys to retain water and salt, which causes you to blow up like a bad-tempered puffer fish. Aldosterone excess can be caused by stress, oestrogen excess, too much dietary salt, or a magnesium deficiency.

While Type-D PMS only affects around 5% of women on its own, it is seen in combination with Type A in around 20% of PMS sufferers. This depression is directly linked to a lack of oestrogen production, in contrast to PMS-A which is attributable to elevated oestrogen levels. Low oestrogen production can be caused by an excess of the adrenal hormones or progesterone, in response to stress. Besides oestrogen and progesterone, another key player involved in pre-menstrual hormonal change is the pituitary hormone prolactin. Elevated prolactin levels are commonly seen in women with PMS, and result in breast enlargement and tenderness in the days before menstruation.

While PMS symptoms can vary, many PMS sufferers share in common an imbalance in the ratio of oestrogen to progesterone in the pre-menstrual days — oestrogen levels are elevated and progesterone levels reduced five to ten days before menstruation. Other common hormonal imbalances seen in women with PMS include elevated prolactin levels, and a sluggish, underactive thyroid (hypothyroidism). Every woman suffering from PMS should have a thyroid test to ensure that undiagnosed hypothyroidism is not at the root of her hormonal problems. The level of aldosterone (the hormone that influences fluid retention) is often elevated as well.

Liver function plays an important part in regulating oestrogen levels. A sluggish and inefficient liver struggling to effectively break down and detoxify oestrogen (often as a result of B-vitamin deficiency) is partly responsible for the excess oestrogen seen in many PMS cases. Increased oestrogen levels themselves aggravate the poor liver detoxification.

Once oestrogen levels become elevated (in relation to progesterone levels), many of the common symptoms of PMS result. Raised oestrogen interferes with the normal production of brain neurotransmitters and endorphins, responsible for regulation of mood. Elevated oestrogen also interferes with the ability to utilise essential hormone-regulating vitamin B6.

Essential fatty acid imbalance is a common causative factor in PMS. Supplementing with the 'right' kind of fatty acids in the form of evening primrose oil has helped many women revolutionise their pre-menstrual week. Evening primrose oil contains a fatty acid called gamma-linoleic acid or GLA. Our diet provides us with the precursor to this essential fatty acid, in the form of linoleic acid, found in meat, vegetable oils, shellfish, vegetables and linseed. The problem is that once we ingest linoleic acid, we then have to transform it into usable GLA — a process that is often very inefficient. A number of common dietary practices can impede the essential fatty acid conversion. These include: a high intake of red meat; a high consumption of processed oils such as those found in margarine, chips, bread, cakes, biscuits and so on; moderate consumption of alcohol; or nutritional deficiencies, especially of zinc, B6 and magnesium. Evening primrose oil, with its pre-formed GLA, can significantly improve PMS symptoms, as will avoiding those foods which impede the conversion of linoleic acid to GLA.

GLA is further converted and used by the body to create prostaglandins (local hormones), one series of which is called PGE1. This particular prostaglandin has a crucial role to play in regulating and balancing the levels of oestrogen, progesterone and prolactin in the second half of the cycle.

Medical treatment

Medical treatment of PMS may include the use of hormonal drugs such as the oral contraceptive pill or synthetic progesterone. Antidepressants and tranquillisers may offer symptomatic relief for anxiety and depression.

The pharmaceutical industry has created a new syndrome to describe severe pre-menstrual mood changes, called 'pre-menstrual dysphoric disorder' (PMDD), for which the recommended drug treatment is antidepressants, especially Prozac.

Self-help treatments

For most women, PMS can be effectively and completely resolved with a combination of lifestyle change, stress management and relaxation, dietary modification, exercise, and nutritional supplementation. Sometimes additional treatment such as acupuncture or herbal medicine may also be required.

Diet and PMS

Diet has everything to do with PMS, and in most cases it is impossible to resolve PMS issues without making some fairly significant dietary changes.

The main unifying aim for all these nutritional changes is to improve the oestrogen/progesterone balance. An optimally functioning liver is an essential part of this process, and so too is a healthy gut with balanced gut flora (friendly gut bacteria). If you have had a history of antibiotic use, it's worth seeing a naturopath for a professional gut-repair programme. This will usually involve a detox diet followed by reinoculation of the gut with a balance of friendly gut bacteria. Once the gut bacteria have been restored to a healthy balance, following the recommendations for the PMS diet will keep the gut balanced. The gut-repair programme will need to be repeated each time you use antibiotics.

The PMS diet is also designed to remove as much 'detox' work as possible from the liver, by eliminating those foods and drinks which place an especially heavy load on the liver. These include alcohol (very top of the list!); processed foods with added chemicals such as preservatives and colourings; unhealthy fats (trans-fats); or excessive amounts of fat.

The PMS diet

If you suffer from PMS, avoid . . .
Some foods are guaranteed to aggravate your PMS problems, and consequently should be avoided whenever possible. They include the following.

✳ **Alcohol.** Alcohol robs your body of B-complex vitamins and magnesium, as well as placing an undesirable detoxification load on the liver, which can contribute to increased oestrogen levels.

✳ **Sugars and sweetened processed foods, and refined (high GI) carbohydrates.** These include some breakfast cereals, snack bars, lollies, chocolate, cakes, white bread, biscuits, and crackers. Simple sugars aggravate the roller-coaster blood-sugar problems common amongst women with PMS. Low blood sugar will itself produce a wide range of symptoms resembling common PMS symptoms, such as irritability, depression, tearfulness, fatigue, headaches, and so on. A diet high in refined sugars and carbohydrates can increase circulating oestrogen levels, thus aggravating PMS. Sugars also increase the excretion of vital hormonal regulating nutrients such as B-complex vitamins (especially B6) and magnesium.

✳ **Saturated fats** including dairy products, red meat and processed foods with a high saturated fat content; and processed fats which contain trans-fats such as margarine, commercial peanut butter, French fries from fast-food chains, and potato chips. Reducing dietary intake of saturated fat (and trans-fats) while increasing dietary fibre leads to a dramatic decrease in oestrogen levels. The easiest way to achieve this goal is to reduce intake of animal products such as meat and dairy, and increase plant foods.

✳ **Synthetic foods** that are highly processed with chemical additives, colourings and preservatives. These place an increased detoxification load on the liver.

✳ **Caffeinated drinks** such as coffee, tea, cola and energy drinks. Caffeine increases the loss of B-complex vitamins and magnesium through the urine, and increases symptoms of anxiety, irritability and breast tenderness. If you drink more than four cups of caffeine-containing beverage a day, you are dramatically increasing the likelihood of suffering from severe PMS. Avoid coffee, tea, caffeinated soft drinks and energy drinks, and chocolate (yes, I know it's cruel). Try drinking filtered water, herbal teas, dandelion tea, or cereal-based coffee substitutes instead, or water-decaffeinated coffee (in moderation) if you just can't adjust to these new drinks.

✳ **Salt and heavily salted foods** such as processed meats, snack foods and cheese. A high-salt diet will aggravate symptoms of bloating, fluid retention and breast tenderness. Too much salt also blocks the conversion of dietary essential fatty acids to gamma-linoleic acid. If you just can't live without the salty taste, try a sodium-free potassium-based salt substitute.

. . . and eat . . .

Eat a vegetarian or semi-vegetarian diet, consuming organic produce whenever possible. Vegetarian women excrete more oestrogen in their stools, and have circulating oestrogen levels half those of meat eaters. If you eat animal proteins, consume moderate amounts of lean meat and fish. Avoid red meat and dairy products as much as possible and eat the following.

✳ **Fresh fruits and vegetables**, preferably organic. Aim for 9 servings a day. Fruits and vegetables boost dietary fibre levels and promote the excretion of oestrogen from the bowel, as well as helping to keep gut flora healthy.

✳ **Cold-water fish** such as salmon, sardines, herrings, mackerel, snapper and hapuka. These fish are especially rich in omega-3 essential fatty acids. Our diets tend to have an excess of omega-6 fatty acids, and an imbalance in the omega-6 to omega-3 ratio contributes to production of prostaglandins which aggravate menstrual problems, including PMS.

✳ **Whole grains** such as wholemeal bread; cooked grains for breakfast including rolled oats, soya flakes, buckwheat, millet and barley; brown or basmati rice. These foods are rich in B-complex nutrients and magnesium. They are also high in fibre and increase gut excretion of oestrogen.

✳ **Nuts and seeds** — just make sure they are fresh, and don't overdo them or you'll blossom in size.

✳ **Daily servings of healthy fats** to boost omega-3 fatty acids. Plentiful servings of the right kinds of fats are essential for a healthy hormone balance. Cook with cold-pressed virgin olive oil, and use flax oil or avocado oil on salads. Avocado, fish, and nuts and seeds also supply healthy fats.

✳ **Phyto-oestrogen-rich foods.** These include soya milk, tofu, miso, nuts, seeds, legumes, beans, and a range of vegetables (see list of phyto-oestrogen foods in Chapter 6). Phyto-oestrogens (which are much weaker than oestrogen made in the body) bind to oestrogen receptors on cells, blocking the ability of human oestrogen to bind with these receptors. Thus they have an anti-oestrogenic effect in women with PMS.

Nutritional supplements

Dietary deficiencies of magnesium, B-vitamins (especially B6), vitamin E, zinc, and essential fatty acids are especially implicated in female hormonal imbalance.

Magnesium deficiency is a strong causal factor for PMS, and is very common amongst Western women. This deficiency is aggravated by the use of diuretics which many PMS sufferers use to reduce bloating and swelling. Interestingly, many of the symptoms of magnesium deficiency are also the symptoms of PMS; for example fatigue, insomnia, irritability, heart palpitations, blood-sugar swings and sugar cravings.

PMS-A is believed to result from an excess of oestrogen, which can lead to a relative deficiency of brain dopamine. Magnesium deficiency also depletes brain dopamine levels, as well as impairing oestrogen metabolism, thus contributing to an escalation of circulating oestrogen levels.

Supplementing with magnesium helps to stabilise blood-sugar levels as well as enhancing the liver's ability to break down oestrogen. Magnesium deficiency also alters the secretion of insulin, the hormone that regulates blood sugar, thus contributing to the symptoms of PMS-C. PMS-H is associated with elevated aldosterone levels (a hormone secreted by the adrenal glands), an imbalance of which can be triggered by low magnesium levels.

Along with magnesium, B-vitamins — especially B6 — are vital for restoring balance to female hormones. B-vitamins help normalise glucose metabolism, assist the liver with inactivation of hormones, and stabilise brain chemistry. B6 is also important for the metabolising of essential fatty acids, as well as functioning as a natural diuretic, and helping to preserve blood levels of magnesium. B6 deficiency is common in women. Many women have a low dietary intake, which is further compounded by the B6-depleting effects of alcohol, coffee consumption, smoking and the contraceptive pill. The most common signs of B6 deficiency are anxiety, depression, loss of sense of responsibility, and insomnia — all classic PMS symptoms.

Clinical trials going back as far as 1942 prove that B6 supplementation significantly alleviates PMS problems, with dramatic mood improvement in around 85% of women. For PMS, B6 (along with a combined B-complex) is used in the range of 50–100 mg a day. B6 supplementation should be limited to 50 mg in any one dose. Higher doses may be used under the supervision of a health professional.

B6 and magnesium have an intimate relationship, with adequate magnesium essential for efficient utilisation of B-complex. B6 supplementation is thought to actually increase the levels of magnesium within the body's cells.

Women with PMS often have low zinc levels. Zinc is a vital nutrient for the proper action of sex hormones, and is involved in regulating prolactin levels. Zinc deficiency increases prolactin levels, and supplementing with zinc decreases prolactin. Since many PMS sufferers are found to have abnormally high prolactin levels, correcting zinc deficiency is vital. Where high prolactin is a feature, zinc supplements in the range of 30–40 mg a day are required.

Essential fatty acids are vital for normal hormonal health, and supplementing with evening primrose oil is a popular and often effective therapy for PMS sufferers. Many PMS sufferers have abnormally low levels of the essential fatty acid GLA (gamma-linolenic acid). The body can manufacture its own GLA from linoleic acid in the diet, but only if there are healthy amounts of zinc, B6 and magnesium . . . which is frequently not the case in PMS sufferers. Evening primrose oil (as well as blackcurrant and borage oil) contains GLA in a 'preformed' state, and is thus a useful way of ensuring that adequate levels are achieved.

Extra nutritional supplements can be added if needed, depending on which particular type of PMS you suffer from. While PMS-A and PMS-B in particular benefit greatly from B-complex and magnesium, PMS-B would benefit from additional zinc (to 50 mg a day) and vitamin C (up to around 3000 mg a day during the second half of the cycle); PMS-C may need essential fatty acids (evening primrose oil, 3000 mg a day throughout the month) and a chromium supplement (200 mcg a day) to help normalise carbohydrate metabolism and blood-sugar levels. A high-potency multi-mineral and multivitamin complex makes a useful supplemental base to which other nutrients can be added.

Exercise away your PMS

Here's another great reason to become a fit and active woman (if you're not already one): women who exercise regularly suffer far fewer problems with PMS than their sedentary peers. Simply going for a brisk walk several times a week, or taking up a sport like tennis, badminton, netball or jogging, is a significant part of your self-help programme for PMS.

Exercise works in several ways. Working muscles stimulate the movement of lymphatic fluid (the body's waste disposal unit), as well as stimulating blood circulation and oxygenation of the brain (for mood improvement). Improved blood circulation helps to reduce fluid retention, puffiness, poor concentration and mood disorders. Vigorous aerobic activity stimulates the flow of 'feel good' endorphins, leaving you feeling relaxed and unwound at the end of your workout. Exercise also helps to regulate insulin levels and carbohydrate metabolism, preventing the blood-sugar fluctuations that are partly responsible for your PMS mood swings. The stress hormones cortisol and adrenalin are also lowered with vigorous exercise. Aim for at least 45 minutes of aerobic activity four or five times a week for maximum benefit.

Relax!

It may sound ironic telling you to 'relax' when you're feeling so strung-out, but it really is a vital part of beating PMS. Most people have to actively learn how to relax, and the best time to start is during the two or three weeks when you haven't got PMS. The progressive relaxation and simple meditations outlined in Chapter 4 are an easy place to start.

Alternatively, you may find that doing yoga or tai chi, deep breathing, meditation, visualisation, walking on the beach, or listening to beautiful music are more relaxing for you. Once you have found your particular key to relaxation, use it regularly, especially during your PMS days!

Herbal medicine and PMS

There are a number of herbs which are effective in rebalancing female hormones and reducing PMS. Of these, the most commonly used herb is *Vitex* or chaste tree. *Vitex* helps to rebalance oestrogen and progesterone levels, correcting a relative progesterone deficiency. It is often fast acting, but to ensure permanent improvement, *Vitex* should be continued for at least 6–12 months. *Vitex* helps to regulate the menstrual cycle and is especially useful for reducing pre-menstrual acne, fluid retention, breast tenderness and mood swings.

Dong quai, black cohosh, and liquorice root all exert a hormonal effect and are variously used for the treatment of PMS. Calming herbs such as valerian, oats, kava, motherwort, and lemon balm are sometimes used for symptomatic relief of anxiety and tension.

Acupuncture for PMS

The energy imbalances which lead to PMS are extremely common in Western women. Usually, there is a condition of stagnation or blockage of the energy in the liver meridian. Classic liver qi stagnation symptoms include irritability, mood swings, breast tenderness and lumps, abdominal distension and hormonal migraines. When kidney and spleen energy is weak, the PMS symptoms are more likely to be fatigue, general bloating, aches and pains and chronic depression. Acupuncture can be extremely effective at relieving the symptoms of PMS.

Natural progesterone cream

Natural progesterone cream is useful for addressing the oestrogen dominance which is common in PMS sufferers. Salivary progesterone levels should be monitored before and during use. (See Chapter 5.)

Thrush

Thrush is the common name for a type of yeast infection affecting the mouth, anus or vagina, caused by an overgrowth of the *Candida albicans* yeast. It is an extremely common, and often infuriatingly stubborn, problem to treat, and is the cause of much female suffering, trips to the doctor and sabotaged sex lives.

Causes

A healthy vagina has an efficient self-regulating system that maintains a slightly acidic pH. This acidic environment prevents harmful bacteria from flourishing and causing vaginal infections.

Not all bacteria cause problems. *Lactobacilli* bacteria are a very important part of the vaginal pH regulatory system. The cells that make up the walls of the vagina store sugar (in the form of glucose), and as these cells are sloughed off, their sugar stores are released into the vagina. Sugar is a nectar for a whole host of undesirable bacteria and fungi. In a healthy vagina, however, the friendly *Lactobacilli* turn this sugar into weak lactic acid, thus maintaining an acidic environment hostile to the 'undesirables'.

The organism that causes *Candida* is often present in a healthy vagina, as a one-celled fungus which doesn't make a nuisance of itself. If the acidity and bacterial balance in the vagina is upset, the fungal form may change into long branches of yeast cells, which proliferate and become *Candida*. At ovulation and menstruation the vagina naturally becomes more alkaline, and consequently more prone to infection.

Many women notice maddening vaginal itching during pregnancy, resulting from the increased vaginal alkalinity caused by hormonal changes. Use of the oral contraceptive pill can also predispose you to ongoing thrush problems. Diabetic women, with their higher than usual blood-sugar levels, are especially vulnerable to vaginal thrush. Chronic thrush sufferers should always have a diabetes test, as this may be an early sign of an undiagnosed diabetic condition.

The widespread and frequent use of broad-spectrum antibiotics is a major causative factor in a large proportion of vaginal yeast infections. Broad-spectrum antibiotics kill a wide spectrum of both beneficial and pathogenic bacteria alike. Once friendly bacteria are killed off in sufficient numbers, the *Candida* spores flourish without constraint.

It's not just antibiotics that can upset the delicate self-regulatory ecology of the vagina. Feminine hygiene products such as douches and deodorant sprays are both unnecessary and can actually disrupt the normal vaginal environment, causing maddening vaginal itching, and even thrush. Frequent douching tends to dry out the protective mucous secretions in the vagina and upset the pH balance, sometimes paving the way for an attack of vaginal thrush. In general, douching is not necessary with a healthy vagina, except for brief periods while you have thrush, when douching with antifungal substances may be appropriate.

If you are prone to vaginal infections, even the way you dress can worsen your problems. Tight jeans may look great, but they can play havoc with your health. Yeast infections thrive in hot, moist environments, and tight jeans which prevent air circulation around the genitals create just such an environment. Choose cotton pants instead of nylon pants, which hinder air circulation around the genitals. Avoid wearing nylon pantihose whenever possible, instead wearing 'knee highs' or even stockings and suspender belts!

Dietary choices can significantly influence your susceptibility to thrush. An overabundance of refined, high-Glycaemic-Index carbs such as sugars, white flour and alcohol can also increase susceptibility to vaginal fungal infections. Women who are iron-deficient also tend to suffer from more vaginal thrush.

Symptoms

Itching, itching and more itching. If you have thrush, you will know about it. The vagina, labia and even the top of the thighs become reddened, irritated and madly itchy. There may be a yeasty-smelling, cottage-cheese-like vaginal discharge, too. Sometimes there is no discharge, and instead the vagina feels dry.

Medical treatment

Antifungal creams and pessaries are available over the counter at the pharmacy. They are available in both single-dose and multiple-dose courses. A single dose is usually as effective as the longer courses of treatment. Many of the vaginal treatments weaken condoms and diaphragms, so check that you are using a safe product if this is your form of contraception.

DiFlucan One is a single-dose oral antifungal capsule. Its efficacy is equivalent to that of the vaginal products. It cannot be used during pregnancy, and possible side effects include headaches and gastrointestinal upsets.

Pharmaceutical antifungals are usually very effective at getting rid of an acute infection. However, many women find that their problems return within 12 weeks, necessitating another course of treatment. If symptoms persist after treatment, or recur again quickly, it is important to see your doctor for a test to determine if your symptoms are the result of thrush or of another vaginal infection.

Dietary change

Dietary modification plays a vital role in overcoming chronic vaginal thrush problems. Be prepared for some serious limitations.

Sugars and refined carbohydrates are first on the hit list. Throw away the chocolate bars, biscuits and cakes. Even dried fruits and fruit juice are too high in sugar. Gone too are honey, jams, alcohol and sweetened processed foods.

Yeasted foods are also a no-no. This means no leavened bread, although Lebanese and pita breads are safe. Avoid using brewer's yeast as a supplement, or drinking beer, and make sure that your nutritional supplements are yeast-free. Vegemite and some crackers also contain yeast. Rice crispbreads and Ryvitas are yeast-free, as is the heavy German rye bread called pumpernickel. Vinegar-containing foods such as sauces, pickles and mayonnaise are also on the hit list.

Other forbidden foods include cheese, mushrooms and melon (all of which contain some type of fungus that tends to aggravate thrush), and mouldy nuts (which, by the way, are highly carcinogenic and should never be eaten at all).

So what *can* you eat?

Despite initial appearances, this is not a food-free diet. Choose from a wide range of raw or cooked vegetables; fish, chicken, eggs, red meat, dairy products, nuts and seeds (as long as they are fresh); lentils, brown or basmati rice, beans, and whole grains. Fruit can be eaten in moderation, while avoiding the sweeter varieties of fruit, and melons.

Try to include plenty of unsweetened *Lactobacillus acidophilus* yoghurt (that is, yoghurt containing a live culture). This will implant the friendly bacteria into the bowel, and help control any overgrowth of *Candida* fungus living there. In turn, this makes cross-infection from the bowel to the vagina less likely.

Onions and garlic contain antifungal chemicals, and should be used daily if possible.

Nutritional supplements

A number of supplements and herbs are appropriate for the treatment of *Candida*. These include the following:

* A high-quality probiotic powder or capsule containing *Lactobacillus acidophilus*.

* High-potency garlic capsules or tablets.

* High-potency B-complex, vitamins C and A, and zinc to strengthen the immune system and restore normal health to the mucous membranes lining the vagina.

* Caprylic acid. Caprylic acid is a fatty acid found in the oil of coconuts and palm nuts, butter fat and some vegetables. Caprylic acid is a useful part of a nutritional and anti-fungal regime.

* Pau D'Arco (taheebo) tea is a natural antifungal and can be taken as a beverage every day.

* Kolorex is an antifungal product made from New Zealand native herbs. For chronic *Candida* it can be taken orally, as well as used as a local cream for vaginal use.

If you suffer from more than the occasional vaginal thrush episode, it is advisable to consult a naturopath for a more sophisticated treatment approach, rather than self-medicating at each new acute episode.

Local therapy

There are a number of different options for local treatment of vaginal thrush. One of the cheapest and easiest options (but unfortunately rather smelly) is simply to use a garlic clove as a pessary. Peel a garlic clove carefully, taking care not to nick it with your fingernails. Insert the clove high into the vagina at bedtime . . . and remember to remove it the following morning. If you feel nervous about ever finding it again, you can thread a piece of cotton through the clove as a drawstring.

Alternatively, douche with garlic juice! Peel two smallish cloves of garlic and blend with a cup of warm water (in a food processor or blender). Leave the thoroughly blended solution to sit for five minutes before carefully straining through a piece of muslin. Add another cup of water to the strained liquid. Soak a tampon in the mixture and insert high into the vagina. Leave the tampon in place for several hours. Change the garlic tampon three times daily. Garlic treatment may need to be continued for three to eight days depending on the severity of the infection.

A tampon soaked in *Lactobacillus* yoghurt is another traditional naturopathic therapy for thrush. The *Lactobacilli* change the pH of the vagina, making it less hospitable for the *Candida*. This treatment is gentle and often effective, but results can be a little slow. Change the yoghurt-soaked tampons three times a day (and wear a pad to prevent embarrassing mess).

Tea tree oil is a powerful antifungal and antibacterial. Use diluted oil as a douche and to wash the external genitals to lessen vaginal itching. To make a douche solution, add one teaspoon of oil to two litres of tepid water, and douche twice daily. As an external wash, simply add five or six drops of oil to a bowl of warm water. Squat over a bowl in the shower or bathtub, and repeatedly splash the external genitals with the tea-tree oil solution. Gently pat dry.

For those times during your course of treatment when itching and burning drive you mad, the following local applications will give you some respite from your suffering. If you are at home, try taking a saline bath. Into a bath of tepid water, add half a cup of salt. Bathe for as long as is comfortable, and try to encourage the water into the vagina. Salt baths can be taken several times daily if needed.

Calendula lotion can be applied to the external vagina, either full strength or diluted in water. Chickweed ointment is also useful to apply around the outside of the vagina to sooth the itching.

Simple self-help tips

* Avoid tight-fitting trousers, nylon pants and pantihose. Always wear cotton pants and crotchless pantihose or stockings and suspenders. Go without underwear whenever you can!

* Don't douche unless you have to (that is, when you have an infection).

* After a bowel movement, always wipe from front to back to avoid transferring bacteria from the anus to the vagina.

Acupuncture

Traditional Chinese medicine describes chronic thrush as damp heat, usually resulting from an imbalance in both the liver and spleen meridians. Regular acupuncture treatment to cool the heat and disperse the damp can help resolve both acute and chronic thrush problems.

Abbreviations

2,4-D	2,4-dichlorophenoxyacetic acid, herbicide
ALA	alpha-linolenic acid
ASC-US	atypical squamous cells of undetermined significance
BHC	benzene hexachloride, pesticide
BMD	bone mineral density
BMR	basal metabolic rate
BP-3	benzophenone-3
BPA	bisphenol-A, plastic additive
CIN	cervical intraepithelial neoplasia
CoQ10	coenzyme Q10
CPSII	Cancer Prevention Study II
CT scan	computed tomography (also CAT scan)
D and C	dilatation and curettage
DDE	breakdown product of DDT
DDT	dichloro-diphenyl-trichloroethane, pesticide
DGLA	dihomo-gamma-linolenic acid
DHA	docosahexaenoic acid
DIM	di-indolylmethane
DNA	deoxyribosenucleic acid
DXA	dual-energy X-ray absorptiometry
EFA	essential fatty acid
EGCG	epigallocatechin gallate
EPA	eicosapentanoic acid
EPIC	European Prospective Investigation into Cancer and Nutrition
ERT	oestrogen-only replacement therapy
FBD	fibrocystic breast disease
FSH	follicle-stimulating hormone
GI	Glycaemic Index
GLA	gamma-linolenic acid

GTF	glucose tolerance factor
HCB	hexachlorobenzene (perchlorobenzene), fungicide
HDL	high-density lipoprotein
HERS	Heart and Estrogen-Progestin Replacement Study
HIV	human immunodeficiency virus
HPV	human *Papilloma* virus
HRT	hormone replacement therapy
HSIL	high-grade squamous intraepithelial lesion
HSV	herpes simplex virus
I3C	indole-3-carbinol
IUCD, IUD	intrauterine contraceptive device, intrauterine device
LDL	low-density lipoprotein
LETZ	loop excision of the transformation zone of the cervix
LH	luteinising hormone
LSA	linseed, sunflower, almond
LSIL	low-grade squamous intraepithelial lesion
MRI	magnetic resonance imaging
OCP	oral contraceptive pill
PCBS	polychlorinated biphenyls, banned coolant
PCP	pentachlorophenol, pesticide/herbicide/fungicide etc.
PMDD	pre-menstrual dysphoric disorder
PMS	pre-menstrual syndrome
POS	polycystic ovarian syndrome
PVC	polyvinyl chloride
RDI	recommended daily intake
REM	rapid eye movement
RNA	ribosenucleic acid
SAM-e	S-adenosyl-methionine
STD	sexually transmitted disease
UTI	urinary tract infection
WHI	Women's Health Initiative

Appendix:
Useful contacts

Holistic health registers and services

Antara Association Inc.
Antara Free Natural Health Clinic
(offering free holistic treatment to those unable to afford it)
www.antara.co.nz
Ph (09) 834 7987

Breast Thermography
Thermography NZ
www.thermographynz.co.nz
Ph (07) 578 5899

Integrated Medicine Health Trust
IM Health
www.imhealth.org.nz
Ph (09) 489 9362

Intravenous Vitamin C therapy
Chelation therapy
Centre for Advanced Medicine
www.camltd.co.nz
Ph (09) 524 7743

Natural Hormone Therapy
Patient Advocate Ltd
www.naturalhormonetherapy.co.nz
Ph (09) 639 0905

New Zealand Association of Medical Herbalists
www.nzama.org.nz
Ph (09) 855 6724

New Zealand Chiropractic Association
www.chiropractic.org.nz
Ph (09) 360 2089

New Zealand Health Charter
Private Box 302305, North Harbour, Auckland
www.healthcharter.org.nz
Ph (09) 414 5501

New Zealand Homoeopathic Society
www.homoeopathica.org.nz
Ph (09) 630 5458

New Zealand Register of Acupuncturists
The Registrar, PO Box 9950, Wellington 6001
www.acupuncture.org.nz
Freephone 0800 228 786

New Zealand Society of Naturopaths Inc.
www.naturopath.org.nz

Osteopathic Society of New Zealand
www.osnz.org
Ph (03) 313 5086

Support groups and health information

Alcohol Drug Association New Zealand (ADANZ)
www.adanz.org.nz
Ph (03) 379 8626
Freephone helpline: 0800 787 797

Alcoholics Anonymous
www.alcoholics-anonymous.org.nz
Freephone 0800 229 675

Breast Cancer Foundation
    see New Zealand Breast Cancer Foundation

Breast Cancer Network New Zealand Inc.
(breast cancer prevention through the precautionary principle)
www.bcn.org.nz
Ph (09) 526 8853

Breast Health New Zealand
(resources for women with breast cancer)
www.breast.co.nz

Breast Screen Aotearoa
(for information on free mammograms)
Freephone 0800 270 200

Cancer Society of New Zealand
www.cancernz.org.nz
Freephone 0800 226 237

Cervical Screening
(National Cervical Screening Program)
Freephone 0800 729 729

Eating Disorders Association NZ
anorexia@xtra.co.nz
Ph (09) 818 9561

Endometriosis Foundation
www.nzendo.co.nz
Ph (03) 379 7959
Freephone 0800 733 277

Family Planning Association
(free consult for people under the age of 22)
www.fpanz.org.nz
Ph (04) 384 4349

Fertility NZ
www.fertilitynz.org.nz
Freephone 0800 333 306

Herpes Foundation
www.herpes.org.nz
Freephone 0508 111 213

La Leche League (for breastfeeding support)
www.lalecheleague.org.nz
Ph (09) 846 0752

Lifeline (online counselling services)
www.lifeline.org.nz
Freephone 0800 111 777

Miscarriage Support Auckland Inc.
www.miscarriagesupport.org.nz
Supportline (09) 378 4060

New Zealand Breast Cancer Foundation
www.nzbcf.org.nz
Freephone 0800 902 732

New Zealand Endometriosis Foundation
www.nzendo.co.nz
Ph (03) 379 7959
Supportline 0800 733 277

National Heart Foundation of New Zealand
www.heartfoundation.org.nz
Ph (09) 571 9191

New Zealand Single Parents
www.nzsingleparents.com

Natural Fertility New Zealand
www.naturalfertility.co.nz
Freephone 0800 178 637

Osteoporosis New Zealand
www.bones.org.nz
Ph (09) 499 4862

Parents Centres New Zealand Inc.
www.parentscentre.org.nz
Ph (04) 233 2022

The Post Natal Psychosis Charitable Trust
www.pnpsupport.org.nz
Ph (09) 449 1011

Pregnancy Counselling Services
www.pcs.org.nz
Freephone 0800 633 328

Preventing Violence in the Home
(domestic violence prevention service)
www.dvc.org.nz
Freephone 0508 384 357

Rape Crisis
www.rapecrisis.org.nz
Ph (09) 360 4001 (office), (09) 360 4004 (crisis)

Stillborn and Newborn Death Support
SANDS
www.sands.org.nz

Woman's Health Action Trust
(high-quality information and education on women's health issues)
www.womens-health.org.nz
Ph (09) 520 5295

Women's Refuge
www.womensrefuge.org.nz
Ph (04) 802 5078

Further reading

Useful websites

General and nutrition

www.Drweil.com (Dr Weil is an integrative medical doctor)

www.westonprice.org (nutrition/fats)

www.lef.org (life extension foundation – nutrition)

www.aima.net.au (Australian Integrative Medicine)

www.mercola.com (general holistic health)

http://www.mercola.com/
www.gilliansanson.com
(investigative look at current women's health issues)

www.susanweed.com (herbal medicine for women)

www.healingfoodsreference.com (healing through nutrition)

www.whfoods.com (nutrition and wholefoods)

Breast cancer

www.breastcancernetwork.org.nz

www.breastcancerfund.org

www.breastcancerorg.com

www.ssellman.com (female hormonal issues and the environment)

www.nomorebreastcancer.org.uk

www.aicr.org (American Institute for Cancer Research — diet and nutrition for cancer prevention)

www.cancernutritioninfo.com

www.dslrf.org (Dr Susan Love's website)

Menopause

http://www.powersurge.com/ and
www.sacredcycle.com
  (looking at the deeper spiritual transformations that occur
  during menstruation and menopause)

www.naturalhormonetherapy.co.nz
  (a New Zealand clinic specialising in natural hormone
  replacement therapy)

www.johnleemd.com
  (website for the pioneer of natural progesterone cream)

Bibliography

Battaglia, Salvatore. (2005) *The Complete Guide to Aromatherapy.* Perfect Potion, Brisbane.

Beijing College of TCM (compilers). (1980) *Essentials of Chinese Acupuncture.* Compiled by Beijing College of TCM. Foreign Languages Press, Beijing.

Beliveau, Richard and Gingras, Denis. (2006) *Foods That Fight Cancer: Preventing and treating cancer through diet.* Allen and Unwin, New South Wales.

Bradley, Dinah. (1999) *Hyperventilation Syndrome.* Tandem Press, Auckland.

Castro, Mieranda. (1992) *Homoeopathy for Mother and Baby.* MacMillan, London.

Colgan, Michael. *Hormonal Health.* Apple Publishing, Vancouver.

Conley, Edward. (2006) *The Breast Cancer Prevention Plan.* McGraw-Hill, New York.

Elias, Jason and Ketcham, Katherine. (1995) *In the House of the Moon: Reclaiming the feminine spirit of healing.* Hodder and Stoughton, Rydalmere, New South Wales.

Fisher, Carole and Painter, Gillian. (1996) *Materia Medica of Western Herbs for the Southern Hemisphere.* Self-published, Auckland.

Flaws, Bob. (1991) *Arisal of the Clear: A simple guide to healthy eating according to traditional Chinese medicine.* Blue Poppy Press, Boulder, Colorado.

Flaws, Bob. (1993) *Fulfilling the Essence: A handbook of traditional and contemporary Chinese treatments for female infertility.* Blue Poppy Press, Boulder, Colorado.

Flaws, Bob and Wolfe, Honora. (1983) *Prince Wen Hui's Cook: Chinese dietary therapy.* Paradigm Publishing, Brookline, Massachusetts.

Haas, Elson M. (1992) *Staying healthy with nutrition.* Celestial Arts, Berkeley, California.

Hay, Louise. (1988) *You Can Heal Your Life.* Specialist Publications, Concord, New South Wales.

Kaptchuk, Ted. (1988) *Chinese Medicine: The web that has no weaver.* Century, London.

Kenton, Leslie. (2002) *Age Power.* Vermilion, London.

Lark, Susan. (1990) *The Menopause Self Help Book.* Celestial Arts, Berkeley, California.

Love, Susan M. (2000) *Dr Susan Love's Breast Book.* Merloyd Lawrence Books, Cambridge, Massachusetts.

Lu, Henry C. (1986) *Chinese System of Food Cures.* Sterling, New York.

Murray, Michael and Pizzorno, Joseph. (1998) *Encyclopedia of Natural Medicine.* Three Rivers Press, New York.

Plant, Jane. (2000) *Your Life in Your Hands: Understanding, preventing and overcoming breast cancer.* Virgin, London.

Radd, Sue and Setchell, Kenneth. (2002) *Eat to Live: A phytoprotection plan for life.* Hodder, Sydney.

Reader's Digest. (2005) *Nature's Medicines.* Reader's Digest, Ultimo, New South Wales.

Reid, Julie. (2000) *Subfertility: A natural approach to getting pregnant.* Tandem Press, Auckland.

Rosenthal, M. Sara. (1997) *The Gynecological Sourcebook.* Lowell House, Los Angeles.

Sanson, Gillian. (2001) *The Osteoporosis 'Epidemic'.* Penguin Books, Auckland.

Sears, Barry. (1997) *Mastering the Zone.* Regan Books, New York.

Seligman, Martin E. (1992) *Learned Optimism.* Random House, Milsons Point, New South Wales.

Seligman, Martin E. (2002) *Authentic Happiness.* Random House, Milsons Point, New South Wales.

Shanghai College of Traditional Chinese Medicine. (1974) *Acupuncture: A comprehensive text.* Translated by John O'Connor and Dan Bensky. Eastland Press, Shanghai.

Statham, Bill. (2002) *The Chemical Maze.* Possibility.com, Ringwood, Victoria.

Thorne Research. (2002) *Alternative Medicine Review.* Thorne Research, Dover, Idaho.

Tierra, Lesley. (1992) *The Herbs of Life.* The Crossing Press, Freedom, California.

Ting-liang, Zhang. (1991) *A Handbook of Traditional Chinese Gynaecology.* Blue Poppy Press, Boulder, Colorado.

Tipping, Colin C. (2000) *Radical Forgiveness: Making room for the miracle.* Gateway, Malaysia.

Wharton, Lynda. (1993) *Be Well Naturally.* Tandem Press, Auckland.

Journal articles

Aggarwal, B. et al. (2005) Curry spice may curb breast cancer spread. *Clinical Cancer Research, 11,* October 15.

Ahlgren, M. (2004) Growth patterns and the risk of breast cancer in women. *New England Journal of Medicine,* October 14.

Anderson, I. et al. (1988) Malmao mammographic screening trial. *British Medical Journal, 297:* 943–8.

Berry, D.A. et al. (2005) Effects of screening and adjuvant therapy on mortality from breast cancer. *New England Journal of Medicine, 355:* 1784–92; 1846–7.

Blumenthal, J.A. et al. (1999) Effects of exercise training on older patients with major depression. *Archives of Internal Medicine, 159,* October: 2349–56.

Boonen, S. et al. (2005, online) Effects of osteoporosis treatments on risk of non-vertebral fractures: review and meta analysis of international studies. *Osteoporosis International.* (Published online 29 June.)

Borugian, M. et al. (2004) Insulin macronutrient intake and physical activity. *Cancer Epidemiology, Biomarkers and Prevention, 13(7):* 1163–72.

Bougnoux, P. et al. (1994) Alpha linolenic content of adipose breast tissue. *British Journal of Cancer, 70(2),* August: 330–4.

Charlier, C. et al. (2003) Breast cancer and serum organochlorine residues. *Occupational and Environmental Medicine, 60:* 348–51.

Clark, L.C. et al. (1991) Distribution of selenium and molybdenum and cancer mortality in Niigata, Japan. *Archives Environmental Health, 46:* 37–42.

Clark, L.C. et al. (1996) Effects of selenium supplementation for cancer prevention in patients with carcinoma of skin. *Journal of the American Medical Association, 276*: 1957–63.

Cohen, A. (1963) Fats and carbohydrates as factors in atherosclerosis and diabetes in Yemenite Jews. *American Heart Journal*, 65: 291.

Collaborative Group on Hormonal Factors in Breast Cancer. (1996) *Contraception, 34*: S1–S106.

Collaborative Group on Hormonal Factors in Breast Cancer. (1997) *Lancet, 350*(9084), October 11: 1047–59.

Couch, F.J. et al. (2001) Cigarette smoking including risk for breast cancer in high risk breast cancer families. *Cancer Epidemiology, Biomarkers and Prevention, 10*: 327–32.

Cramer, D. (2001) Caffeine consumption and estradiol levels. *Fertility and Sterility, 76*: 723–9.

Deuble, L. et al. (2000) *Environmental pollutants in meconium in Townsville, Australia.* Department of Neonatology, Kirwan Hospital, Townsville.

Dunn, A.L. et al. (2005) Exercise treatment for depression. *American Journal of Preventative Medicine, 28*(1), January: 8.

Edinger, J. et al. (2001) Cognitive behavioural therapy for treatment of chronic primary insomnia. *Journal of the American Medical Association, 285*: 1856–64.

Elmore, J. et al. (2005) Efficacy of Breast Cancer Screening in the community according to risk level. *Journal of the National Cancer Institute, 97*(14), July 20: 1019.

Ernster, V.L. et al. (1996) Incidence of and treatment for ductal carcinoma in situ. *Journal of the American Medical Association, 275*(12), March 12: 913–8.

Felton, C.V. et al. (1994) Dietary polyunsaturated fatty acids and composition of human aortic plaques. *Lancet, 344*: 1195.

Gapstur, S.M. et al. (2004) Alcohol consumption and the risk of breast cancer in a prepaid health plan. *Journal of the American Medical Association, 286*(17): 2143–51.

Gotzsche, P.C. and Olsen, O. (2001) Cochrane review on screening for breast cancer with mammography. *Lancet, 358*: 1340–2.

Graham, J. et al. (2002) Stressful life experiences and risk of relapse of breast cancer. *British Medical Journal, 324*: 1420–2.

Guthrie, N. (1977) Inhibition of proliferation of estrogen receptor negative MDA-MB-435 and positive MCF7 human breast cancer cells by palm oil, tocotrienols and tamoxifen alone and in combination. *Journal of Nutrition, 127*: S544–S548.

Heerdt, A.D. et al. (1995) Calcium glucarate as a chemopreventative agent in breast cancer. *Israeli Journal of Medical Science, 31*: 101–5.

Hulley, S. et al. (1998) Randomised trial of estrogen and progestin for secondary prevention of heart disease in post-menopausal women. *JAMA, 280*(7), August 19: 605–13.

Ingram, D. et al. (1997) Case controlled study of phyto-estrogens and breast cancer. *Lancet, 350*, October 4: 990–4.

Josefson, D. (2000) High insulin levels linked to death from breast cancer. *British Medical Journal, 320*: 1496.

Keyserlingk, J. (1998) Infrared imaging of the breast. Initial reappraisal using high resolution digital technology in 100 successive cases of stage one and two breast cancer. *Breast Journal, 4*(4), July/August.

Kowalska, E. et al. Increased rates of chromosome breakage in BRCA 1 carriers are normalised by oral selenium supplementation. *Cancer Epidemiology, Biomarkers and Prevention, 14*(5): 1302–6.

Kumle, M. et al. (2002) Use of the oral contraceptive pill and breast cancer risk – the Norwegian Swedish Woman's Lifestyle and Health Cohort Study. *Cancer Epidemiology, Biomarkers and Prevention, 11*, November: 1375–81.

Lee, I-M. et al. (2005) The Women's Health Study. Vitamin E in the primary prevention of cardiovascular disease and cancer. *Journal of the American Medical Association*, 294, July 6: 55–6.

Li, J. et al. (2002) Cancer incidence in parents who lost a child. *Cancer, 95*: 2237–42.

Malhotra, S. (1968) *Indian Journal of Industrial Medicine, 14*: 219.

Mann, G. (1994) Metabolic consequences of dietary trans fatty acids. *Lancet*, 343: 1268–71.

McTiernan, A. et al. (2003) Women's health initiative cohort study. Recreational physical activity and the risk of breast cancer. *Journal of the American Medical Association, 290*: 1331–36.

Miller, A. et al. (2000) Canadian national breast cancer screening study. Screening for breast cancer. Recommendations and rationale. *Journal of the National Cancer Institute, 92,* September 20: 1490–9.

Molyneux, S. et al. (2004) Bioavailability of CoQ10 supplements in New Zealand. *New Zealand Medical Journal, 8*(117), October 8: 1203.

Mondloch, Michael et al. (2001) Does how you do depend on how you think you'll do? *Canadian Medical Association Journal,* 165(2).

Narod, S.A. et al. (2002) Oral contraception and the risk of breast cancer in BRCA1 and BRCA2 mutation carriers. *Journal of the National Cancer Institute, 94*(23): 1773–9.

Neilson, N.R. et al. (2005) Self-reported stress and risk of breast cancer: prospective cohort study. *British Medical Journal, 331,* September 10: 548.

Nystrom, L. et al. (2002) Long-term effects of mammographic screening: undated overview of the Swedish randomised trials. *Lancet, 359,* March 16: 909–19.

Olsen, A.H. et al. (2005) Breast cancer mortality in Copenhagen after introduction of mammography screening: cohort study. *British Medical Journal, 330,* January: 220.

Perumal, S.S. et al. (2005) Combined efficacy of tamoxifen and CoQ10 on the status of lipid peroxidation and antioxidants in DMBA induced breast cancer. *Molecular Cell Biochemistry, 273*(1–2), May: 151–60.

Rose, G. et al. (1983) UK heart disease prevention project. *Lancet, 1*: 1062–65.

Schairer, C. et al. (2000) Menopausal estrogen and estrogen-progestin replacement therapy and breast cancer. *Journal of the American Medical Association, 283*(4): 485–91.

Shrubsole, M. et al. (2001) Dietary folate intake and breast cancer risk. Results from Shanghai breast cancer study. *Cancer Research, 6*(19): 7136–41.

Thomas, D.B. et al. (1997) Randomized trial of breast self examination in Shanghai. *Journal of the National Cancer Institute, 89*: 355–65.

Thune, I. et al. (1997) Physical activity and the risk of breast cancer. *New England Journal of Medicine, 336*: 1269–75.

Torgerson, D.J. and Bell-Syer, S.E. (2001) Estrogen treatment of patients with established post-menopausal osteoporosis. *Journal of the American Medical Association, 285*(11), June 13: 2891–97.

United States Preventative Services Task Force. (2002) Screening for breast cancer: recommendations and rationale. *Annals of Internal Medicine, 137*(5), September 3: 344–6.

Velicer, C. et al. (2004) Antibiotic use in relation to the risk of breast cancer. *Journal of the American Mdecial Association, 291*(7), February 18: 827–35.

Wolff, J. et al. (1999) The effect of exercise training programs on bone mass. *Osteoporosis International 9*:1–12.

Wolff, M.S. et al. (1993) Blood levels of organochlorine residues and risk of breast cancer. *Journal of the National Cancer Institute, 85*: 648.

Wolk, A. et al. (1998) A prospective study of association of monounsaturated fats and other types of fat with risk of breast cancer. *Archives of Internal Medicine, 158*, January: 41–5.

Wu, A. et al. (2002) Adolescent and adult soy intake and risk of breast cancer in Asian Americans. *Carcinogenesis 23*(9), September: 1491–6.

Yusef, S. et al. (2004) Effect of potentially modifiable risk factors associated with myocardial infarction in 52 countries (the INTERHEART study). *Lancet*, issue 9438: 937–52.

Zhang, S.M. et al. (2003) Plasma folate, vitamin B6, vitamin B12, homocysteine and risk of breast cancer. *Journal of the National Cancer Institute, 95*, March 5: 373–380.

Zhong, S. et al. (1999) Dietary carotinoids and vitamins A, C, E and risk of breast cancer. *Journal of the National Cancer Institute, 91*: 547–56.

Index